Traian Enache, Ion Andrei Mueller-Funogea,
Peter Petros, Klaus Goeschen, Cătălin Copăescu,
Emmanuel Delorme, Sidi Muctar,
Andrei Manu-Marin, Marcel Moisa, Mihai Ionică

PELVIC FLOOR DISORDERS
Rational Diagnostic and Surgical Management

ISBN: 978-3-11-068360-8
https://doi.org/10.2478/9783110683615

Authors

Traian Enache
MD, PhD, Obstetrics and Gynecology, "Prof. Dr. Panait Sirbu" Clinical Obstetrics and Gynecology Hospital, Bucharest, Romania

Ion Andrei Mueller-Funogea
MD, PhD, Obstetrics and Gynecology; Pelvic surgeon; Head of Department of Obstetrics and Gynecology; Centre of Continence and Pelvic Diseases, Sf. Maria Hospital, Rochusstr. 2, 40479 Dusseldorf, Germany

Peter Petros
Professor, DSc DS (UWA), PhD (Uppsala), MB BS MD (Syd), FRCOG (Lond), FRANZCOG; Hon. Professor, University of NSW Professorial Dept. of Surgery, St. Vincent's Hospital, Sydney; Adjunct Professor, University of Western Australia School of Mechanical and Chemical Engineering, Perth WA

Klaus Goeschen
Professor Dr. Med., KVINNO-Centre Hannover, University of Hannover, Germany

Cătălin Copăescu
Assoc. Prof. of General Surgery, *Carol Davila* University of Medicine and Pharmacy, Bucharest, Romania; Coordinator, Department of Minimally Invasive Surgery, Regina Maria Ponderas Academic Hospital, Bucharest, Romania

Emmanuel Delorme
PhD, urologist, Private Hospital Sainte Marie, 71100 Chalon sur Saone, France

Sidi Muctar
MD, Urology and Urogynecology; Coordinator – Centre of Continence and Pelvic Diseases, Saint Mary Hospital, Rochusstr. 2, 40479, Dusseldorf, Germany

Andrei Manu-Marin
MD, urologist, Evo Med, Centre of Diagnostic and Treatment of Urinary Disorders, Bucharest, Romania

Marcel Moisa
MD, PhD, Obstetrics and Gynecology; MD, General Surgery; *Prof. Dr. Panait Sirbu* Clinical Obstetrics and Gynecology Hospital, Bucharest, Romania

Mihai Ionică
1st Degree Researcher, Centre of Medical and Military Scientific Research Bucharest, Romania; Assoc. Prof. Department of Technology, Electronics and Reliability, Faculty of Electronics, Telecommunications and Information Technology, "Politehnica" University, Bucharest, Romania

Collaborators

Andreea-Beatrice Enache
MD, PhD, Obstetrics and Gynecology, "Prof. Dr. Panait Sirbu" Clinical Obstetrics and Gynecology Hospital, Bucharest, Romania

Irina Bălescu
MD, General Surgery, Department of Minimally Invasive Surgery, Regina Maria Ponderas Academic Hospital, Regina Maria Hospital, Bucharest, Romania

Maeva Serrand
Service de Gynécologique Obstétrique - CHU Dijon, 2 bd de Lattre de Tassigny, 21000 Dijon, France, serrandmaeva@orange.fr

Translation, proofreading & text editing

Consuela-Mădălina Gheorghe
PhD, Authorized translator, Assist. Prof., Marketing and Medical Technology Department, "Carol Davila" University of Medicine and Pharmacy, Bucharest, Romania

Reviewers

Prof. Christian Karl
MD, PhD, obstetrician and gynaecologist, Aachen, Germany
https://www.sah-eschweiler.de/kliniken-experten/kliniken/frauenheilkunde/team/

Burghard Abendstein
MD, PhD, surgeon, proctologist, gynecologist, Feldkirch, Austria
https://www.landeskrankenhaus.at/leistungsangebot/fuer-patienten/medizinische-fachbereiche/lkh-feldkirch/gynaekologie-geburtshilfe#editor2

Bernhard Lidl
MD, PhD, urologist, and gynecologist, Muenchen, Germany
https://www.qz-ts-muc.de/wer-macht-was/operationen/dr-bernhard-liedl/

Motto
"A surgeon must be both an architect and an engineer.
Architect – to be able to design a surgical
procedure.
Engineer - to be able to perform it."
Peter Petros

Cernavodă Bridge, which was designed and built by the Romanian engineer Anghel Saligny, is one of the first suspension bridges in the world, built on a metallic structure, to which, beams with consoles were used as a world premiere.

At the time it was inaugurated it was considered the longest bridge in Europe and the third in the world.

Traian Enache

Content

1. General considerations   11
2. Evolution of *"Pelvic floor disorder"* concept   12
    2.1. Definition   12
    2.2. History   12
    2.3. 21st century perspectives   17
    2.4. Current quantification of pelvic floor disorders   18
3. Classical anatomy of perineum   19
    3.1. General considerations on perineal anatomy   19
    3.2. Perineal muscles   19
        3.2.1. Upper muscle layer   20
            3.2.1.1. Levator ani muscle   20
            3.2.1.2. Coccygeus muscle   23
        3.2.2. Muscular middle layer   23
        3.2.3. Inferior muscle layer   23
            3.2.3.1. Ischiocavernosus muscle   23
            3.2.3.2. Bulbospongiosus muscle   24
            3.2.3.3. Superficial transverse perineal muscle (transversus perinei superficialis   24
            3.2.3.4. Deep transverse perineal muscle   23
            3.2.3.5. Urethral sphincter muscle   23
            3.2.3.6. External anal sphincter (sphincter ani externus)   23
            3.2.3.7. Rectovaginal muscle   23
    3.3. Connective structure of perineum   23
        3.3.1. Superficial investing fascia of perineum (Gallaudet fascia)   23
        3.3.2. Inferior fascia of urogenital diaphragm (perineal membrane)   25
        3.3.3. Deep perineal fascia (endopelvic fascia, parietal endopelvic fascia)   25
    3.4. Subperitoneal pelvic cavity   25
        3.4.1. Deep perineal fascia (endopelvic fascia, parietal endopelvic fascia)   26
        3.4.2. Visceral pelvic fascia (Fascia pelvis visceralis)   26
            3.4.2.1. Pubocervical fascia   26
            3.4.2.2. Rectovaginal fascia (Denonvillier's fascia)   26
        3.4.3. Lax connective tissue   27
            3.4.3.1. Fibrovascular membranes   27
            3.4.3.2. Secondary spaces   27
    3.5. Anatomical landmarks with practical application   28
        3.5.1. Urethra support means   29
        3.5.2. Ureterovesical junction   29
        3.5.3. Arcus tendineus fasciae pelvis   30
        3.5.4. Ischial muscle spindles   30
        3.5.5. Sacrospinous ligament 31
    3.6. Applied histology of pelvic organs and perineal tissues   32
        3.6.1. Histology of bladder   34
4. Perineal physiology and physiopathology   34
    4.1. Introduction to *"Integral Theory System"*   34
    4.2. Elements of dynamic and functional anatomy   35
        4.2.1. Structure of connective tissue 35
        4.2.2. Perineal muscle structure according to Integral Theory System   37
    4.3. Physiology of pelvic floor   38
        4.3.1. Biomechanics of vagina   38
        4.3.2. Biomechanics of bladder   40
        4.3.3. Biomechanics of the human uterus   40
        4.3.4. Biomechanics of rectum   42

4.3.5. Urethral physiology – micturition and urinary retention   42
4.3.6. Anal physiology – defecation and fecal retention   44
4.4. Perineum physiology - vector forces imbalance   45
    4.4.1. Pathogenesis of pelvic floor disorders and of evacuation and continence disorders   45
    4.4.2. Physiopathology of pelvic floor disorders   48
        4.4.2.1. Mechanisms for the appearance of anterior prolapse (cystocele)   48
        4.4.2.2. Mechanisms for the appearance of uterine prolapse   49
        4.4.2.3. Mechanisms for the appearance of vaginal vault prolapse and vaginal prolapse   52
        4.4.2.4. Mechanisms for the appearance of posterior vaginal wall prolapse (rectocele)   52
    4.4.3. Physiopathology of stress urinary incontinence   53
    4.4.4. Physiopathology of anorectal dysfunction   55
    4.4.5. Physiopathology of rectal prolapse   56
5. Clinical and paraclinical diagnosis of pelvic floor disorders   57
5.1. Semiology of pelvic floor disorders   58
    5.1.1. Symptoms   58
        5.1.1.1. Stress urinary incontinence   58
        5.1.1.2. Urinary urge and urge urinary incontinence   59
        5.1.1.3. Pollakiuria   62
        5.1.1.4. Nocturia   62
        5.1.1.5. Bladder voiding disorders   63
        5.1.1.6. Fecal incontinence   64
        5.1.1.7. Constipation   65
        5.1.1.8. Vaginal discomfort and other symptoms associated with pelvic organs prolapse   65
        5.1.1.9. Pelvic pain and dyspareunia   65
    5.1.2. Objective examination   94
        5.1.2.1. Clinical diagnosis of stress urinary incontinence (SUI)   94
        5.1.2.2. Clinical diagnosis of anterior vaginal prolapse (cystocele)   96
        5.1.2.3. Clinical diagnosis of uterine prolapse   97
        5.1.2.4. Clinical diagnosis of vaginal vault prolapse   99
        5.1.2.5. Clinical diagnosis of posterior vaginal wall prolapse (rectocele)   100
5.2. "Posterior fornix" syndrome   101
    5.2.1. Urinary urge   102
    5.2.2. Bladder voiding disorders   103
    5.2.3. Nocturia   103
    5.2.4. Pelvic chronic pain   104
5.3. Clinical diagnosis algorithm according to „*Integral Theory System*"   104
5.4. Paraclinical investigations in pelvic floor disorders   106
    5.4.1. Urodynamic investigations   108
        5.4.1.1. Diurnal urinary frequency   108
        5.4.1.2. Urinary flow rate   109
        5.4.1.3. Study of urethral function   111
        5.4.1.4. Classification of static urethral profile disorders   113
        5.4.1.5. Cystometry   114
        5.4.1.6. Videourodynamic tests   120
        5.4.1.7. Outpatient urodynamic tests   120
        5.4.1.8. Neurophysiological tests   121
    5.4.2. Ultrasound   121
    5.4.3. Radiological examinations   123
    5.4.4. Imaging examinations   124

6. Conservative treatment of pelvic floor disorders   125
    6.1. Medical evaluation   125
    6.2. Physiotherapeutic evaluation   126
    6.3. Kinesiotherapeutic treatment   126
    6.4. Stress urinary incontinence   126

7. Surgical treatment of pelvic floor disorders   128
    7.1. General principles of surgical treatment of pelvic floor disorders   128
    7.2. Surgery for anterior compartment   131
        7.2.1. Classical surgical procedures   131
            7.2.1.1. Kelly Procedure   131
            7.2.1.2. Marshal-Marchetti-Kranz Procedure and Burch Procedure   134
            7.2.1.3. Direct urethrocystopexy   135
        7.2.2. Surgical techniques using alloplastic material   136
            7.2.2.1. Retropubic suburethral sling   136
            7.2.2.2. Tissue fixation system for the treatment of stress urinary incontinence   137
            7.2.2.3. Transobturator suburethral tape   141
            7.2.2.4. Mini-sling   152
    7.3. Middle compartment surgery   153
        7.3.1. Classical surgical procedures   154
            7.3.1.1. Anterior colporrhaphy   154
            7.3.1.2. Paravaginal defect repair   158
        7.3.2. Surgical techniques using alloplastic material   160
            7.3.2.1. Transobturator four-arms mesh in surgical repair   160
            7.3.2.2. Tissue fixation system for the middle compartment   166
            7.3.2.3. Anterior pelvic organ prolapse repair using a six tension-free strap, low-weight transvaginal mesh: OPUR® kit   168
    7.4. Posterior compartment surgery   177
        7.4.1. Classical surgical procedures   177
            7.4.1.1. Posterior colpoperineorrhaphy   177
            7.4.1.2. Surgical treatment of vaginal vault prolapse   182
            7.4.1.3. Surgical treatment of elitrocele   187
            7.4.1.4. Colpocleisis   191
            7.4.1.5. Recovery after vaginal disorders   195
            7.4.1.6. Bilateral plication of the puborectal muscles: a new surgical concept for treating gaping genital hiatus   198
        7.4.2. Surgical techniques using alloplastic material   202
            7.4.2.1. Posterior intravaginal mesh   203
            7.4.2.2. Posterior intravaginal mesh with bilateral sacrospinous fixation   206
            7.4.2.3. Posterior "patch" with sacrospinous fixation   218
            7.4.2.4. Posterior patch, homograft with sacrospinous fixation   226
            7.4.2.5. Pericervical cerclage with sacrospinous fixed mesh   228
            7.4.2.6. Tissue fixation system for the posterior compartment   233
            7.4.2.7. Surgical treatment with posterior vaginal wall prolapse (rectocele) "bridge"   235
            7.4.2.8. Perineal body restoration   238
            7.4.2.9. Uterosacral ligaments restoration   240
    7.5. Laparoscopic surgery in pelvic floor disorders   249
        7.5.1. Laparoscopic treatment of uterine and vaginal vault prolapse – sacrocolpopexy   249
        7.5.2. Laparoscopic rectopexy   255
        7.5.3. Laparoscopic Burch surgery   262

8. Postoperatory complications 266
    8.1. Complications regarding the synthetic materials used 266
        8.1.1. Erosions 266
        8.1.2. Mesh infections 269
        8.1.3. Mesh retraction 269
    8.2. Complications regarding the technique used   269
        8.2.1. Hemorrhage and hematoma 269
        8.2.2. Pelvic suppurations 270
        8.2.3. Injuries of adjacent organs 270
    8.3. Other postoperatory complications 271
        8.3.1. Dyspareunia 271
        8.3.2. Chronic pelvic pains 272
        8.3.3. Urinary retention 272
        8.3.4. Other urinary symptoms 272
        8.3.5. Urinary infection 272
        8.3.6. Relapse of pelvic floor disorders or of stress urinary incontinence 273
        8.3.7. Pelvic deep vein thrombosis 273
    8.4. "Syndrome of tethered vagina" 273
9. 21st century perspectives 288
References 289

1. General considerations

Pelvic floor disorders represent one of the public health issues with a major impact on the quality of life and the integration in society (**Enache T. & Enache A., 2012**). The global incidence of this pathology is difficult to ascertain, but, for example, most of the epidemiological data in the USA appreciate that almost 11%, some of the studies even mentioning 19%, of the women come to a point when they need surgery for this disease (**ICS., 2010**). This pathology, which is situated at the border of three disciplines, such as Gynecology, Urology, and Proctology, needs a complex approach for both the understanding but more for the application of an efficient treatment (**Enache T.,** *et al.,* **2014**). The symptoms include a broader spectrum, such as the following: stress urinary incontinence, bowel incontinence, difficulties in the evacuation of feces and urine, nocturia, pelvic pains, sexual dysfunctions. The anatomical defects associated to these types of symptoms are the following: urethrocele, cystocele, rectocele, enterocele, and uterine prolapse (**Enache T.,** *et al.,* **2013**). An objective evaluation can be made by a sectorial analysis of these affections (**Enache T.,** *et al.,* **2015***a*).

Among all the affections mentioned, stress urinary incontinence is the most frequently met and was the most studied, that is why it has a special status, benefiting from a superior statistics and more efficient, standardized, and cheaper therapeutic methods. Its prevalence among women in Europe and the U.S.A. varies between 5 and 69%. However, its maximum incidence is in the postmenopausal period, especially if there is at least one pregnancy in the medical history. Taking into account that the life expectancy in the occidental world is raising, this percent can reach up to the population of 90 to 80 years old (**Lazarou G., 2013**).

Other studies performed in different countries mention the incidence of bowel incontinence to be between 1.4 and 11% (**Lazarou G., 2013**). The prevalence of symptomatic uterine prolapse is reported to vary between 7 and 23%. However, the small percentage would be due both to a high amount of asymptomatic patients and to some less studied cases in literature (**Lazarou G., 2013**), because many symptoms are not traditionally correlated to the pelvic floor disorders such as micturition imperiosity, nocturia, sacrum pains, dyspareunia, etc. (**Enache T.,** *et al.,* **2012**). Moreover, a problem arises, whether classical pathogenic associations, such as the hypertrophic elongation of the cervix in the case of uterine prolapse, is not in fact a reversible disorder, which establishes a new therapeutic conduct (**Enache T.,** *et al.,* **2015***b*).

In some studies undergone in the U.S.A. and U.K., the incidence of the patients who benefit from surgery varies between 1.9 and 4.9/1000 of women/year (**Lazarou G., 2013**). More studies performed in the U.S.A. mention costs of over 20 billion dollars annually for the treatment of stress urinary incontinence and of over 1 billion dollars for the treatment of uterine prolapse, which represent direct and indirect expenses. The classical reconstruction surgical techniques are encumbered by a very high rate of relapse (30-52%) (**Rosenman A.E., 2017**), which generate additional costs.

If as far as the previous disorders are concerned, the surgical techniques tend to become more and more standardized, the treatment of the lower compartment disorders still represent a subject of dispute in the academic environment (**Enache T.,** *et al.,* **2016***a*). There are schools with tradition in laparoscopy, which propose this first-degree approach, as well as voices who consider the vaginal approach better (**Stoica R.A. & Enache T., 2012**). The surgical reconstruction of the uterosacral and cardinal ligaments raises many technical problems due to the deep anatomical disposal at the pelvis level (**Enache T.,** *et al.,* **2013**). Regarding the vaginal prolapse treatment, there are many ideas, but, currently, no gold standard approach has been imposed (**Enache T.,** *et al.,* **2013**). The book presents a proposal of a simplified correction technique of vaginal prolapse, which reduces the risk of postoperatory accidents and incidents, with favorable results, and, for which, a Patent was obtained (**Enache T.,** *et al.,* **2016***b*).

This way, the major impact of this pathology can be noticed, through a high prevalence in the general population, with important material consequences on the health systems. Even if, most often, there are no life-threatening risks, the affected patients suffer from a significant alteration of the quality of life, with important social and economical implications.

In addition, we consider that a fair knowledge of both the physiology and physiopathology and of the necessary therapeutic methods is of paramount importance for the understanding and establishment of an efficient treatment conduct.

2. Evolution of the *"pelvic floor disorder"* concept
2.1. Definition

Pelvic floor disorders include a wide variety of perineal affections that seem to have, as a common denominator, an acquired laxity of the musculoskeletal system, which makes up the pelvic floor.

This concept is new and it tries to comprise all the anatomoclinical entities in a standardized way, to facilitate, on one side, the description of the lesions and on the other, to favor scientific communication.

At present, there is no consensus regarding terminology (**Messelink B, 2005**), and, at the same time, literature has some examples of two essential notions necessary for the understanding of this pathology.

a) Pelvic floor disorders represents a notion that describes the relations between the pelvic organs and the pelvic floor. The main organs are the bladder, uterus and vagina, rectum and the contents of the pouch of Douglas. Beside these organs, both ureters and different vascular and nervous elements have a certain connection at the pelvis level. However, the pelvic floor is the one that makes up the complex anatomical structure of the pelvis.

b) The pelvic floor represents the caudal delimitation of the pelvic excavation, which is a complex musculoskeletal structure that in the case of women is crossed by three ducts: urethra, vagina, and anal canal.

c) The fiber conjunctive component makes the connection between the organs and the muscles.

Through relaxation and contraction, the muscular component has two main roles:
i) of supporting the pelvic organs and
ii) of taking part in the main functions of the neighborhood organs: micturition and urinary continence, defecation and fecal continence, takes part in the sexual activity and has an obstetrical role.

These findings have led to the appearance of static and dynamic anatomy notions (**Petros P.P., 2010**).

The pelvic floor disorders are characterized by different degrees affection of the structures specific for the pelvic floor, which leads to the appearance of some anatomoclinical entities, among which the most frequent are the following: stress urinary incontinence, faecal incontinence, and pelvic organs prolapse. Besides, these are associated with the concept of *"old perineal tear"* in classic gynecology. However, the notion is unspecific and does not express the complexity of the disorders and consecutively of the symptoms.

The most recent studies describe five groups of symptoms associated with pelvic floor disorders: urinary, intestinal, vaginal (prolapse) symptoms, sexual dysfunctions, and pelvic pains (**Abrams P.,** *et al.,* **2002; Thompson W.G., 1999; Whitehead W.E.,** *et al.,* **1999; Fall M.,** *et al.,* **2003; Bump R.C., 1996**).

2.2. History

Although the concept of *"pelvic floor disorder"* is relatively new, it represents the last attempt of systematization of the perineal pathology. Some of the symptoms and anatomical defects that can be found in this category have been known from antiquity.

The first time uterine prolapse was mentioned is met in the oldest medical document, the *Egyptian Kahun Gynecological Papyrus* – around 1835 B.C., and the first therapeutical methods were mentioned in another papyrus, Ebers, around 1550 B.C., which presented *"ground oil (oil), manure mixed with honey and applied and massaged on the body of the patient"* as remedies for uterine disorders (**Bump R.V., 1996**).

1000 years later, Hippocrates (460-377 B.C.) and his followers launched the concept according to which, the uterus (womb) is *"an animal within an animal"*, which must be treated with fumigations in order for it to retract (**Douglas J.A.**, **1730**; **Lazarou G.**, *et al.*, **2007**).

One of Hippocrates's disciples, Polybus, who was the author of the first Treaty of Gynecology entitled *"On the diseases of women"*, mentioned the use of astringent solutions applied locally, sponges soaked in vinegar or pomegranate extract, among the remedies for uterine prolapse.

In case these therapeutic measures were unsuccessful, a so-called "succussion splash" was chosen, which presupposed the hanging of the female patient upside down and her continuous movement until the reduction of the prolapse. Afterwards, the patient was laid on the bed and tightly tied up by her legs for 3 days (**Downing K.T.**, **2012**, **Lazarou G.**, *et al.*, **2007**).

The most famous gynecologist in Antiquity, Soranus (1st century B.C.), had the first scientific approach, insisting on the necessity of reducing the prolapse, for which he used a wool pad to put on hold (**Downing K.T.**, **2012**).

In 98 B.C., it was Soranus who first described the necessity of removing the prolapsed uterus, which had become necrotic (**Lazarou G.**, *et al.*, **2007**).

However, with all these incontestable therapeutic progresses, the anatomical knowledge has remained poor, first due to the interdiction of dissection of human corpses by the Romans.

Galen's description of the uterus, according to which, it is bicornuate, was just an extrapolation of the discoveries made on animals.

In the Middle Ages, Medicine went through a regression period, anatomy was no longer studied, so that, the conclusion that the uterus has seven compartments, three on the left side, where the female fetuses developed, three on the right side, where male fetuses developed and one in the middle, where hermaphrodite fetuses developed.

In 1603, Roderigo de Castro recommended the burning with a hot iron of the prolapsed uterus, so that it retracted in the vagina (**Ricci J.V.**, **1950**; **Gombrich E.H.**, **2005**).

Even if during Renaissance, artists such as Leonardo da Vinci have undergone studies on human corpses, they were not taken into consideration by the medical world.

It was not until the 16th century that Andreas Vesalius made a full description of the whole female genitalia in his book *"De Corporis Humanis Fabrica"*, in which he also included the ligaments of the uterus, benefiting from the anatomical pictures that are famous even today, which belong to Jan Stephen van Kalkar, and which definitely changed the perceptions regarding anatomy from Galen's time (**Speert H.**, **1973**). The first vaginal hysterectomy was performed and described by Giacomo Berengario da Capri in 1507 (**Downing K.T.**, **2012**). What is interesting is that one of the first successful hysterectomies performed was made by a 46-year-old peasant woman, whose name was Faith Haworth, and, whose hysterectomy was invalidated due to a total uterine prolapse, to which she self-tapped the herniated form. The hemorrhage stopped fast enough, but she remained with a serious sequelae: vesicovaginal fistula (**Sutton C.**, **1997**).

The technical difficulties of that period, including the asepsis and antisepsis have made this method impossible to apply on a large scale. Towards the end of the 16th century, Ambroise Paré (1514-1590), a military surgeon to the Court of the King of France, invented the pessary, made up of brass and waxed cork, which had a wire attached, so that it could be taken out easily (**Par´e A.**, **1649**).

One of the first descriptions of the uterosacral ligaments belongs to Philip Verheyn and dates from 1708 (**DeLancey J.O.**, **1992**). Having the title *"uteri connexio"*, Verheyn underlined that the uterine cervix is connected with the vaginal fornix, posterior to the rectum and anterior to the bladder (**Verheyn P.**, **1708**).

In 1727, René-Jacques de Garengeot designed the vaginal speculum, which offered the possibility of analyzing and differentiating the various types of *"vaginal prolapses"*, probably assimilated with cystocele and rectocele (**Downing K.T.**, **2012**).

In 1730, James Douglas made his first adequate description of the peritoneum, thus opening the path towards retro and subperitoneal surgery (**Douglas J.A.**, **1730**).

Remarkable progresses were registered in the 19th century; this also being the moment the first perineal surgical systematic correction attempts appeared.

In 1813, Conrad Langenbeck successfully achieved his first vaginal hysterectomy, which was scheduled for uterine pathology and, was successful, despite the lack of anaesthesia and surgical asepsis (**Langenbeck C.J.M., 1817**).

In 1847, Anders Adolf Retzius defined the same space, thus opening the path towards the prevesical and preperitoneal surgical approach (**Retzius A.A., 1849**).

In 1853, the anatomist Hyrtl from Vienna underlined, especially in his paper "*Handbuch der topographischen Anatomie*", the fact that except for the round ligaments, there are also peritoneal sheaths, which stretch from the bladder to the uterus and which are called "*ligamenta vesico-uterina*", as well as sheaths that stretch from the rectum to the uterus, called "*ligamenta recto-uterina*". These ligaments contain very strong connective fibers, thus being able to fix the uterus to its place (**Hyrtl J., 1853**).

In 1877, Leon Clement LeFort described his method of accomplishing the partial "colpocleisis", a surgical technique that can be used even today in some selected cases of total uterine prolapse (**Sîrbu P., 1981**). The most important drawback of this technique is the impossibility of sexual activity afterwards, as well as the impossibility of exploring the uterus, because it remained on the spot. However, the technique was improved by Goodel and Power, by the excision of a triangular membrane of vaginal mucosa.

The year 1895 brought a very important accomplishment, which opened the path towards the understanding of the pelvic floor disorders. Alwin Mackenrodt's paper, in which he described the causes and the treatment methods of uterine prolapse, by highlighting the role of the connective tissue and the cardinal ligaments, bears his name (**Mackenrodt A., 1895**).

Subsequently, Archibald Donald and William Fothergill described the surgery in Manchester, which was associated with anterior colporrhaphy and posterior colpoperineorrhaphy, and the connection between the parametrial and paravaginal tissues.

This has become the most common technique of solving the uterine prolapse (**Fothergill W.E., 1915**). Through an analogy with the Greek architecture, Donald believed that the uterus represented the key to the pelvic floor. This idea was resumed at the beginning of the 21st century with biophysical arguments and is the starting point of a new theory.

Simultaneously with Donald, Watkins proposed the vesicovaginal interposition of the uterus as a treatment method for uterine prolapse and cystocele (**Watkins T.J., 1899**).

However, the second half of the 19th century was marked by Hugh Lenox Hodge's theory, which recommended as a main treatment method of uterine prolapse, the mechanical reduction with the pessary (**Judd J.P., *et al.*, 2010**).

At the beginning of the 20th century, David Gillman proposed the first ligamentotaxis as a treatment for uterine prolapse and immediately afterwards John M. Baldy and John Clarence Webster (1902) simultaneously described the procedure (further known as Baldy-Webster procedure) of sheathing the uterosacral ligaments to correct the uterine retroversion, these being considered a cause for uterine prolapse (**Baldy J.M., 1902**).

An important step was made in 1912 by Alexis Moschcowitz by defining the rectal prolapse as a form sliding hernia through a pelvic fascial defect, which he corrected by occluding the pouch of Douglas with non-resorbable encirclement sutures.

The gynecologists have taken this technique for elitrocele prophylaxis after hysterectomy (**Moschcowitz A.V., 1912**).

The difficulty of finding an efficient method of treatment for uterine prolapse was due to the deficient understanding of the means that sustained the pelvic organs.

In 1907, the Austrian gynecologist Josef Halban and the anatomist Julius Tandler from the University of Medicine in Vienna published the paper "*Anatomie und Atiologie der Genital prolapse beim Weibe*".

According to their theory, the endopelvic fascia was able to sustain the normal weight, but unable to sustain an additional loading. This way, the *levator ani* muscle became essential in pelvic floor disorders (**Halban J., 1907**).

In 1914, Symington (**Symington J., 1914**) described for the first time in his book *"Quain's Elements of Anatomy"*, the fact that a muscular tissue with tight topographic connections with *"plexus pelvicus"* was present in the *"uterosacral ligaments"*.

In 1917, Blaisdell confirmed in one of his complex works about the macroscopic and microscopic structure of "plicae sacro-uterinae", that the smooth muscle cells (myocytes) are an integral part of these structures (**Blaisdell F.E., 1917**).

An important step was made by Bonney, who published in 1934 the paper entitled "The Principles that should Underlie all Operations for Prolapse" (**Bonney V., 1934**).

His conclusions were based on the classification proposed by DeLancey in 1992 (**DeLancey J.O., 1992**), who mentioned three levels of pelvic support. As a result of some studies on cadavers, two years later, in 1936, Mengert came to the conclusion that the main pelvic support of the uterus were the parametrial and paravaginal tissues (**Mengert W.F., 1936**).

The first vaginal hysterectomy for the treatment of uterine prolapse was performed by Chopin, in New Orleans, in 1861 (**Choppin S., 1866**), but his result was not taken into consideration until the beginning of the 20th century.

In 1915, C.H. Mayo published his own vaginal hysterectomy technique (**Mayo C.H., 1915**), and three years later, Bissel proposed the association of hysterectomy with anterior and posterior colporrhaphy (**Bissell D., 1918**).

In 1937, Baer and col. published a paper in which it was admitted that vaginal hysterectomy is a standardized surgery, which has become a chosen technique in (uterine) prolapse, thus replacing the vesico-vaginal interposition of the uterus (**Baer J.L., et al., 1937**).

In 1938, Martius, one of the most famous German gynecologists, published the observation that uterosacral ligaments are mainly built of smooth muscles that spastically and painfully contract in case of irritation (**Martius H., 1938**).

In the middle of the 20th century, the vaginal vault prolapse had become a very often-met sequel of vaginal hysterectomy. The correction trials of this complication started in 1927, when Miller described a method of reducing the occurrence of vaginal vault prolapse by its transperitoneal iliococcygeus suspension or, according to the local anatomy, its anchoring to both sacrospinous ligaments (**Miller N.F., 1927**).

In 1946, Heinrich Martius, one of the most famous German gynecologists, considered as premise in his gynecology manual that "the utero-vaginal prolapse can lead to incontinence, voiding disorders, postmiction residues, pollakiuria and nocturia".

Moreover, he made the following remarks regarding the pelvic pains associated to the uterine prolapse (**Martius H., 1946**).

"In case of vaginal or uterine prolapse, severe pain might appear at the lower abdominal level or at the posterior pelvic area, which is induced by a marked tension of the prolapsed organs on the plexus sacralis. The symptoms are not only correlated with the prolapse degree but also mostly with the sensitivity of the female patients affected.

Almost every woman presents at least a small degree of pelvic organ descent, after a birth. A major pelvic organs prolapse is noticed in some of them. At the same time, not all the patients experience pain and there is no clear relationship between the prolapse degree and the symptom intensity. Because the pain has a neurological origin, major symptoms can appear even in the case of a minimal prolapse.

The patients complain that their intestines descend, also mentioning the feeling as if they dropped something and connect the back pain with prolapse on their initiative".

In 1950, Campbell detected smooth muscle fibers only on the anterior and medium sides of *"ligamenta sacro-uterina"*, while posteriorly, only lax connective tissue, vessels and nerves could be found (**Campbell R.M., 1950**).

In 1951, Milton McCall performed the posterior culdoplasty, a method also widely used at present (**McCall M.L., 1957**).

However, the most important step was made in 1957, by two English gynecologists, Arthure and Savage, who noticed that vaginal vault prolapse appears after the practice of any hysterectomy technique, thus proposing *"sacrocolpopexy"*, which is also used at present, despite the fact that there are other approaches besides the one initially described (**Arthure G.E. & Savage D., 1957**).

Between 1950 and 1960, the French School proposed two techniques of elitrocele correction, "Laparoscopic douglasectomy" promoted by Jamain and "pouch of Douglas partition", a technique promoted by Marion. However, these techniques were not needed because of the increased intraoperative risks and reproducibility (**Sîrbu P., 1981**). The use of sacrospinous ligaments as anchoring points for the vaginal vault prolapse was first mentioned in 1892, by Zweifel, in Germany (**Zweifel P., 1892**).

In 1950, a German gynecologist, J. Amreich, proposed two techniques of *sacrotuberous anchoring, transgluteal and transvaginal* (**Sederl J., 1958**).

12 years later, in 1962, Sederl and Richter performed the sacrospinous anchoring by using the approach proposed by Amreich (**Richter K., 1968**). This way, the surgical technique, later known as Amreich-Richter, appeared, a technique that has been very successful both in Europe and in the U.S.A., and which is still being used at present as standard surgery for the treatment of vaginal vault prolapse in many centers.

The 20th century marked the beginning of the preoccupations regarding the surgical treatment of stress urinary incontinence (SUI). In 1913, Kelly described the same surgery, which consisted in plication of the pubocervical fascia at the level of the ureterovesical junction, thus resulting a lifting with its consecutive angulation (**Kelly H.A., 1913**). This procedure was the first surgery that had favorable results, however, with a high rate of recurrence. Marion published a similar technique in France, at the same time with Kelly (**Sîrbu P., 1981**).

However, microanatomy and cystomanometry studies demonstrated the inexistence of a urethral sphincter and the performance of urinary continence through the urethral angulation, especially in the medium third (**Sîrbu P., 1981**).

Starting from this observation, a series of surgical procedures, which used suburethral meshes applied on the adjacent anatomical structures have been imagined.

This way, based on Goebbel's researches, in 1917, Stoeckel successfully performed a method of suspending the ureterovesical junction by using a muscle membrane from pyramidalis muscle and rectus abdominis muscle (**Sîrbu P., 1981; Stoeckel W., 1917**).

By applying the same principle, in 1942, A.H. Aldridge performed a suburethral mesh by using strips that were collected from the aponeurosis of the abdominal external oblique muscle (**Sîrbu P., 1981; Aldridge A.H., 1942**).

Aldridge is also the first gynecologist who launched the hypothesis according to which stress urinary incontinence could be connected to obstetrical traumas.

Also in the 1940s, an urologist, Victor Marshall, together with other two gynecologists, Andrew Marchetti and Kermit Krantz performed the suspension of the ureterovesical junction at the level of the periosteum of pubic symphysis and the posterior sheath of rectus abdominis muscle.

The results were better compared to the ones that appeared until then and the Marshall-Marchetti-Kranz surgery has become the main therapeutic method of SUI for the next decades (**Sîrbu P., 1981; Marshall V.F., *et al.*, 1949**).

Figurnov performed the first direct urethrocystopexy in the immediate post-war period. In 1959, Pereyra performed the anchoring of the urethra to the aponeurosis of the external oblique muscle, a surgery that was afterwards modified by Dan Alessandrescu and was made known in that form in Romania (**Sîrbu P., 1981**).

This technique has been very successful, being used even today in many clinics in Romania. The limit of this procedure lies in the fact that due to not being a *"tension-free"* technique, it predisposes to urinary continence followed by its specific complications.

In 1961, John Cristopher Burch modified this technique by performing the suspension to Cooper ligaments, which simplified the surgical technique, thus becoming the gold standard for more than half a century (**Sîrbu P., 1981; Burch J.C., 1961**).

2.3. 21st century perspectives

The beginning of 1990 brought two major changes in approaching the pelvic floor disorders through the appearance of vaginal meshes of alloplastic material and laparoscopic surgery. These two elements opened the way to new perspectives and led to the rethinking of surgery techniques. The idea of fixing the perineal defects originates at the beginning of the 20th century, when grafts collected from fascia lata tensor muscle were used.

The view according to which pelvic floor disorders are some forms of hernia, led to the appearance of an extremely interesting idea of replacing the fascia defects with different forms of auto-, alo-, and xenografts (**Downing K.T., 2012**).

The whole theory of perineum, the way Petros and Ulmsten published it for the first time in Europe, in 1990, represents a complex system of physiological and physiopathological interpretation of the permanent interaction of different pelvic anatomical structures. In addition, the theory presupposes the anatomical integrity of the whole pelvic floor as a "*sine qua non*" condition of performing the functions of perineal organs, thus leading to the insurance of fecal and urinary continence, but also of normal micturition and defecation. In other words, perineal structures act "*synergistically* in a dynamic system" (**Petros P.P., 2001**), in which fascia and ligaments represent transmission paths of the forces of pelvic floor perineal muscles, which finally act on the pelvic cavity organs.

The appearance of some lesions at any level of the above-mentioned structures would lead to a poor transmission of the muscular forces and would negatively influence the emptying and/or continence functions of pelvic cavity organs. The above-mentioned lesions are mostly discreet, often showing a slow degeneration of the molecular structure of the collagen and elastin from ligaments and pelvic fascia. This phenomenon is triggered by the perineum overload by events which lead to the raise of the intra abdominal pressure (such as pregnancy and giving birth, obesity, prolonged physical effort) and which is accelerated by the normal senescence pressure, but also by the appearance of other pathologies, such as asthma, chronic obstructive pulmonary disease, collagenases, diabetes or abdominal-pelvic surgeries. Thus, ligaments and pelvic fascia gradually loose elasticity and resistance and the harmed collagen fibers lose their linear reorganization, organizing transversally, irreversibly losing (partially or totally) the capacity of correctly transmitting the muscle forces. This is the cause for the appearance of some very different symptoms with a highly negative influence on the quality of life of the affected women, being mainly represented by stress urinary incontinence and urinary urge. At the same time with urinary incontinence, there are a series of disorders, usually regarded as having un unclear cause and an interdisciplinary treatment: nocturia, pollakiuria, disorders of bladder or rectal emptying, fecal incontinence, chronic pelvic pains or dyspareunia. The last two symptoms are often met by the gynecologists, urologists, surgeons, or neurologists, being erroneously considered "*symptoms of psychic cause*" and generating serious disorders of the couple life. Thus, the Integral Theory System represents the first unitary physiopathological explanation for the appearance of all these symptoms.

Gynecologists got the idea of polypropylene synthetic meshes from general surgery and, currently, the polypropylene macroporous meshes with a type I monofilament have become a gold standard, thus benefitting from the studies that confirm their maximum biotolerance (**Luijendijk R.W., 2000**).

The appearance of TVT (tension free trans-vaginal tape), as a remarkably successful technique of inserting the suburethral mesh, superior to all the other methods of SUI correction, has demonstrated the potential of the alloplastic grafts in improving the surgical results of these new methods of treatment. In 2001, Petros proposed the infracoccigeal sacrocolpopexy as a method of surgically treating the vaginal vault prolapse, however encumbered by serious frequent complications such as perirectal abscess and rectovaginal fistula (**Petros P.P., 2001**). Von Theobald introduced a mesh that followed both the concomitant therapy of the small bowel prolapse/ vaginal vault prolapse and the rectocele. It is fixed both at the infracoccigeal level and through inferior branches, at the level of the perineum, thus aiming to anchor the whole posterior vaginal wall (**Von Theobald P. & Labbe E., 2008**).

In 2004, Farnsworth introduced the posterior mesh with 6-points fastening 2 upper points of pararectal fixation on the sacrotuberous ligament on each side, 2 middle fixation points on the inferior levator ani muscles of the sacrospinous ligament and 2 inferior anchoring points on the perineum. This system presents a concomitant anatomical or an *"en bloc"* reconstruction, but does not support the principles of Petros' theory anymore, which highlights the functional independence of the perineum levels. Thus, his theory is not respected and this can lead to emptying disorders or bladder and rectal continence. Besides, through the great implanting surface, an excessive scarring can be induced, which indirectly negatively influences the elasticity of the posterior walls of the vagina.

Although at present there are many systems of meshes that are produced by various companies, different problems, which are common in all these techniques have also appeared: surgical techniques are complex, needing both thorough anatomical knowledge as well as sound experience, the late postoperative complications being scarce, however, most of the times, hard to control and fix, such as the case of a chronic pain or rectovaginal fistula. Still, the companies force the implementation of these techniques with the aim of raising the profit.

The improper use of meshes in the therapy of pelvic floor disorders by inexperienced surgeons in the U.S.A. has led to the triggering of an alarm signal by the FDA (food and drug association) in July 2011. Thus, the FDA has registered over 1500 complications between 2008 and 2010; especially mesh erosions and cohabitation pains. These have led to a certain panic in this specialty world community. As a result, for a period of 2 years, these techniques have stagnated (*****., 2008**; *****., 2011**).

In the last years, these techniques have been reapplied but with modified systems (the so-called mini grafts with other non-transfixing anchoring techniques). Surgeries usually take place in specialty units, in which over 200 surgeries are performed per year, called "Pelvic Floor Units". There are still no data in literature to identify an optimum method of vaginal correction of uterine prolapse with alloplastic material and of vaginal vault prolapse. This case imposes the development of researches to find new methods of solving these problems. Thus, the discovery of a new technique of vaginal reconstruction, which lacks major complications, represents an objective of maximum importance.

In the last couple of years, an important progress has been made through the laparoscopic correction of pelvic floor disorders, the surgeries that were laparoscopically performed being the laparoscopic sacrocolpopexy, Burch surgery and last, but not least, and new, the robotic approach (**Judd J.P.,** *et al.,* **2010**; **Tan-Kim J.M.M.,** *et al.,* **2011**).

For the time being, a definitive conclusion regarding a perfect method of choice is difficult to be made. There are pilot studies, with an important subjective component regarding the individual surgical abilities, which, however, do not offer a significant comparison about the efficiency limits of different surgeries applied in vaginal correction.

The researches made in the next years, will have to use the most efficient method, easier to appropriate by the surgeon, cheaper and with minimum postoperatory complications.

2.4. Current quantification of pelvic floor disorders

In October 1995, the International Continence Society (ICS) introduced the POP-Q classification, using clinical criteria. The necessity of introducing this classification was conditioned by the need of finding a unique system of evaluating de pelvic floor disorders.

Thus, the POP-Q classification has become the standard reporting method in literature, being more and more appreciated by clinicians, and, even if it is not unanimously accepted and appreciated, this represents an important step in establishing a common language (**Auwad W.,** *et al.,* **2004**).

The paraclinical means of quantifying the pelvic floor disorders are mostly used for research and not for the current practice. MRI has been used very often in the last studies, but the decubitus necessary for the examination limits the efficiency of the method.

Moreover, the urodynamic samples and ultrasound still have an uncertain role in the evaluation of this pathology.

3. Classical anatomy of perineum
3.1. General considerations on perineal anatomy

Broadly, the perineum is anatomically made up of all the soft parts, which caudally define the pelvic excavation. These are represented by *fascias, muscles, vessels and nerves*, and are crossed by ducts of the urogenital and digestive systems, structures that offer a complex biomechanics, whose understanding is indispensable in a judicial therapeutic approach (**Papilian V., 1993**).

The perineum is a structure that is difficult to define *in vivo*, its anatomy being influenced by the position of the subject. The *classical description* is performed in *dorsal decubitus* position, because the perineum has a rhomboid form. Its defining at the surface of the body is represented by the pubic symphysis, the two ischiopubic rami, the ischial tuberosities, the inferior limits of the gluteus maximus muscles and coccyx (**Papilian V., 1993**). The *linea biischiadica* divides the perineum into two sides: anterior, or the *urogenital triangle* and posterior or the *anal triangle* (**Papilian V., 1993**), Fig. 3.1.

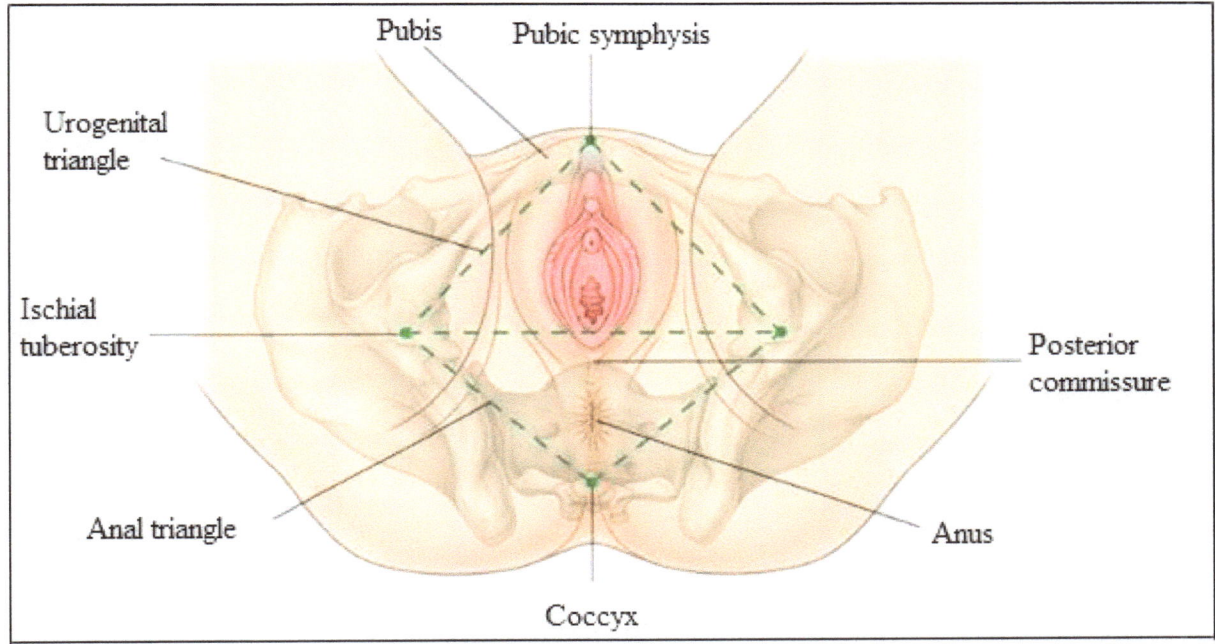

Fig. 3.1. Perineal area in women

In depth, the perineum stretches to the parietal fascia that covers the levator ani muscles and the coccygeus muscles that form the demarcation line with the pelvic subperitoneal space. For didactic reasons, the complexity of the perineum structure imposes a presentation of the constituent elements and afterwards a topographic presentation.

3.2. Perineal muscles

Perineal muscles divide into 3 groups:
a) Pelvic floor muscles;
b) Anterior perineum muscles;
c) Posterior perineum muscles.

Together with these three groups, there are also 2 more important structures, which result from the insertions of different muscle bundles.

Perineal body represents a fibrous condensation formed from the meeting of all the fascias and through the interconnection of the muscles and tendons fibers of the perineum. In a sagittal plane, this is a triangular anatomical space, which is in an anterior report with the vagina, in a posterior report with the rectum (cranially, the two structures intimately adhere) and it is inferiorly delimited by the tegument (**Papilian V., 1993**). There are fascicles of levator ani muscle, deep transverse perineal muscle, superficial transverse perineal muscle, sphincter ani externus and bulbospongiosus muscles, with a very important role in pelvic floor disorders and in obstetrics practice, their damage during birth having a major clinical impact (**Sirbu P.**, *et al.*, **1981**).

Anococcygeal ligament

It is a linear fibrous formation, between the anus and the coccyx. According to the Integral Theory of Petros P., the perineum muscles can be divided from the functional point of view in 3 important groups.

3.2.1. Upper muscle layer
3.2.1.1. Levator ani muscle

Levator ani is a wide, very thin, pair muscle, which realizes a complex space structure, whose role must be understood from the perspective of the surgical approach. Studies regarding the MRI reconstruction of these muscles have shown an irregular, conical architecture, with different rays of curvature between its anterior and posterior segments (**Roshanravan S.M.**, *et al.*, **1976; Aukee P.**, *et al.*, **2004**).

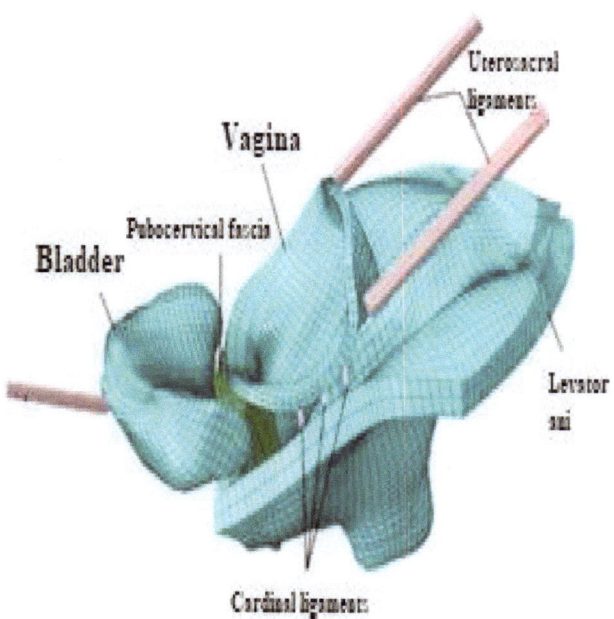

Fig. 3.2. 3D model of levator ani muscle architecture
(according to **Maurer M., 2014**)

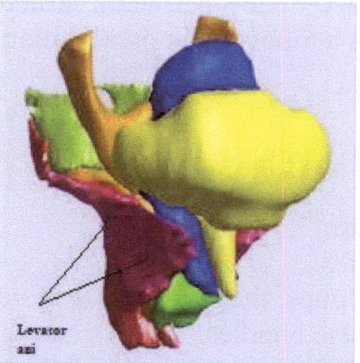

Fig. 3.3. 3D reconstruction of pelvic anatomy – MRI
(according to **Enache T., 2014**)

Its origin can be found along a light curve line with an upward concavity, which starts from the posterior wall of the pubic symphysis, passes over the fascia of the internal obturator muscle – where it realizes a condensation of connective fibers, which is called *arcus tendineus fasciae pelvis*, and reaches the ischial spine, Fig. 3.2 and 3.3. Its role is to lift the pelvic diaphragm, posterior perineum, anal canal, and anus, playing a role of internal anal sphincter and constrictor muscle of the vagina, made up of two different sides: pubic and iliac, Fig. 3.4.

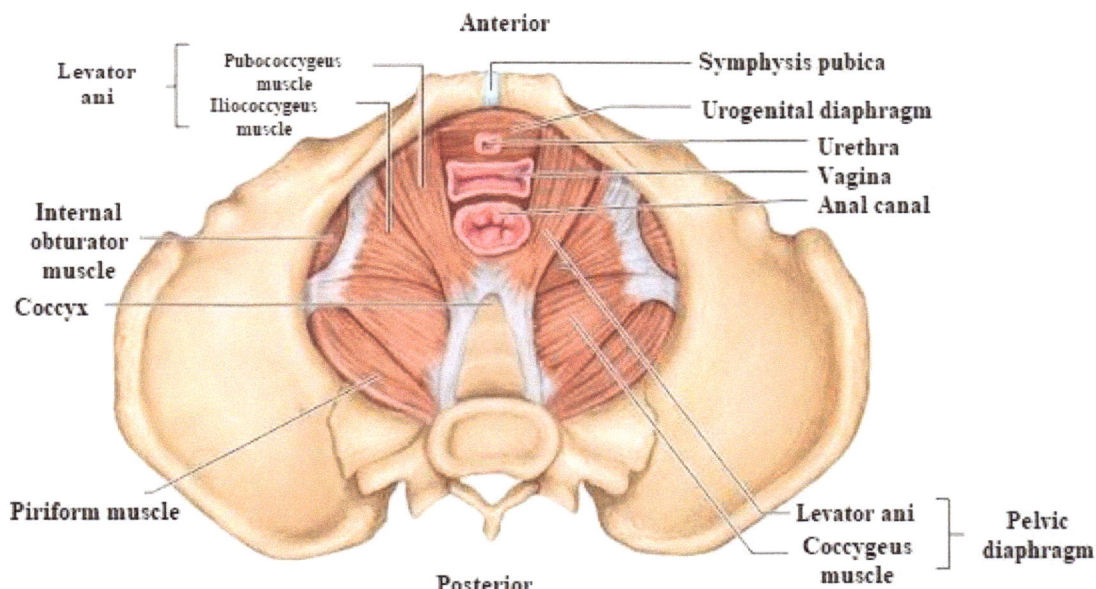

Fig. 3.4. Pelvic diaphragm

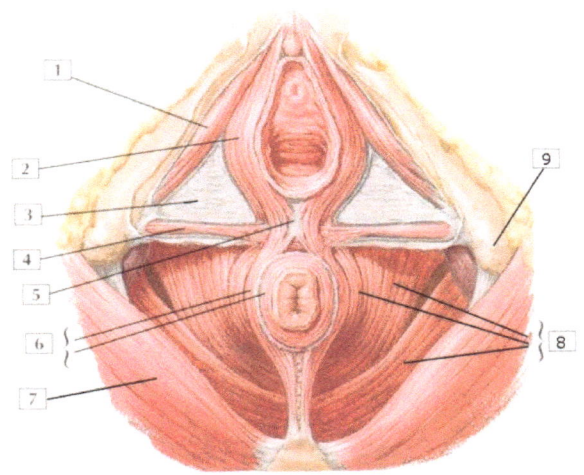

Fig. 3.5. Perineum muscles
(according to **Strohbehn K.**, *et al.*, **1996**)

1 – Ischiocavernosus muscle, 2 – Bulbospongiosus muscle, 3 – Deep transverse perineal muscle, 4 – Deep transverse perineal muscle, 5 – Center tendon of perineum, 6 – External anal sphincter, 7 – Gluteus maximus, 8 – Levator ani muscle, 9 – Ischial tuberosity

Pubic side – with fibers that start from the posterior side of the pubis and from the anterior side of the tendinous arch, which have a posterior, inferior, and medial direction, thus forming the *pubovaginal muscle*. The medial fibers are in contact with the lateral and posterior sides of the vagina, inserting at the level of the perineal body, being strongly connected through connective tissue to it, thus, practically being its component. Vaginal constriction is produced through its bilateral contraction. Medial fibers pass laterally from the vagina and go round the rectum, one side inserting among the rectal muscle fibers, others continuing with the ones on the opposite side, thus forming the *puborectal and puboanal fascicles*.

Lateral fibers insert on the anococcygeal ligament (**Papilian V., 1993; Lupu G., 2005**), forming the *pubococcygeus muscle*. Lateral fascicles intertwine with the iliococcygeus muscle.

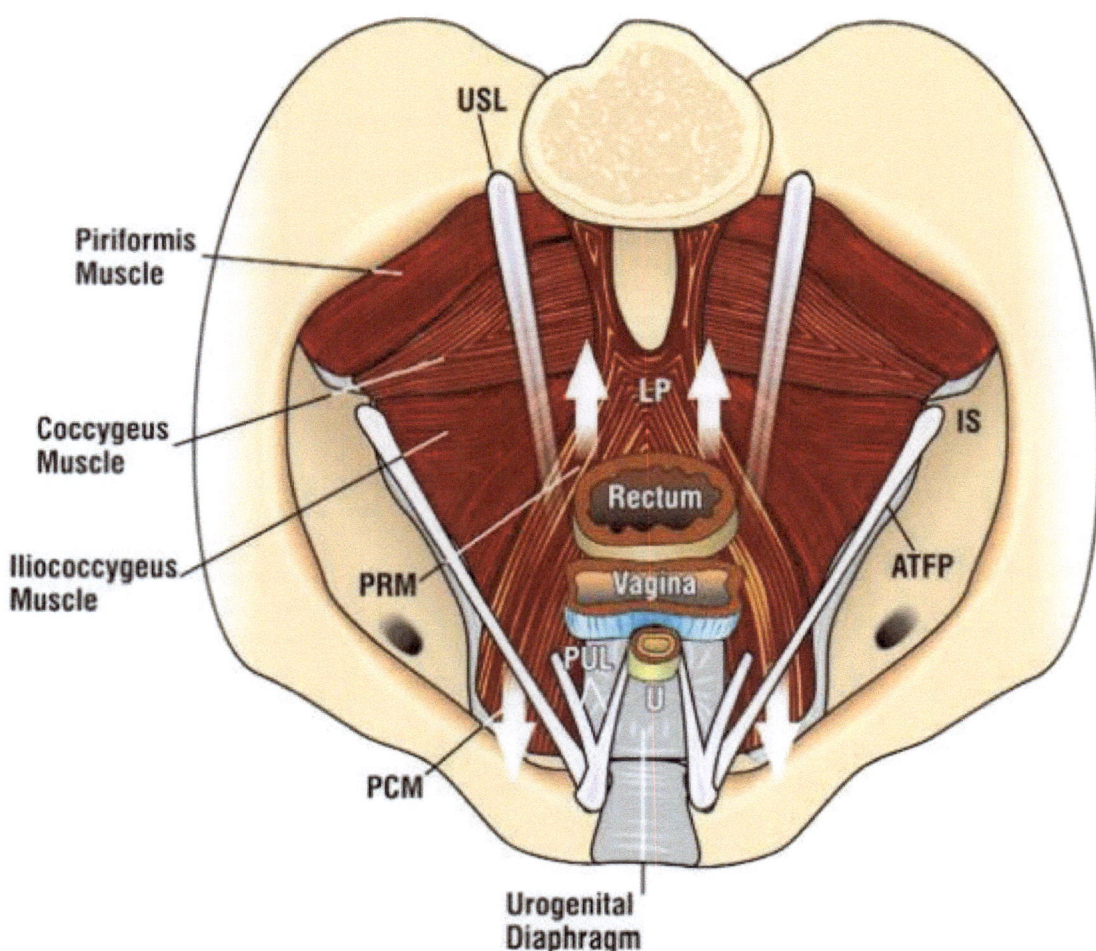

Fig. 3.6. Schematic representation of levator plate
(according to **Petros P., 2011b**)

ATFP = arcus tendineus fascia pelvii, F = fascia, IS = ischial spine, LP = levator plate, PRM = puborectal muscle, PS = pubic symphysis, PUL = pubourethral ligament, S = sacrum, U = urethra, USL = uterosacral ligaments

Puborectal muscle has an important role in pelvic floor anatomy. It starts from the internal side of the superior pubis and medially from the pubococcygeus muscle, being inserted on the anterior and lateral wall of the rectum, crossing all the three muscle layers. The muscle is vertically oriented and plays a quite important role in the voluntary contraction of the perineum, during Kegel exercises, lifting the levator plate during its contraction.

Its form is of a fan, dividing its fibers into two categories:
- superior fibers will divagate, compared to the longitudinal fibers of the rectum, inserting laterally on a fibrous membrane and medially creating a fibrous tendinous arch, which will insert posteriorly on the rectovaginal fascia and on the perineal body;
- inferior fibers will descend together with the longitudinal rectal fibers, to the level of the perianal tegument, thus inserting at this level.

i) *Iliac side* – the iliococcygeus muscle originates on the posterior side of the tendinous muscle and on the ischial spine, and is inserted on the posterior side of the anococcygeal ligament and coccyx.

The pubococcygeus muscle together with the iliococcygeus and puborectal muscles represents the so-called *levator plate* described by Petros, which has an important functional role.

The levator ani muscle is covered by 2 fascias: superior fascia of pelvic diaphragm and its inferior fascia.

3.2.1.2. Coccygeus muscle

It represents a musculotendinous structure that takes part in the formation of the posterior side of *pelvic diaphragm*. It is triangular, originates on the ischial spine, and is inserted on the edges of the coccyx and sacrum vertebrae (S4).

3.2.2. Muscular middle layer

The muscular middle layer is made up of the longitudinal anal muscle (LAM), an inconsistent anatomical structure formed from the fibers of the puborectal and puboanal muscles and interposed between the circular layers of the internal (IAS) and external (EAS) anal sphincters (**Strohbehn K.,** *et al.***, 1996**). It extends from the level of the anorectal junction along the anal canal, receiving fibers from the innermost part of the puborectalis and the puboanalis muscles, and terminating with seven to nine fibro-elastic septa, which traverse the subcutaneous part of the external anal sphincter, reaching the perianal dermis. With the fibers oriented inwards, LAM exerts pulling on the bladder, keeping it closed during physical effort and moving it inferiorly to allow micturition. Being situated at the level of the external anal sphincter, LAM will also determine the posterior angulation of the rectum during its contraction (Fig. 3.7).

3.2.3. Inferior muscle layer

The inferior muscle layer is made up of the muscles inserted on the perineal membrane, the urogenital diaphragm muscles, the external anal sphincter, and the post levator plate, a tendinous structure that may contain striated muscle fibers with insertion at the level of the external anal sphincter. It mainly represents an anchoring and stabilization plane of the inferior sides of the urethra, vagina, and anus (Fig. 5.5).

3.2.3.1. Ischiocavernosus muscle

Originates on the medial side of ischial tuberosity and the ischiopubic ramus and covers the free surface of the roots of cavernous body of clitoris, its role being of compressing them through its contraction (**Lupu G., 2005**), but also of stabilizing the perineal membrane, by stretching the external urethral meatus through the pulling exerted on the adjacent bulbocavernosus muscle (**Strohbehn K.,** *et al.***, 1996**).

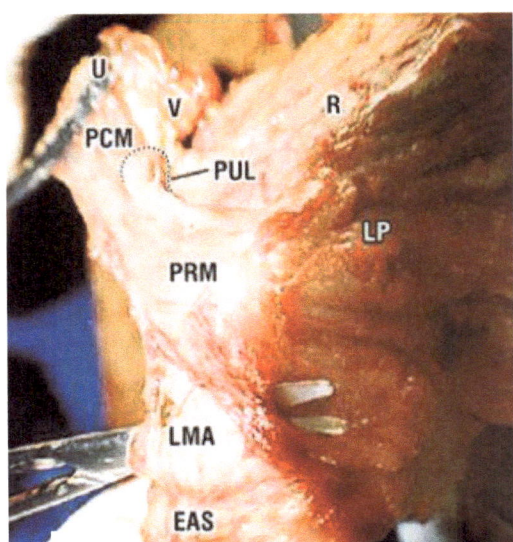

Fig. 3.7. Anatomic specimen that shows the presence of the longitudinal anal muscle
(according to **Petros P., 2011***b*)

EAS = external anal sphincter, LMA = longitudinal anal muscle, LP = levator plate, PCM = pubococcygeus muscle, PRM = puborectal muscle, PUL = puborectal ligament, R = rectum, U = urethra, V = vagina.

3.2.3.2. Bulbospongiosus muscle

It represents a thin paramedian muscle that covers the external side of the vestibular bulb and the greater vestibular glands (Bartholin). The two bulbospongiosus muscles connect posteriorly at the level of the perineal body and are fixed in the posterior side at the level of the anovulvar median raphe. They terminate at the anterolateral side of the vaginal aperture and are fixed at the clitoris level, through two fascicles inserted on its dorsal side and on the suspensory ligament of clitoris. Through its contraction, it compresses the soft structures, which it covers, anchors the distal plane of the urethra (Petros) and contributes to the constriction of the vagina in the anterior plane (**Papilian V., 1993**).

3.2.3.3. Superficial transverse perineal muscle (transversus perinei superficialis)

Its origin is on the internal side of the ischial tuberosity, it passes more or less transversely and ends at the level of the perineal body, which it can put in tension through its bilateral contraction. It can also lack, both unilaterally and bilaterally, being replaced by fibrous tracts (**Papilian V., 1993**).

3.2.3.4. Deep transverse perineal muscle

It is located on the medial side of the ischium and inserts at the level of the perineal body, fixing it and having the role of supporting the pelvic floor (**Papilian V., 1993**).

3.2.3.5. Urethral sphincter muscle

It is a muscle which spreads along the whole urethra and which is hard to be evidenced macroscopically. In the upper segment, where the urethra does not adhere to the vagina, the sphincter totally surrounds it. In the upper segment where the organs adhere, the muscle has a semicircular form, its margins being inserted in the vagina. These fascicles make up the urethrovaginal muscle (**Papilian V., 1993**).

3.2.3.6. External anal sphincter (sphincter ani externus)

It is a well-developed layer of voluntary striated muscle, which originates on the anococcygeal ligament, from which the fibers split into two halves that surround the rectum and then insert on the central tendon. Some of the muscular fibers continue with the bulbospongiosus muscles. It is made up of 3 tissues (subcutaneous, superficial and deep), but, fibers from the next muscular groups also participate in its structure: bulbospongiosus, puborectalis muscles, and puboanalis muscles. Recently, a new fascicle of muscular fibers with a longitudinal trajectory and which has been called *longitudinal anal muscle* has been described (**Petros P., 2011***b*). Its structure represents a functional connection of two muscular systems with different structures and topography (**Papilian V., 1993**).

3.2.3.7. Rectovaginal muscle

It connects the two organs and is located above the perineum center (**Papilian V., 1993**). Moreover, it is enclosed in the rectovaginal septum.

3.3. Connective structure of perineum

It is represented by perineal fascia and ligaments.

3.3.1. Superficial investing fascia of perineum (Gallaudet fascia)

It is a subcutaneous conjunctive form that covers the subjacent areas of the urogenital region. The fascia is laterally delimited by ischiopubic rami, anteriorly by the pubis and posteriorly by the posterior edge of deep transverse perineal muscle, at this level connecting with the inferior fascia of the urogenital diaphragm (**Papilian V., 1993**).

3.3.2. Inferior fascia of urogenital diaphragm (perineal membrane)

It has a triangular form, similar to the previous and it also stretches between the two ischiopubic rami. It is made up of two foils between which the deep transverse perineal muscle can be found. Vestibular (vaginal) bulbs and roots of clitoris adhere to it. Prior to the urethra, the two foils adhere and form a fibrous and resistant condensation called *transverse ligament of perineum (ligamentum transversum perinei)* (**Papilian V., 1993**).

3.3.3. Deep perineal fascia (endopelvic fascia, parietal endopelvic fascia)

It is a fibrous tissue that covers the superior side of the pelvic floor muscles. It inferiorly limits (or, according to some authors, it is included in) the subperitoneal pelvic cavity. Moreover, it represents a lower continuation of transversus abdominis muscle fascia (**Papilian V., 1993**), Fig. 3.8.

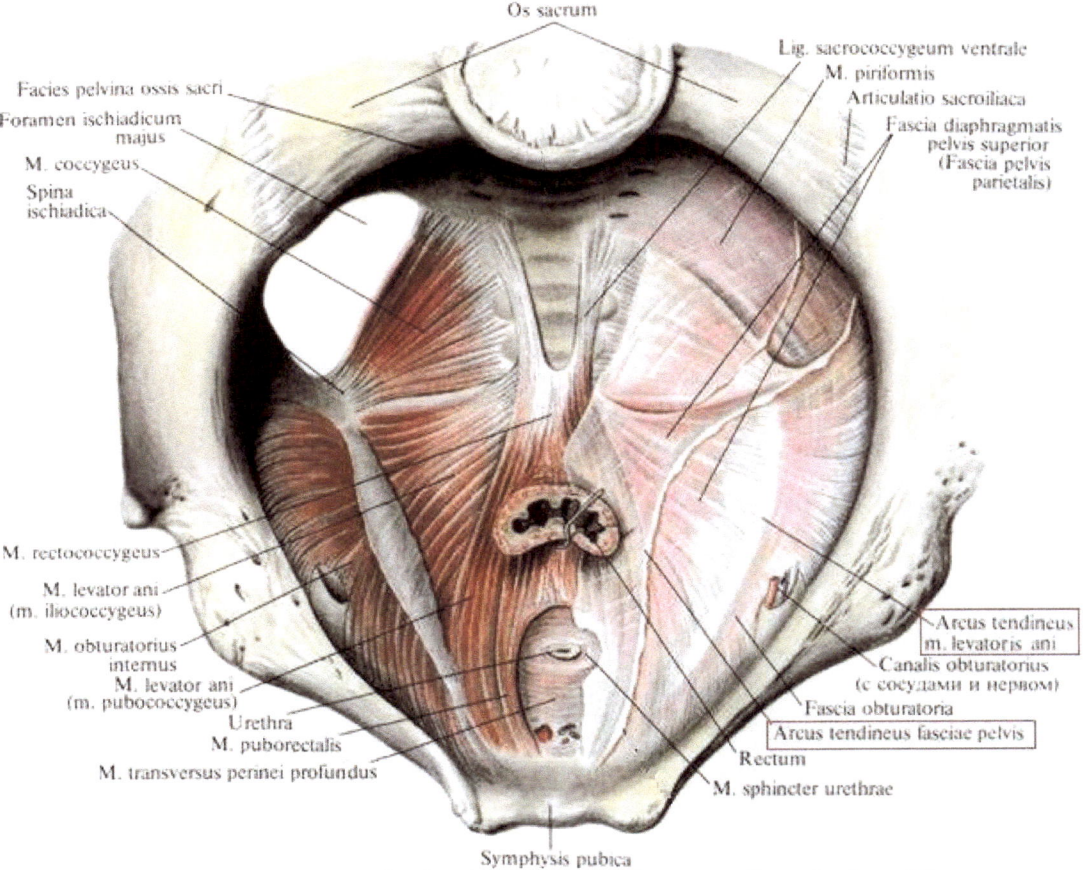

Fig. 3.8. Anatomy of endopelvic fascia and of *arcus tendineus fasciae pelvis*
(according to **Sinelnikov, 1981**)

Internal obturator muscle fascia presents a fibrous condensation - *arcus tendineus levator ani,* which divides the fascia into two: the lower one takes part in delimiting the ischioanal fossa and the upper one is part of the endopelvic fascia.

At the level of levator ani muscles, the parietal fascia presents a condensation of conjunctive fibers – *arcus tendineus fasciae pelvis,* which adheres to levator ani muscles fascia and should not be confused with arcus tendineus levator ani. This structure is very important in pelvic floor disorders because it represents a strong means of lateral anchoring of parietal fascia (**Narducci F., *et al.,* 2000**).

3.4. Subperitoneal pelvic cavity

It is represented by the extraperitoneal space, which is delimited by the osteo-muscular walls of pelvic excavation and the pelvic peritoneal space, in which the bladder, uterus and vagina, rectal ampulla, as well as vessels and nerves can be found from front to back. It is made up of a thick connective tissue that is part of the extraperitoneal fascia (fascia extraperitonealis) and which divides in three elements.

3.4.1. Deep perineal fascia (endopelvic fascia, parietal endopelvic fascia)
It was presented in subchapter 3.3.3.

3.4.2. Visceral pelvic facia (Fascia pelvis visceralis)
It covers the pelvic organs such as bladder, vagina, cervix, and rectum, forming its own sheaths. The tissue that covers the vagina is also called *paracolpos*, and the one covering the cervix, *paracervix*.

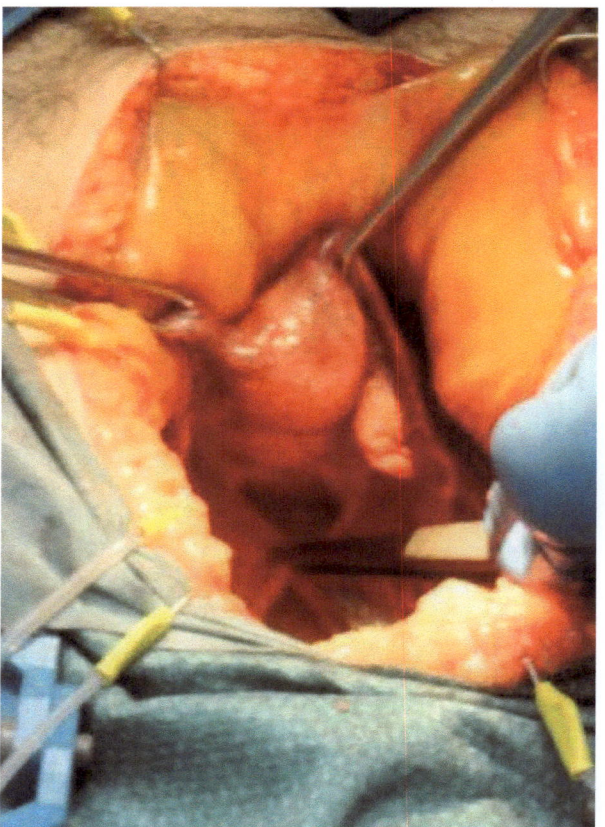

Fig. 3.9. Uterosacral ligaments (recto-uterine ligaments) in a cadaver
(according to **Enache T., 2014**)

3.4.2.1. Pubocervical fascia
These structures interconnect at the level of the vesicovaginal junction and form a very strong structure. Laterally, the fascia inserts at the level of the arcus tendineus fasciae pelvis, posteriorly its fibers intertwine with the paracervix and insert in the cervix, and, anteriorly, the fascia inserts in the pubis, covering the urethra.

3.4.2.2. Rectovaginal fascia (Denonvillier's fascia)
Denonvillier's fascia spreads from the level of corpus perineum in the inferior side to the pouch of Douglas, being attached to the uterosacral ligaments and the pericervical fascia structures. Together with the pubocervical fascia, Denonvillier's fascia represents a stand for the upper vagina. In addition, in the case of uterine prolapse that relapses after the uterosacral ligaments *"strengthening"*, the restoration of the above-mentioned fascia to their initial position is also necessary, by fixing them inferiorly and laterally to the uterosacral ligaments and superiorly and laterally to the cardinal ligaments.

3.4.3. Lax connective tissue

It fills the empty spaces between the viscera and the pelvic walls. Moreover, it condenses, especially around the vessels, due to pulsations that induce tissues vibrations. It also contains smooth muscle fibers that form *fibrovascular membranes*, among which *secondary spaces* are delimited.

3.4.3.1. Fibrovascular membranes

Their muscular fibers adhere to the venous walls of pelvic plexus, thus having a role in adjusting the pelvic venous circulation.

a) Sacral recto genital-pubic lamellas – also called "hypogastric sheaths" are sagittally oriented, originating on the anterior side of the median sacral crest, having a posterior-anterior path and a tight report with the lateral sides of the rectum, vagina, and bladder. The anterior part inserts into the pubic bones. They correspond to the lateral, hypogastric and obturator sacral arteries. Moreover, they are better represented posteriorly, being known as *uterosacral ligaments*, Fig. 3.9., while anteriorly, *pubovesical ligaments*, and pubocervical fascia are met. Cranial, they are covered by peritoneum and caudal, they are inserted at the level of arcus tendineus fasciae pelvis (**Papilian V., 1993; Narducci F., et al., 2000**).

Pubovesical ligaments – are fibromuscular rings that sustain the anterior wall of the bladder and prevent its movement posteriorly during micturition. Their insertion at the level of the bladder, on a wide area with a thickened aspect, is sometimes called Gilvernet pre-cervical transverse arch (Gilvernet trigonalis loop) (Petros P.).

b) Lateral ligaments of rectum – accompany the middle rectal arteries and frontally head from the sacral recto genital-pubic lamellas to the lateral sides of rectal ampulla and its fascia.

c) Rectovaginal septum (Fascia of Otto) – is a thin fibrous structure, which can also be found frontally.

d) Umbilical prevesical fascia (Fascia umbilicalis) – is found on the superior umbilical and vesical arteries (**Papilian V., 1993**).

3.4.3.2. Secondary spaces

Are a connective tissue delimited by fibrovascular lamellae.

a) Pararectal spaces

b) Retrorectal (presacral) space

c) Parameter – is the space at the level of the broad ligaments, crossed by very important elements such as uterine arteries, ureters, veins, lymphatic arteries nerves. At this level, there is a fibrous condensation with a transversal aspect and a powerful anchoring on the paracervix, which is less clearly delimited at the level of the lateral wall of the pelvic excavation. It is one of the most important means of supporting the uterus, also called *Mackenrodt's transverse cervical ligaments*. Caudal, they are not inserted on the deep perineal fascia, Fig. 3.8.

d) Prevesical space – ranges cranial to the navel, being delimited by the navel arteries (**Aukee P., et al., 2004**).

DeLancey divided the pelvic subperitoneal space into three levels of uterovaginal support, in 1992. *Level I* (the upper part) is assigned to the apical support means of paracolpos: uterosacral ligaments and, to a lower degree, Mackenrodt's transverse cervical ligaments. *Level II* – the lateral anchoring of the paracolpos to the pelvic wall represents the medium supporting part of the vagina. Anteriorly to the vagina, the paracolpos is made up of the adventitia of the vagina and the pubocervical fascia, which extends laterally and is inserted on the *arcus tendineus fasciae pelvis*. Posteriorly to the vagina, it is represented by the rectovaginal fascia.

Level III – is the distal part of anchoring of the vagina, which is directly made anteriorly, to the urogenital diaphragm and posteriorly, to perineal body (**DeLancey J.O.L., 2002**), Fig. 3.10. and Fig. 3.11.

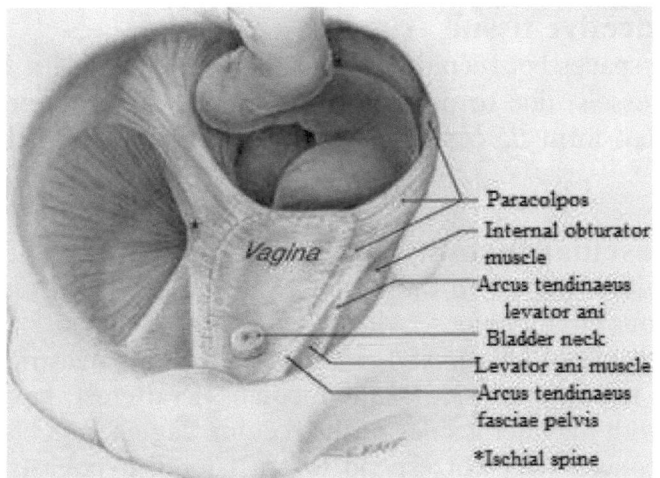

Fig. 3.10. Cervix and upper part of the vagina supporting means
(according to **DeLancey J.O.L., 2002**)

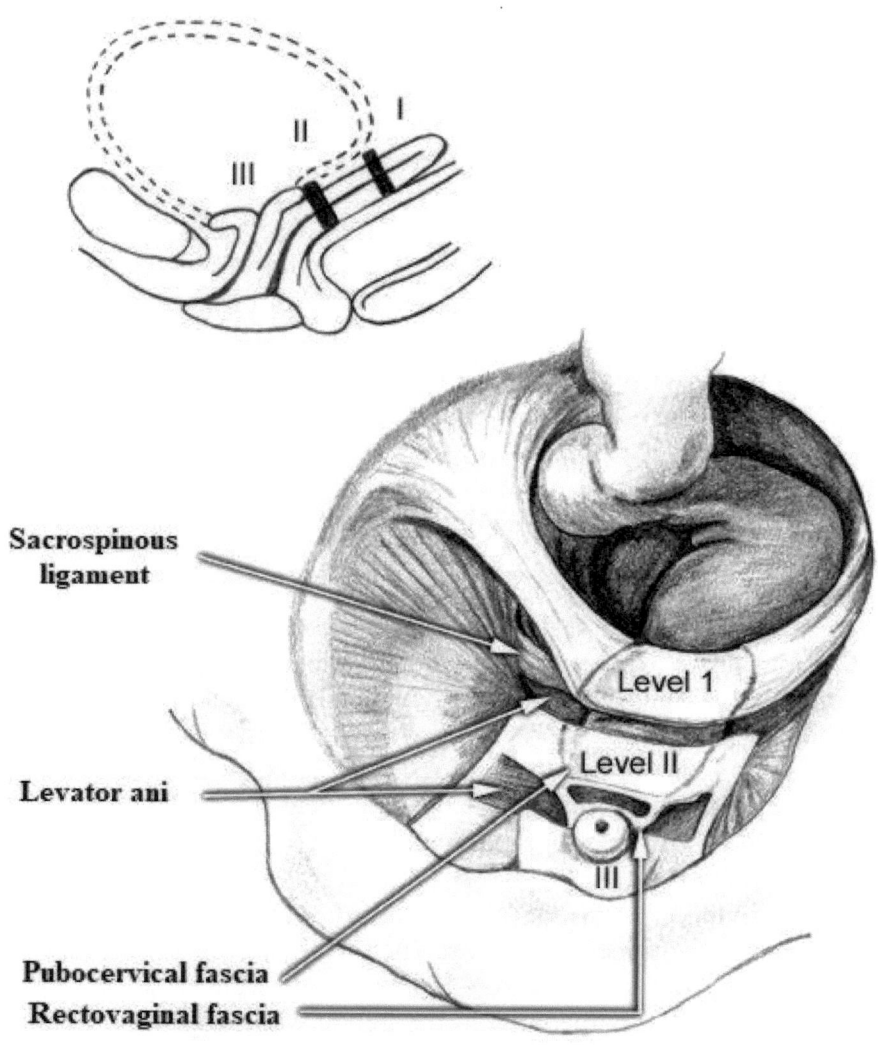

Fig. 3.11. Levels of biomechanical support of pelvic fascia
(according to **DeLancey J.O.L., 2002**)

3.5. Anatomical landmarks with practical application

There are some elements that must be precisely identified in the current surgical practice. Due to the anatomical structure, the perineum is a hardly accessible space, some of the elements cannot be seen, but can only be spotted. This way, their presentation becomes imperative not only from the teaching point of view, which means the correct understanding of the pelvic floor disorders, but mostly for the surgical technique.

3.5.1. Urethra support means

In the subdiaphragmatic part, the urethra is strongly anchored anteriorly through two ligaments:

a) Pubourethral ligament

b) External urethral ligament – is a lateral and posterior extension of the suspensory ligament of the clitoris, Fig. 3.12.

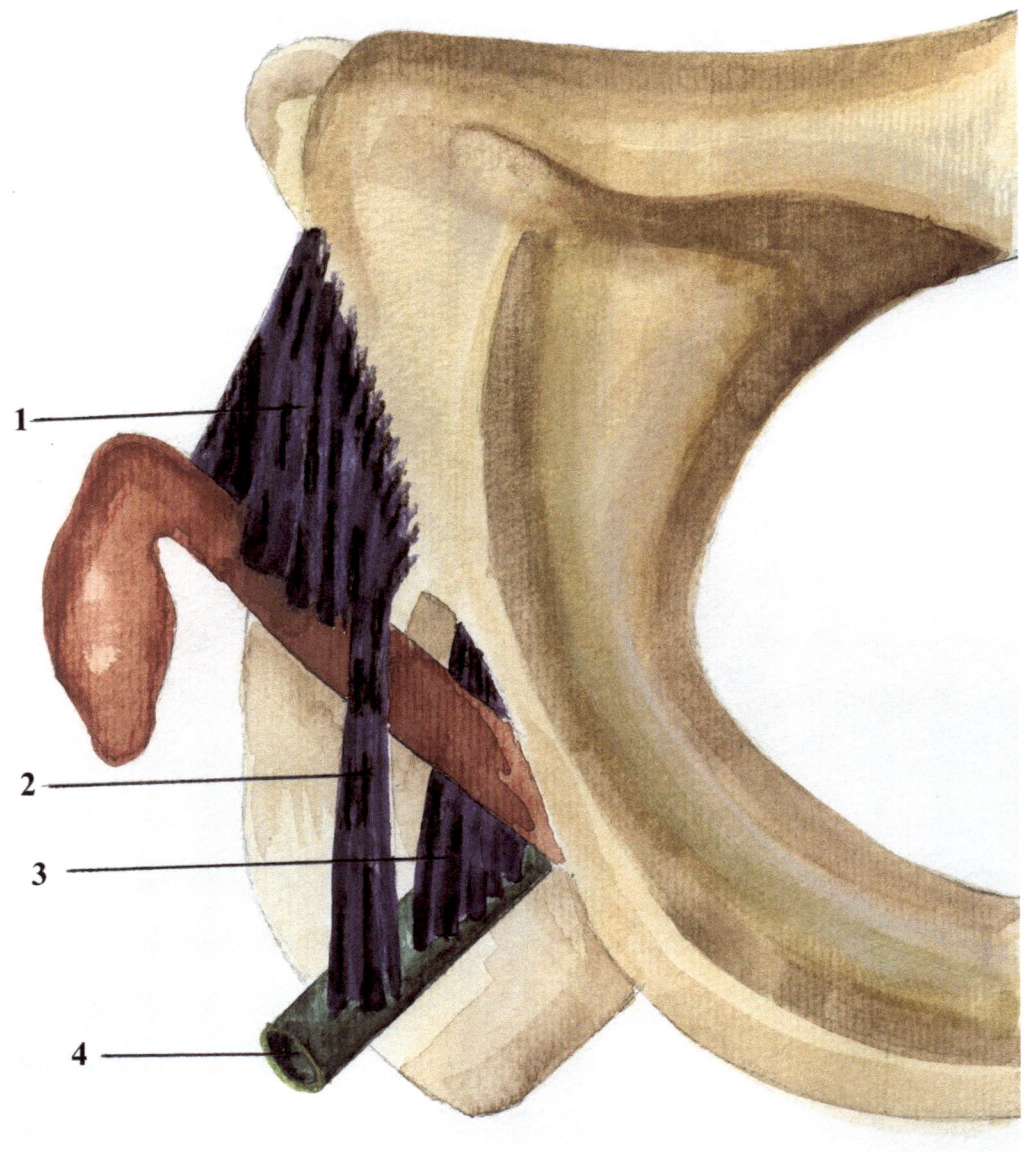

Fig. 3.12. Urethra support means (*drawing by Vanessa Mureşan*)
1 Suspension clitoris ligament, 2 External urethral ligament, 3 Pubourethral ligament, 4 Urethra

3.5.2. Ureterovesical junction

Its clinical spotting is done by mounting a Foley catheter, while inflating the autostatic balloon catheter and its dragging until it blocks at the level of the bladder.

Then the balloon is palpated through the vaginal mucosa, thus identifying the junction. This maneuver is very important because it allows the avoiding of the vaginal trigone of Pawlick, which is homologous to Lieutaud's trigone that corresponds to Foley balloon catheter.

This area which has an embryological origin, different from the rest of the bladder, has a rich network of nerves, thus, must be avoided during the surgical maneuvers (**Kamina P., 2000**), Fig. 3.13.

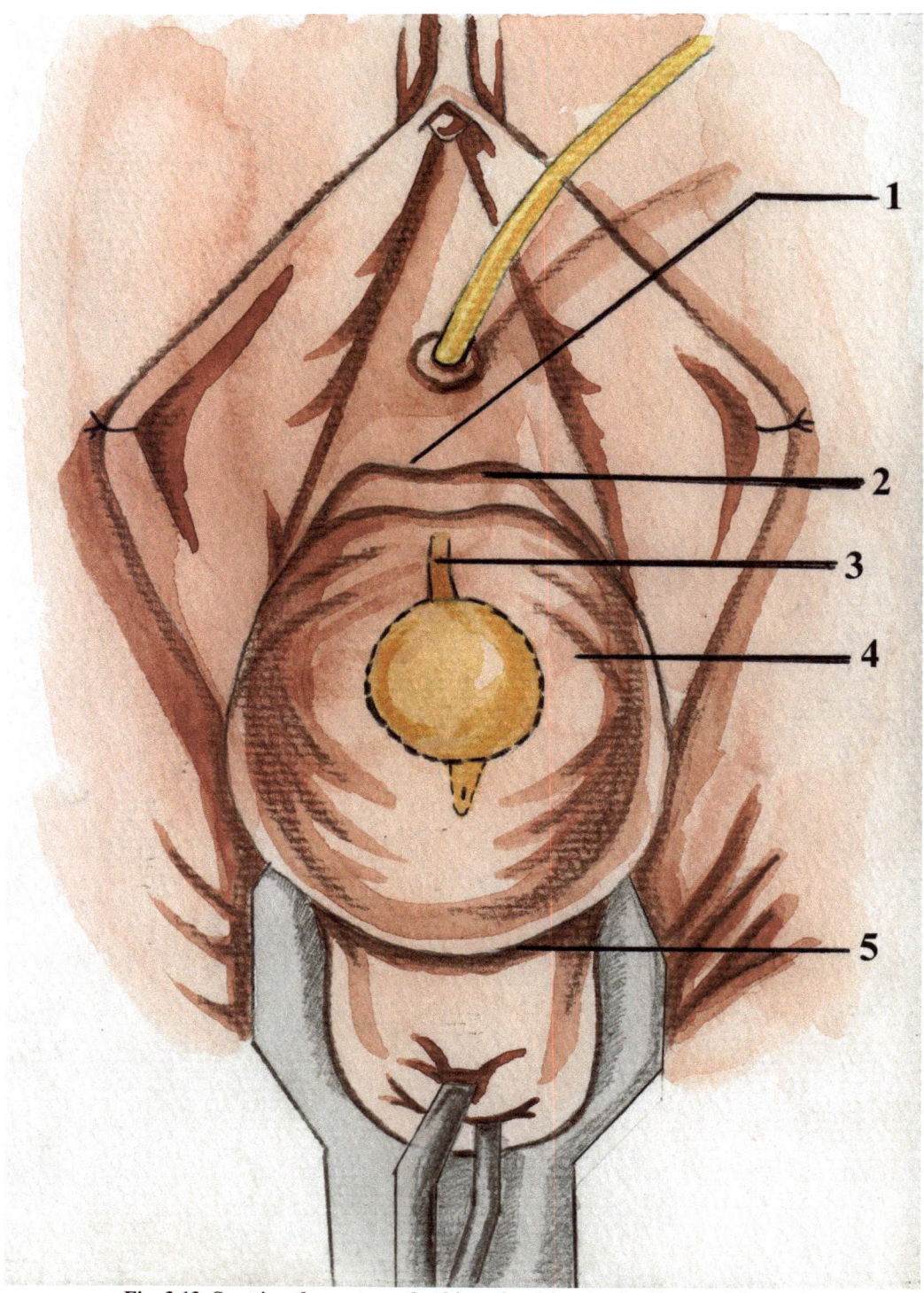

Fig. 3.13. Spotting the cystourethral junction (*drawing by Vanessa Mureşan*)
1 Vaginal covering, 2 Infra-urethral channel, 3 Catheterized urethra, 4 Vesico-vaginal channel,
5 Cervico-vaginal channel

3.5.3. Arcus tendineus fasciae pelvis

It has a theoretical and practical importance, being a mandatory element when looking for the internal side of the internal obturator muscle that covers the obstructed hole (**Narducci F.,** *et al.,* **2000**). This structure is palpated like a fiber cord at the level pof the posterior side of the pubis.

3.5.4. Ischial muscle spindles

Represent one of the most important landmarks of perineal surgery, which are only accessible to digital exploration and are located in the median third of the pelvic excavation, at the level of its lateral wall. During the surgical techniques that use this landmark, it is important to note the ratio with the internal pudendal arteries that posteriorly surround the spindle in their way from the cranial to the caudal, a moment in which they change direction to enter the Alcock canal (**Berek & Novak's, 2012**; **Thompson J.R.**, *et al., * **1999**), Fig. 3.14.

3.5.5. Sacrospinous ligament

It is a triangular ligament, with its top inserted on the ischiatic muscle spindle and its base heading along the lateral sides of the sacrum and coccyx. It is located on the posterior side of the coccygeus muscle, towards its superior edge. According to some anatomists, the sacrospinous ligament is only the posterior tendinous side of this muscle, which is palpated starting from the ischial spine towards posterior and cranial (**Berek & Novak's, 2012**; **Roshanravan S.M.**, *et al.,* **1976**), Fig. 3.15.

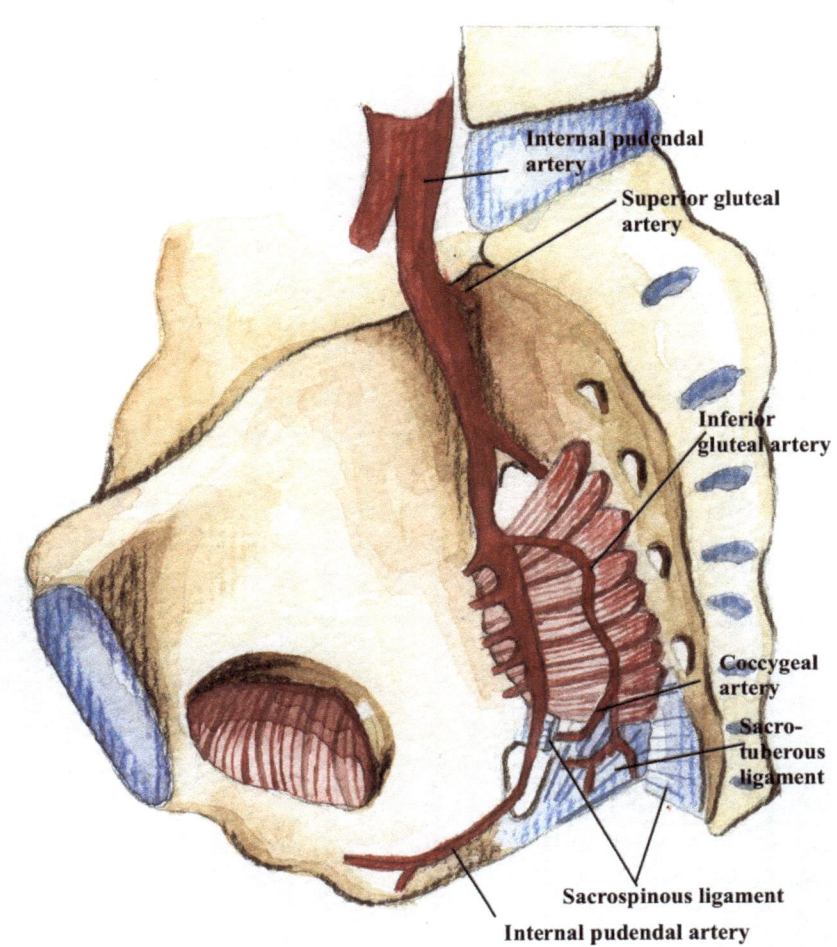

Fig. 3.14. **Ischial spine and its ratio with the internal pudendal artery**
(*drawing by Vanessa Mureşan*)

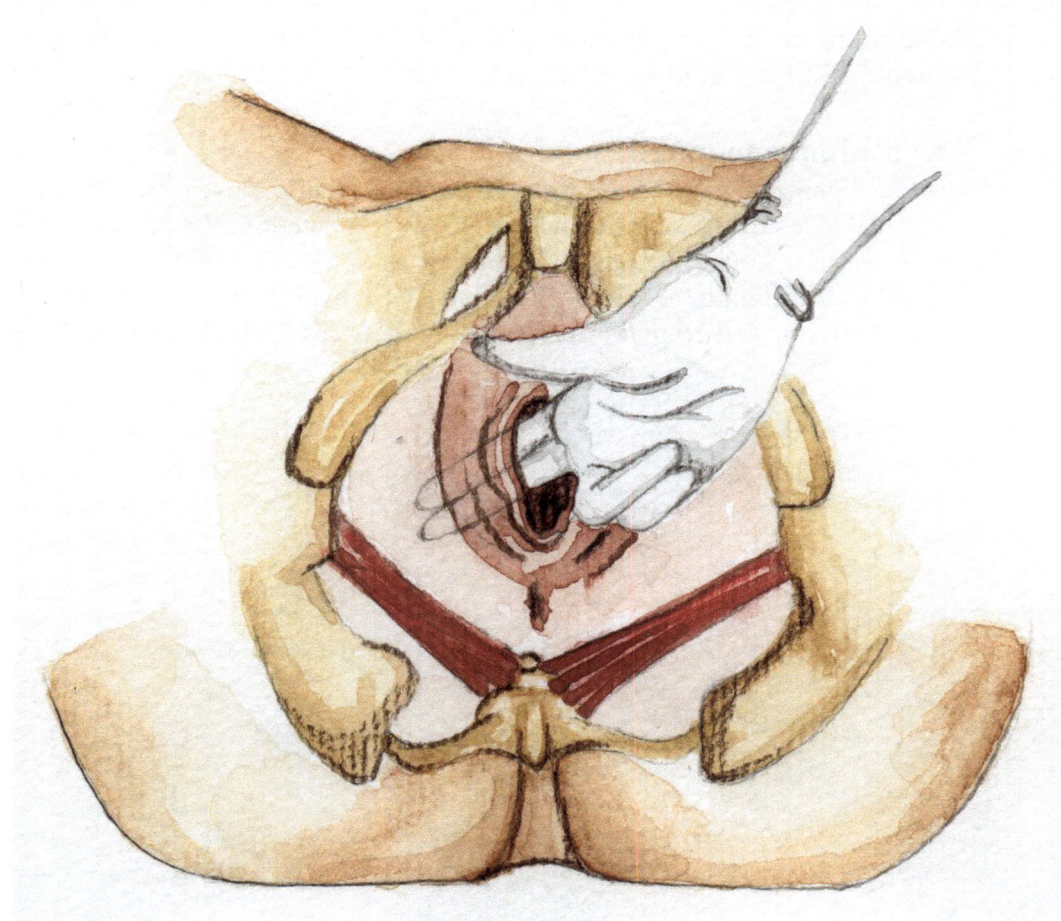

Fig. 3.15. Spotting the sacrospinous ligament
(*drawing by Vanessa Mureşan*)

3.6. Applied histology of pelvic organs and perineal tissues

The main pelvic organs, such as the urethra, vagina, and rectum are similar to some elastic membranes, which do not have an intrinsic ability of sustaining themselves. Thus, the function of the pelvic organs is conditioned by the integrity of the ligaments, fascias and muscles around them, more exactly by their biochemical composition, stiffness, and direction of exerting their force, Fig. 3.16.

Although the muscular lesions obviously lead to the weakening of their contractile properties, the elastic properties of the connective tissue are the ones that ensure continence, fact that was demonstrated by the success of the surgeries based on the strengthening or the functional replacing of the pelvic ligaments (especially the uterosacral ligaments).

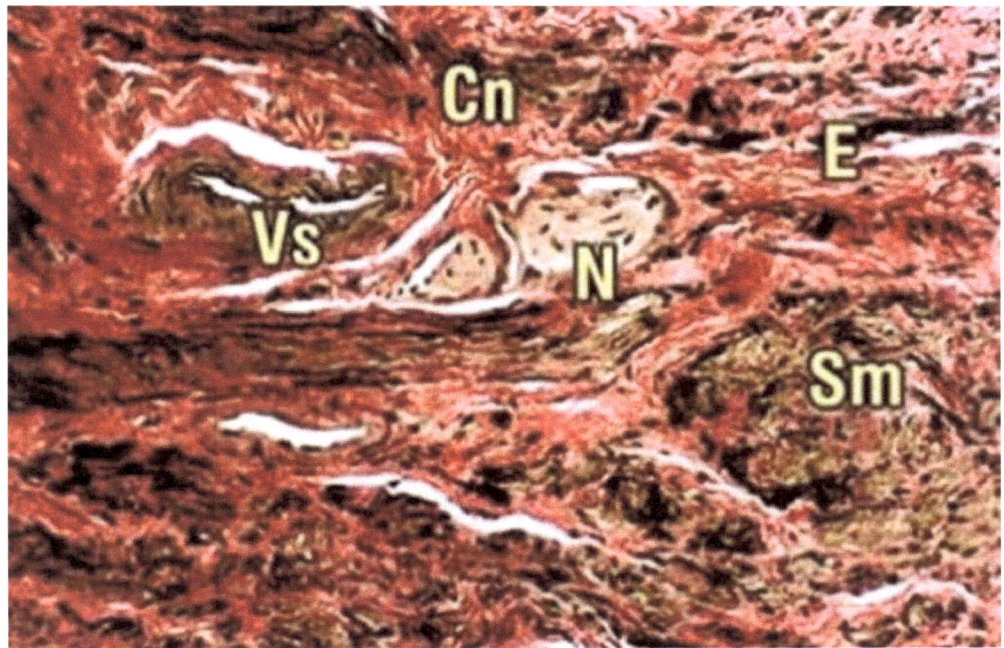

Fig. 3.16. Histological section through the pubourethral ligament
(according to **Petros P., 2011***b*)
Cn = collagen, E = elastin, N = nerve fiber, Sm = smooth muscle, Vs = vessel

Collagen and elastin modify after pregnancy and vaginal birth, but also during the normal process of senescence, weakening the pelvic floor and leading to incontinence in time. The reconstruction of the initial structure of the collagen fiber is only partly possible, leading to a suboptimal transmission of the vectors of muscles strength throughout some fascias and ligaments, whose structural integrity has been compromised.

The structure of the connective tissue varies according to age and hormonal intake. It mainly consists in three biochemical compounds: glycosaminoglycans, basic matrix, elastin, deforming, and collagen, structural stiffness. The understanding of the biomechanics of collagen fibers is mandatory: at rest, the collagen fibers form the letter "S". The moment a ligament is tensioned, the collagen fibers expand and act like a stiff bar, thus preventing the excessive elongation of the muscle fibers and ensuring their optimal contractility.

However, the collagen form at rest alters with age, when less and less intermolecular bridges are formed, thus "*blocking*" the collagen in its at rest state, such as the case of the fibers which are transversally arranged and diminishing the resistance of the tissues to 60% of their potential value (**Perumal S.,** *et al.,* **2008**). The regular contribution of estrogen can prevent the structural and functional impairment of the collagen fibers to some extent, which is why the estrogen that is applied intravaginally is recommended after menopause. The decrease of the elastin level is a well-known component of the aging process and represents an explanation for the involuntary losses of urine in female patients suffering from a low urethral pressure. Moreover, hormone depletion also decreases the turgor of the tissue. Through a cumulative effect, these modifications lead to the poor anchoring of the vagina at different degrees, starting from a discrete lateral fascial defect and ending with the total uterine prolapse.

Another category of modifications also appears during pregnancy, when collagen suffers a depolymerization due to the action of the placental hormones, allowing the vaginal distention during birth. However, laxity also extends at the level of the suspensory ligaments, weakening the support means of the pelvic organs and often leading to stress urinary incontinence during pregnancy. This laxity may also be the cause for pelvic pains, felt like a bilateral pulling in the inferior abdomen, through the loss of sustaining the nerves fibers at the level of the ligaments in the rear compartment. The moment the vaginal birth takes place, the obstetrical traumatisms can lead to the stretching or even the separation of the ligaments from their insertion places, making the surgical reconstruction of the injured tissue mandatory (**Petros P., 2011***a*).

3.6.1. Histology of bladder

The bladder is made up smooth muscle fibers, which overlap forming three layers: longitudinal - external, circularly - middle and plexiform - internal. This muscle architecture has a role due to the way the fibers organize near the neck of urinary bladder.

The longitudinal, eternal fibers concentrate on the anterior and posterior sides of the urinary bladder, condensing into two fascicles: longitudinal anterior and posterior. At the level of the base of the bladder, the lateral parts of the longitudinal posterior fascicles unite to form a posterior concave loop, also called the loop of detrusor urinae muscle. The plexiform internal fibers also have a longitudinal direction, converging to the urinary meatus and prolonging towards the urethra. The disposal of these two types of fibers ensures the dilation of the neck of urinary bladder, thus making the micturition possible.

The circular fibers in the middle layer of the detrusor urinae muscle are caudal oriented and anterior at the level of the neck of urinary bladder, organizing in concentric rings in the rear plan, which become more and more dense at the level of the vesicourethral opening (ostium urethrae internum). They will form a constriction system that will press the neck of the urinary bladder, thus ensuring continence.

4. *Perineal physiology and physiopathology*
4.1. Introduction to *"Integral Theory System"*

Prof. Peter Papa Petros in collaboration with Prof. Ulf Ulmsten from the University in Uppsala have set the theoretical bases of *"Integral Theory System"* (**Petros P. & Ulmsten U.I., 1990; Petros P., 2010**).

As the name suggests, the *"Integral Theory System"* creates a dynamic and interconnected anatomical background to understand the function and dysfunction of perineum (**Petros P., 2010**). The *"Integral Theory System"* defines the pelvic floor as a syncytial system, based on vector equilibrium in which muscles and connective tissue take part and which has a nervous component. The newly formed system represents the sum of all the elements involved. Among them, the connective tissue is the most vulnerable.

The main principle of the theory is that *"the restoration of the form (structure) implicitly leads to the restoration of the function"* (**Petros P., 2010**).

In 1993, the theory was reformulated:

"Symptoms such as stress urinary incontinence, urinary urge and abnormal bladder emptying, derive from the laxity of the vagina or its support elements and cause an alteration of the connective tissue."

Structure and form

The structure and form are shown from the interaction of the muscles and ligaments on the pelvic organs. Both the vagina and the ligaments must be stretched as much as possible in order to offer the necessary resistance to sustain different organs and to counterbalance the abdominal pressure. Thus, it makes sense that the relationships between the different structures are not static, but in a continuous modulation of forces, which vary continuously. An imbalance of forces can tension this system in one way or another, thus affecting the form, support and/ or function of the organs (**Petros P., 2010**).

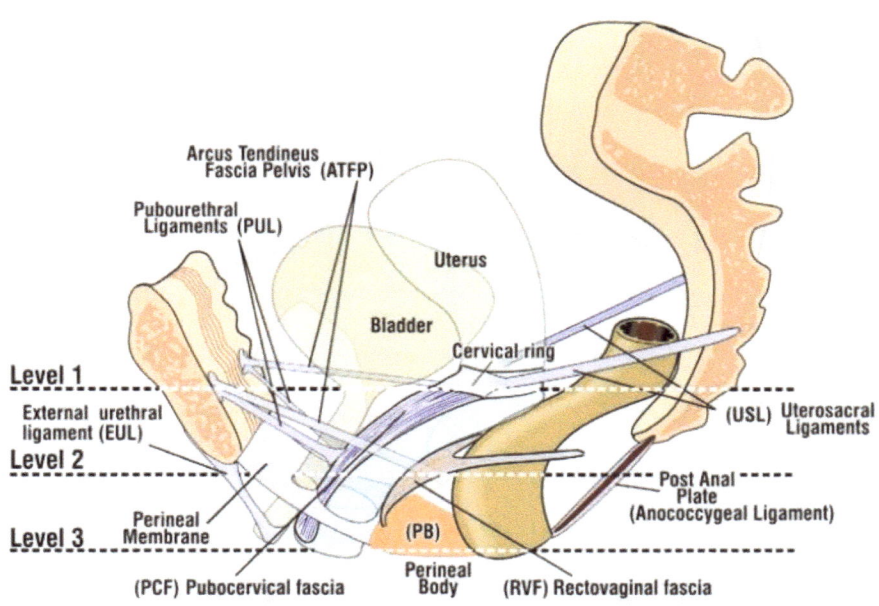

Fig. 4.1. Pelvic connective tissue
(according to **Petros P., 2010**)

Function and dysfunction

The "*Integral Theory System*" describes the normal the bladder and anorectal functions as having two stable states: closed, continence and open – micturition, defecation. The maintenance of these states is the result of the vector equilibrium of forces that act at the level of the perineum (**Petros P., 2010**).

4.2. Elements of dynamic and functional anatomy

The perineal dynamics influences the function of the pelvic organs. The anatomical reports modify according to the resting state or increased tonus, as well as the orthostatic or clinostatic position. In addition, the concept of dynamic anatomy appears. The perineal dynamics determines the function of the perineal organs.

4.2.1. Structure of connective tissue

Together with the bones, the connective tissue represents the structural component of the perineum and organises in ligaments and fascias. It is mainly made up of collagen and elastin; components that change their structure both during pregnancy and with age (**Kerkhof M.H.,** *et al.,* **2014**). These modifications can lead to the alteration of the form and subsequently of the function of the organs.

Collagen is the main structural component of ligaments. They cannot be reconstructed through suture, but through the synthesis of new collagen filaments that must be induced by the insertion of some fragments of alloplastic material so that it could lead to their reconstruction.

The role of elastin is very important in the conformation of the vagina. Elastin offers the vagina a low energy structure that sustains the bladder and contributes to the closure of the urethra.

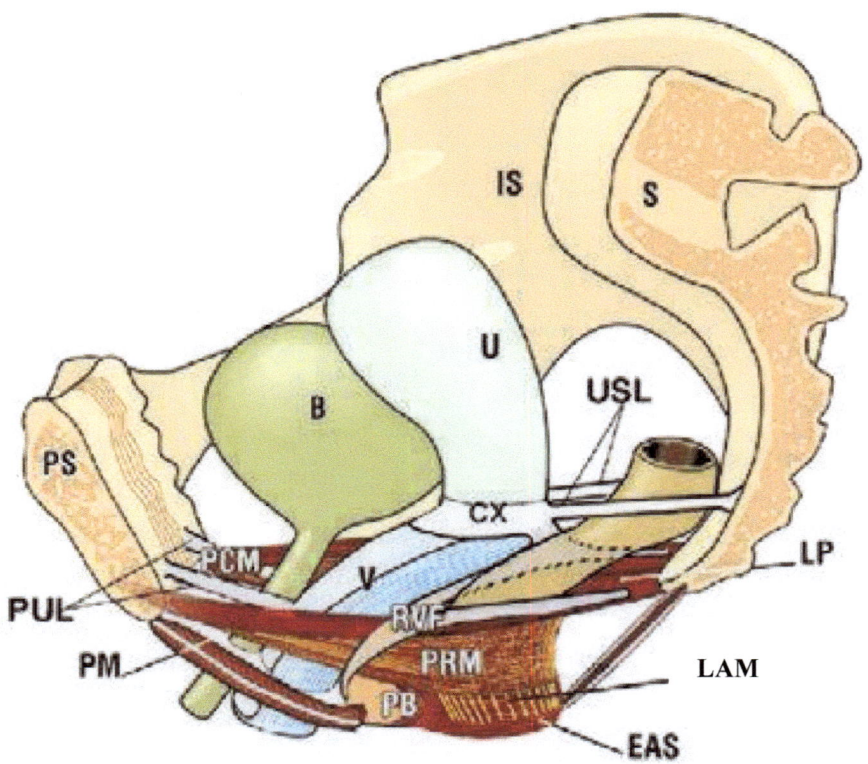

Fig. 4.2. Muscle and connective structure of perineum
(according to **Petros P., 2010**)

IS – ischium, S – sacrum, U – uterus, B – bladder, PS – pubis, CX – cervix, USL – uterosacral ligaments, RVF – rectovaginal fascia, PB – perineal body, PUL – pubourethral ligaments, PRM – puborectalis muscles, LAM – longitudinal anal muscle, LP – levator plate, EAS – external anal sphincter, PCM – pubocervical muscles

The muscle vectors that lead to the closure of the urethra and the anus are transmitted via the vagina. The vaginal mucosa excision during the classical procedures leads to the stiffening of the vagina through a decrease in elastin quantum and the scaring tissue that it induces. Moreover, the alloplastic materials placed on extensive surfaces induce the stiffening of the vagina (**Yamada H., 1970**).

There are some key elements regarding dynamics, in the anatomy of perineum, Fig. 4.1. and 4.2., (**Petros P., 2010**; **Zacharin R.F., 1963**).

a) Pubourethral ligaments (PUL) and external urethral ligaments (EUL).
b) Arcus tendineus fasciae pelvis (ATFP).
c) Uterosacral ligaments (USL).
d) Pubovesical ligament (PVL), described by Ingelman-Sundberg, in 1949, which inserts at the level of the pre-cervical arch of the bladder and gives stiffness to the anterior bladder wall. During effort, the pubovesical ligament helps fixing the neck of urinary bladder, which has a role in urinary continence.
e) Gilvernet pre-cervical transverse arch is a thickened part of the anterior bladder wall on which pubovesical ligaments insert. Its role is to limit the posterior pulling of the anterior bladder wall and to ensure a normal micturition.
f) Vesical trigone – although it has a muscular structure, it behaves like a ligament from a functional point of view, uniting with the bladder on the vaginal wall, which has a role in urinary continence.
g) Lateral extensions of vaginal fascia to arcus tendineus fasciae pelvis. They merge with the pubocervical and rectovaginal fascia.
h) Pubocervical fascia - (PCF) – inserts at the level of paracervix.
i) Rectovaginal fascia.
j) Paracervix.
k) Perineal body.

4.2.2. Perineal muscle structure according to Integral Theory System

Although classical anatomy proposes a topographical description, from the dynamic point of view it can be divided into three layers (**Petros P., 2011c**).

a) Superior layer – placed horizontally. It is represented by the pubococcygeus muscles, that are the anterior component and the levator plate (LP) (**Petros P., 2010**), by the posterior fascicles of levator ani muscles – posterior component. This layer has a role of supporting the pelvic organs and an important role in closing and opening the urethra, vagina, and anus.

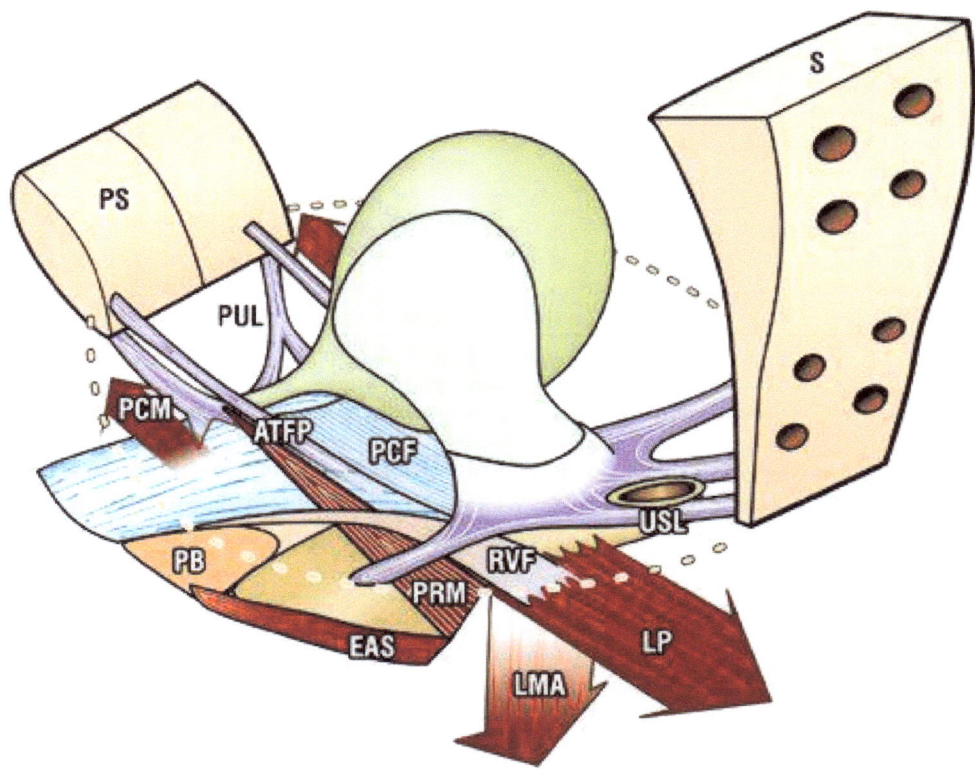

Fig. 4.3. Deep fascia and tension muscular mechanisms
(according to **Petros P., 2010**)

USL – uterosacral ligaments, RVF – rectovaginal fascia, PB – perineal body, PUL – pubourethral ligaments, PRM – puborectalis muscles, LMA – longitudinal anal muscle, LP – levator plate, EAS – external anal sphincter, PCM – pubocervical muscle, PCF – pubocervical fascia, ATFP– arcus tendineus fasciae pelvis

b) Vertical middle layer. It is represented by the longitudinal muscle of the anal canal (LAM). Through its contraction, the rectum presents a lower pulling, thus representing the vector component with a downword positioning of the pelvic muscles (**Petros P., 2010**).

c) Oblique lower layer. It is made up of the anterior perineal muscles and has a role of stabilizing the lower parts of the urethra, anus, and vagina.

The function of this layer depends on the integrity of the perineal body (**Petros P., 2010**).

According to Petros (**Petros P., 2011c**), the puborectal muscle (PRM) has a special role, it is interfacing, located obliquely, vertical than the rest of the levator ani muscles, its role being of lifting the whole levator plate. It represents the voluntary component activated during tenesmus treatment (Kegel exercises).

The muscles together with the ligaments and the perineal fasciae create a complex biomechanical mechanism, which ensures both the support function of pelvic organs, continually adapting to the pressure variations of the peritoneal cavity and to the adopted position, and, at the same time, ensures the extremely important functions of urinary retention and bladder and rectum emptying.

Analyzing the force directions of different muscle groups and the anchoring mode of the connective tissue, Peter Petros made a vector diagram that synthesizes their disposal. The tensioning of all the above-mentioned structures, Fig. 4.3, represents the key to pelvic floor (**Petros P., 2010**).

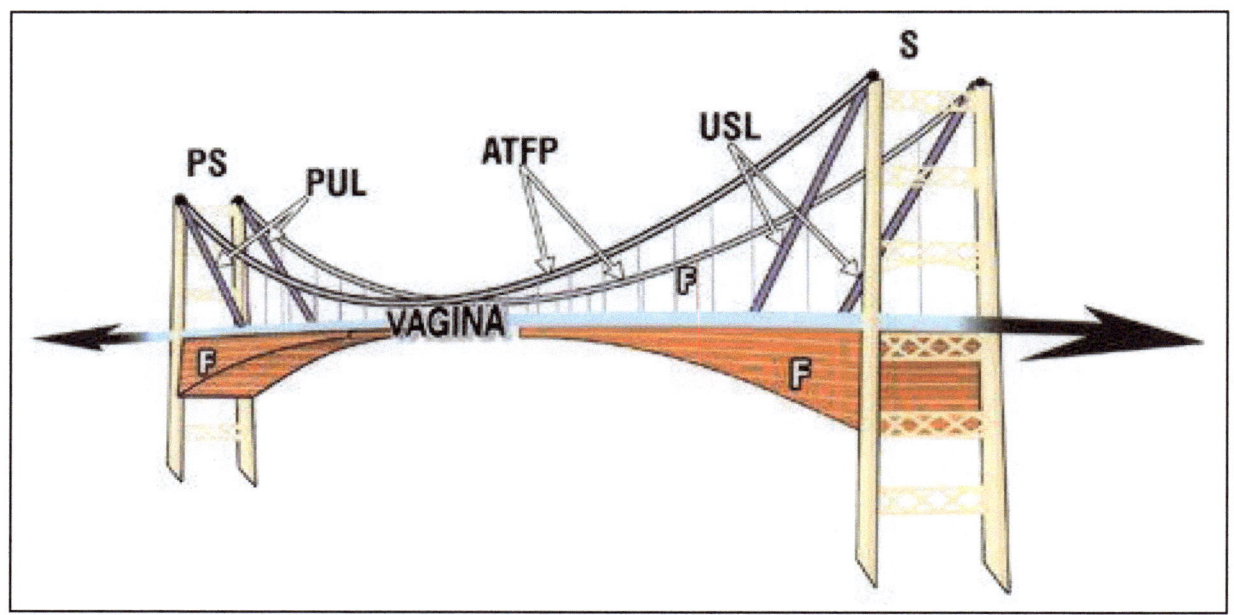

Fig. 4.4. Suspension bridge analogy
(according to **Petros P., 2010**)
USL – uterosacral ligaments, ATFP – arcus tendineus fasciae pelvis, PUL – pubourethral ligaments, S – sacrum, PS – pubis symphysis, F – fasciae

By analogy, the structure can be compared to the architecture of a suspended bridge. The weakening of any resistance element (ligament) can produce an imbalance with consequences both in the form and in the functioning of the whole system, Fig. 4.4.

4.3. Physiology of pelvic floor

The pelvic floor muscles work in a coordinated manner to stretch and angulate the pelvic organs backwards or downwards, to be compressed by the abdominal press but the pelvic floor to be maintained. The most important problem of maintaining the pelvic floor is the occlusion of the levator hiatus, the main role being taken by the vagina, which is attached to the bone walls through ligaments

4.3.1. Biomechanics of vagina

Recent imaging studies have demonstrated (**Durnea C.M.**, *et al.*, **2014**) that *"in vivo"*, while standing, the vagina does not have the oblique position described in classical anatomy. It maintains an oblique position in 1/3 caudally and in 2/3 cranially, it is horizontally oriented, Fig. 4.5. From the biophysical point of view, the vagina acts as an elastic membrane, tensioned by antagonistic muscle forces.

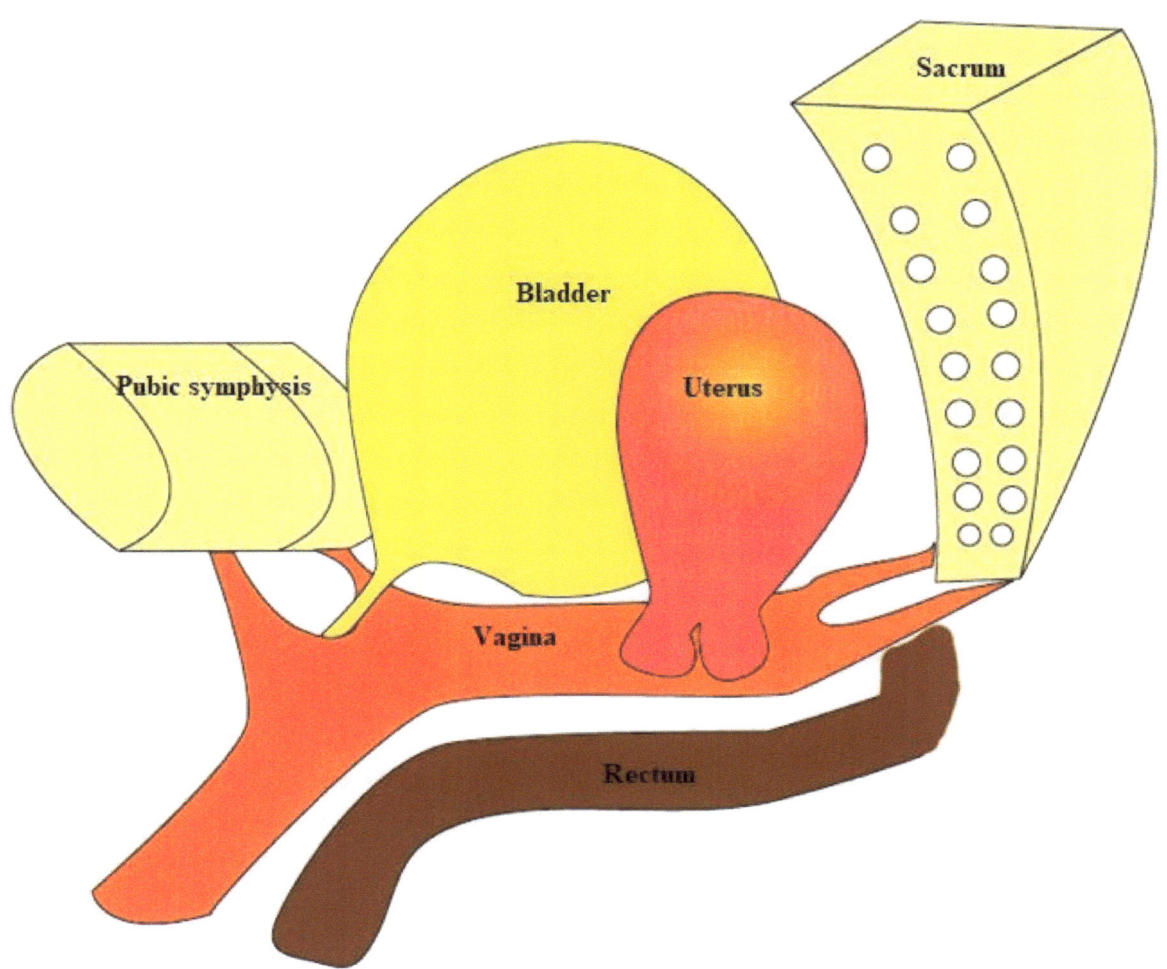

Fig. 4.5. Biomechanics of the vagina in orthostatism
(according to **Durnea C.M.**, *et al.*, **2014**)

Its resistance is given by the fascial connective tissue, adventitia, which connects it to different organs and through which the main structure with collagen fibers offers a limited extensibility. The elastic component is the elastin, which has the ability to return to the initial dimensions after the muscular tension stopped, and secondly, determines the anorectal and urethra closing with a minimal effort (**Petros P., 2010**).

Structure modifications according to the age
The elasticity of the vagina is a key element in pelvic organs function. The stiffening of the vagina with age (due to the reduction of the elastin fibers and the continuous tensioning of the collagen fibers) interferes with perineal physiology. Moreover, inter- and intramolecular bridges of the collagen fibers form with age, which lead, in time, to a raise in stiffness of up to 400% (**Yamada H., 1970**). The result is an incomplete obliteration of levator hiatus with a disruption of the organs' retention function (**Petros P., 2011***c*, **Karam J.A.**, *et al.*, **2007**).

Structure modifications induced by pregnancy
The connective tissue is sensitive to the hormones specific to pregnancy. Collagen goes through a depolymerization process and raises the percent of glycosaminoglycans (hyaluronic acid), decreasing the percent of proteoglycans (decorin) (**Zacharin R.F., 1963**). The result is an increased elasticity and a more lax anchoring of the connective elements to allow the pelvic ligaments dilation during birth. The frequent occurrence of intrapartum uterine prolapse is explained by the laxity of the connective tissue. Moreover, the appearance of stress urinary incontinence is observed, but all these modifications are transient and rapidly reversible (**Cunningham F.**, *et al.*, **2010**; **Karam J.A.**, *et al.*, **2007**; **Rechberger T.**, *et al.*, **1988**).

4.3.2. Biomechanics of bladder

The bladder is very closely connected to the vagina at the level of Lieutaud's trigone, which is correspondent to the vaginal trigone of Pawlick.

The area is very important during surgical treatment from the practical point of view due to the membranous structure of the bladder wall and the rich innervation at this level. The surgical intervention should avoid the trigone area. While standing, the bladder is supported by the vagina through its horizontal position. The support elements are the connective tissue of the vesicovaginal fascia (Halban's fascia), which is part of the pubocervical fascia. Laterally, this fascia is inserted on the pelvic wall, at the level of arcus tendineus fasciae pelvis. Its downwards or upwards tensioning triggers only the bladder mobilization.

The bladder dynamics has an important role in micturition and urinary retention, Fig. 4.11. (**Dietz H.P.,** *et al.,* **2003; Petros P.** & **Ulmsten U., 1997**).

4.3.3. Biomechanics of the human uterus

The uterus is maintained in an anatomical position by two structures that are inserted at the level of the cervix: *cardinal ligaments and uterosacral ligaments,* Fig 4.6. (**Wagenleuhner F.,** *et al.,* **2013**).

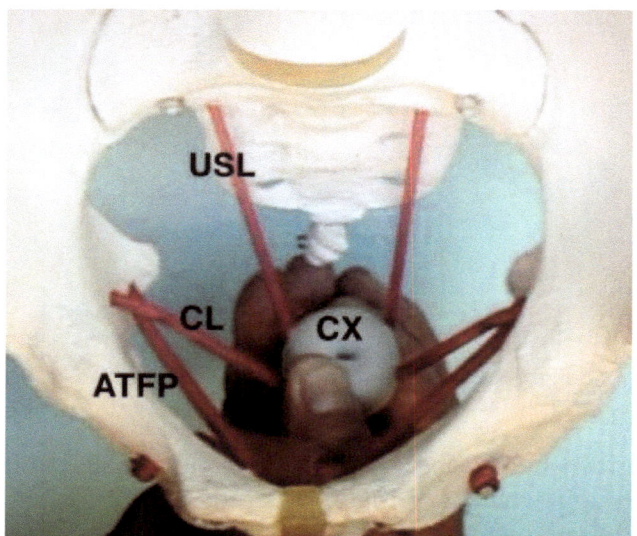

Fig. 4.6. Elements that support the cervix
(according to **Petros P., 2010**)
USL – uterosacral ligaments, CL – cardinal ligaments, ATFP – arcus tendineus fasciae pelvis, CX - cervix

Besides collagen fibers, smooth muscle fibers are also part of their structure, whose contraction determines the cervix retropulsion. Their insertion is through the paracervix. The result is that the cervix and the adjacent connective tissue represent the key element of the downwards anchoring of the pelvic organs.

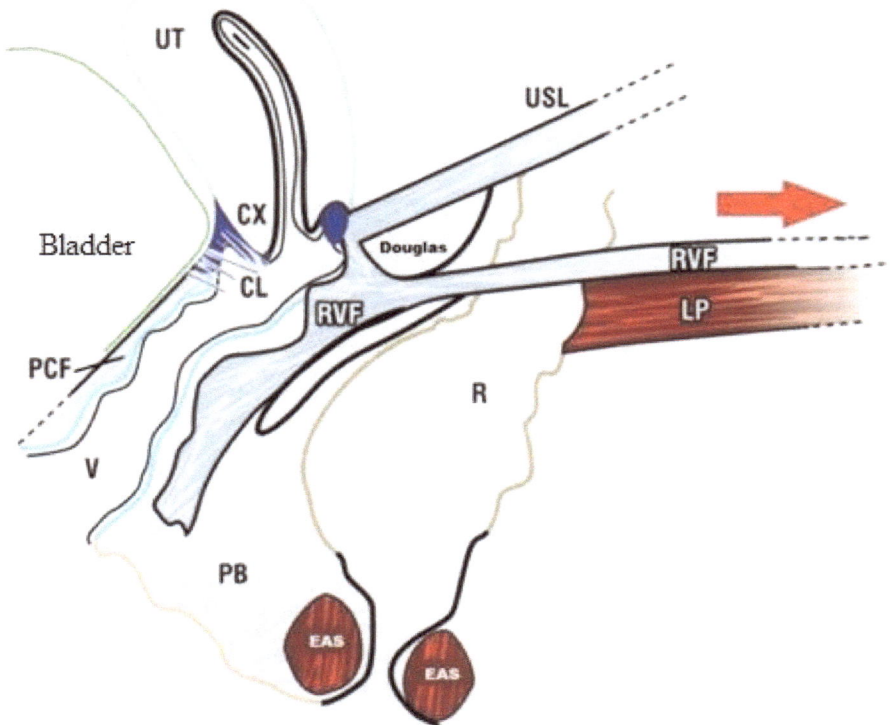

Fig. 4.7. The role of the paracervical ligament apparatus in the downwards anchoring of the pelvic organs
(according to **Petros P., 2010**)
USL – uterosacral ligaments, LP – levator plate, EAS – external anal sphincter, RVF– rectovaginal fascia, CL – cardinal ligaments, PCF – pubocervical fascia, CX –cervix, V – vagina, R – rectum, PB – perineal body, UT - uterus

The paracervix is made up of only pure collagen fibers that offer a high resistance. All the fasciae and ligaments interconnect at this level: pubocervical fascia (with a lateral insertion on ATFP), cardinal ligaments, uterosacral ligaments, and rectovaginal fascia. The latter is very important in the uterine dynamics because it attaches the vagina and the cervix to the perineal body caudally and cranially, it continues with the levator plate fascia (coccygeus and iliococcygeus muscles). Thus, the levator plate contraction is transmitted to the vagina and to the whole connective structure.

From a biophysical point of view, this is the way the downwards vector component of the pelvic biomechanics is transmitted, Fig 4.3. The abdominal pressure increase leads to the reflex contraction of the levator plate with the downwards pulling of the cervix. This way, the abdominal pressure induces the downwards flexion of the uterus and the obturation of the levator hiatus (**DeLancey J.O.L. & Hurd W.W., 1998**).

By making an analogy with the gothic architecture, the cervix-paracervix complex can be compared with the keystone of an ogive, Fig. 4.8. (**Petros P., 2010**). All the important pelvic floor connective structures meet at this level. The correct anatomical position of the uterus is ensured by the integrity of the rectovaginal fascia, cardinal ligaments, and uterosacral ligaments, as well as the contraction of the levator plate, Fig. 4.7.

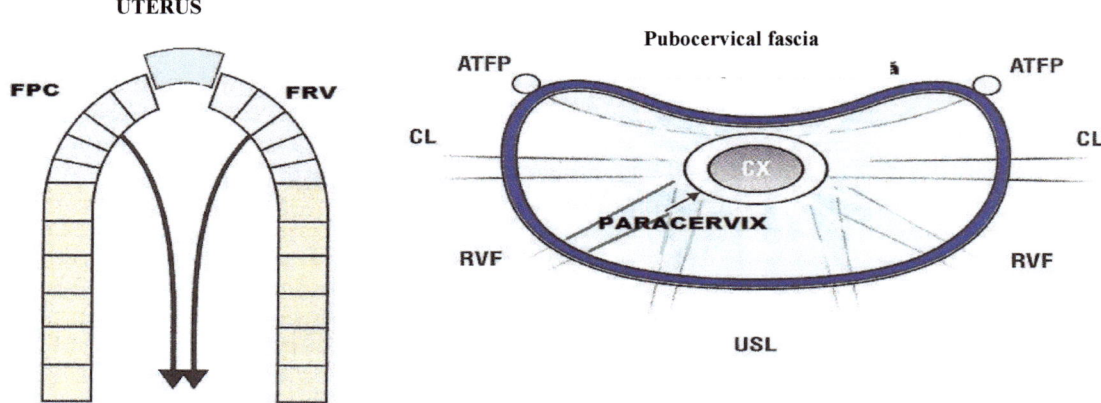

Fig. 4.8. The role of the uterus in pelvic floor (left) and the role of the paracervix in connecting the connective structures of the perineum (right)
(according to **Petros P., 2010**)
ATFP – arcus tendineus fasciae pelvis, CL – cardinal ligaments, CX – cervix, RVF – rectovaginal fascia, USL – uterosacral ligaments, PCF – pubocervical fascia

Uterosacral ligaments contain a very important artery in the vascularization of the uterus and branches that originate in the uterine artery irrigate the other ligament and fascia structures. After a hysterectomy, the vascularization of the fornix of the vagina (fornix vaginae) is diminished, so that the connective tissue suffers some kind of ischemia, decreasing its quality. For this reason, it is often very difficult to identify the uterosacral ligaments in female patients who suffered a hysterectomy (**Petros P., 2001; Petros P., 2000**).

4.3.4. Biomechanics of rectum

At the pelvic level, the rectum creates a curve with the concavity downwards. It changes direction from backwards to downwards at the level of the levator hiatus. The backwards wall of the rectum connects with the vagina below this level. The major role of maintaining the pelvic floor at this level is represented by two structures: *rectovaginal fascia and perineal body*, Fig. 4.7 (**Petros P., 2011c; Hsu Y., et al., 2008**).

4.3.5. Urethral physiology – micturition and urinary retention

Recent urodynamic studies on experimental models (**Petros P., 2011c**) have demonstrated that the mechanism of urinary retention is a combination of the intrinsic muscle forces of the urethra (internal and external sphincters) and the extrinsic forces resulted from the perineal biomechanics. Although it is hard to determine the exact extent to which each of them contributes, it seems that only approximately 1/3 of the maximum pressure at the level of the urethra is developed by the contraction of the intrinsic muscles. The main contribution belongs to the urethra angulation mechanism (similar to a water hose), Fig. 4.9 (**Morren G.L., et al., 2001**).

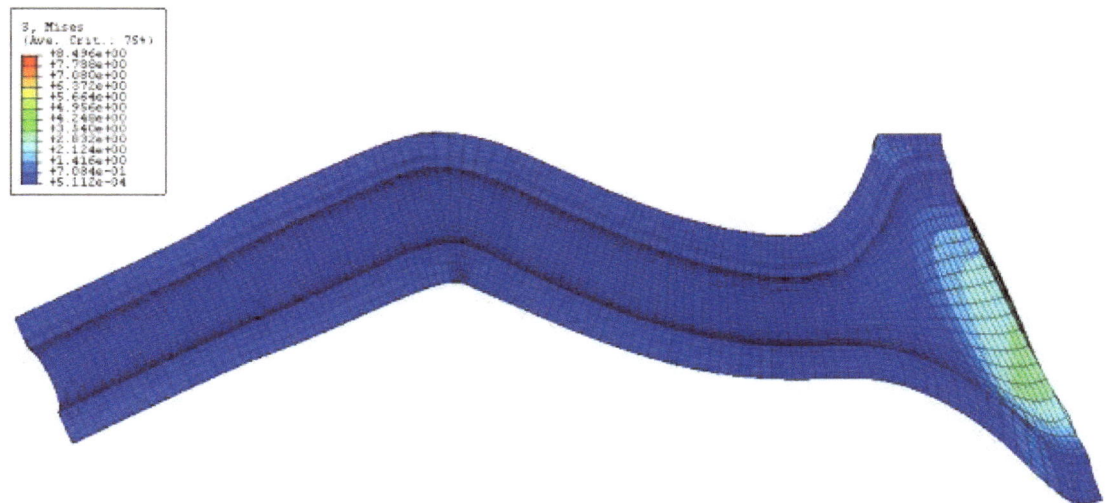

Fig. 4.9. 3D experimental model which reconstructs the angulation of the urethra for urinary retention
(according to **Messner-Pellenc L., Moron C., 2004**)

Three active forces take part in the functioning of the urethra: *downwards component* – levator plate, which acts through the rectovaginal and pubocervical fascia with the consecutive downwards movement of the bladder and urethra, *inferior component* – anal longitudinal muscle, which has the same role as the previous one and the *anterior component* – the pubococcygeus muscle that tensions the urethra backwards through the urethrovesical fascia. The result of the downwards and the backwards components is an inferior caudal oblique vector. The passive tension in the pubourethral ligaments is opposed to this vector (**Petros P., 2010; Panzer J., 2003**).

Urinary retention

It is realized through the contraction of all the muscular forces involved in the process. The result is the downwards pulling of the bladder and the urethra and the infraligamentary urethra antepulsion, so that its angulation occurs, Fig. 4.10. (**Petros P., 2010**).

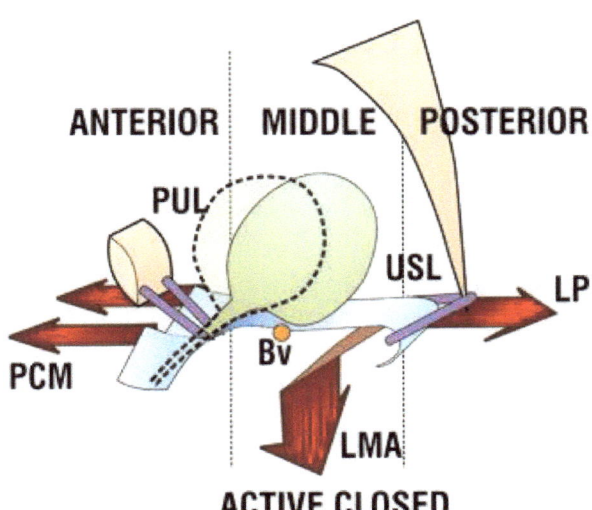

Fig. 4.10. Bladder retention mechanism
(according to **Petros P., 2010**)

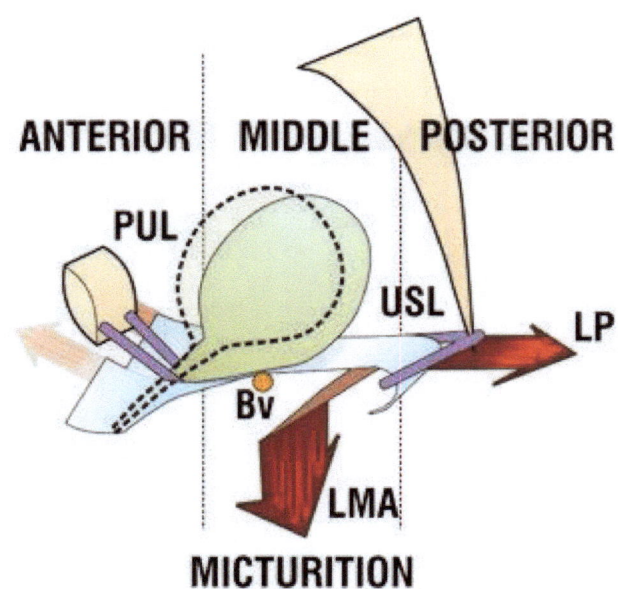

Fig. 4.11. Micturition
(according to **Petros P., 2010**)

Closure at effort
The raise of the abdominal pressure is transmitted at the level of the contents of the bladder and the pressure at the level of the urethra must rise accordingly to prevent the urine leakage. This is represented by the additional angulation of the urethra around the pubourethral ligaments due to the increase of the force developed in the levator plate.

Micturition
It is a process that has an important cortical integration. The moment the bladder volume becomes critical, corresponding impulses are sent to the central nervous system, in the brain bridge and cortex. When the conditions become favorable, efferent impulses are released, which lead to the relaxation of the backwards component of the extrinsic muscles, and the downwards one reduces the tension. Moreover, the action of the intrinsic muscles is cancelled. This way the angulation of the urethra disappears and the conditions necessary for the emptying of the bladder appear, Fig 4.11. (**Petros P., 2010**).

4.3.6. Anal physiology – defecation and fecal retention

Normally, the anal sphincters, the internal, and the external one exclusively control defecation and fecal retention. However, this perspective does not explain the appearance of fecal incontinence in the context of some pelvic floor disorders.

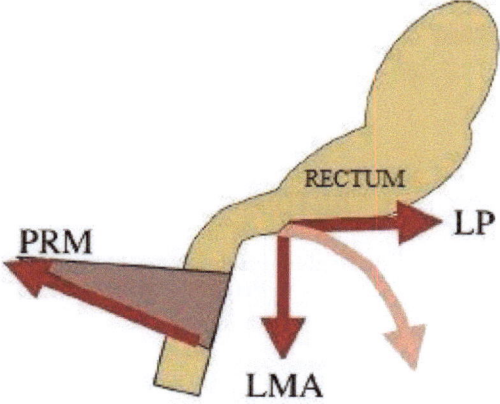

Fig. 4.12. Fecal continence mechanism
(according to **Petros P. 2010**)
PRM – puborectal muscle, LAM – longitudinal anal muscle, LP – levator plate

In 2008, Petros and Swash proposed a new concept a *muscular-elastic sphincter complex* (**Petros P. & Swash M., 2008; Swash M.,** *et al.,* **1985**). The mechanism is similar to urinary retention, the muscle forces taking part in the process being the same, Fig. 4.12. The muscles of the urogenital diaphragm and the external anal sphincter that close the lower half of the anal canal have an important role. The connective tissue is interconnected, thus the muscle tension is transmitted to all the ligaments. The ones vectorially opposing the resultant of these forces are the *pubourethral and uterosacral ligaments*. The fecal retention occurs through the contraction of all these muscle elements and as far as the ligament mechanism is functional. Defecation appears the moment the puborectal muscle and the muscles of the lower half of the anal canal relax. The vector result on the rectum separates the posterior wall and opens the anal canal (**Morren G.L.,** *et al.,* **2001; Petros P., 2010; Petros P., 2011***c*).

4.4 Perineum physiopathology – vector forces imbalance

The main cause for the appearance of pelvic floor disorders is the damage of the connective tissue at many levels. This damage determines a redistribution of the forces resulting from the contraction of the perineal muscles, with the influencing of the anatomy of the pelvic organs and, afterwards, their function (**Petros P., 2010**).

4.4.1. Pathogenesis of pelvic floor disorders and of evacuation and continence disorders.

Because the pelvic organs and vagina need to dilate and contract, they contain significant quantities of elastin, but they are less resistant. The estimated elastic resistance of the pelvic ligaments is of approximately 300 mg/mm^2, and the one of the vagina is of approximately 60 mg/mm^2, (**Yamada H., 1970; Abendstein B., 2008***b*). The elasticity of the vagina is fundamental in the physiology of the pelvic organs and during sexual intercourse.

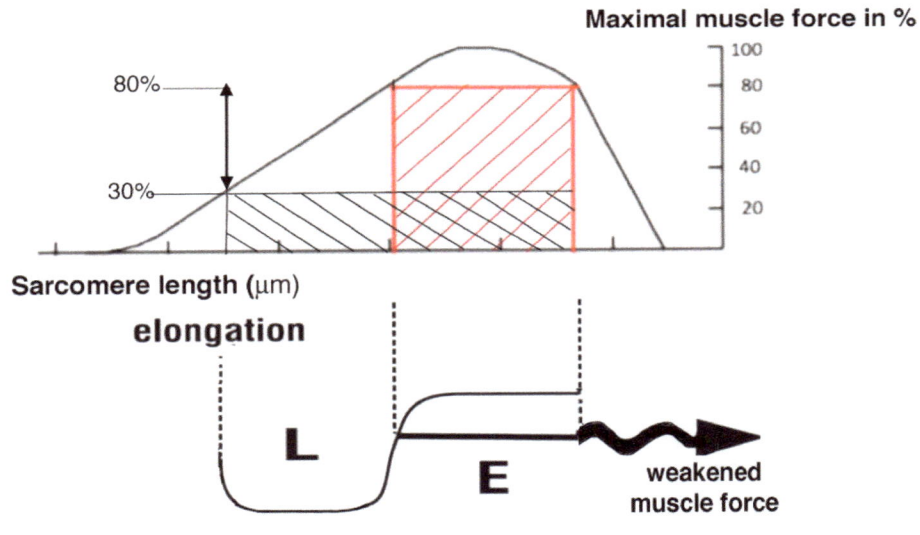

Fig. 4.13. Gordon's Law
(according to **Petros P., 2010**)

The yield of the muscle contraction complies to Gordon's Law, which establishes that the maximum muscle efficiency appears only on the short distance of the sarcomere, Fig. 4.13. If the ligaments elongate more than the distance "*E*", the muscular fibers stretch and their contractile force decreases dramatically. The urethral and anal canals can no longer be adequately closed (incontinence) or opened (emptying disorders) by the muscle vectors. These muscle vectors do not manage to tension the vaginal membrane enough anymore, to sustain the Lieutaud's trigone.

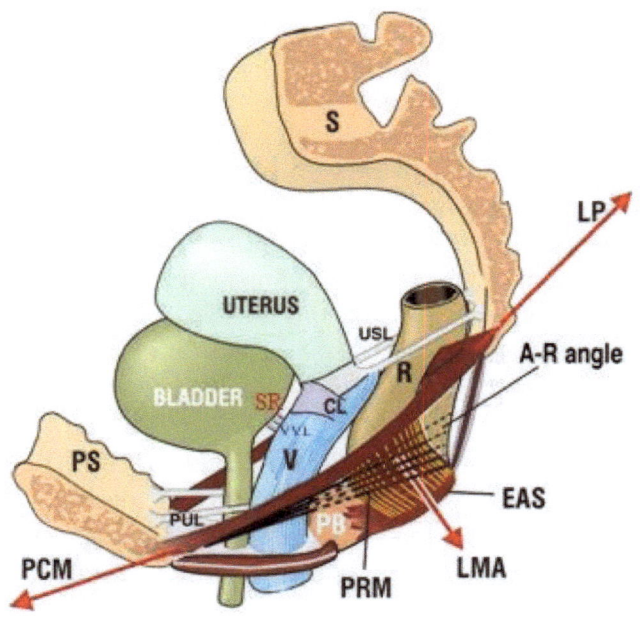

Fig. 4.14. Muscular ligamentous vector layout in the context of the imbalance of the ligament structure
(according to **Petros P., 2010**)
PCM – pubococcygeus muscle; LP – levator plate; LAM – longitudinal anal muscle; PRM – puborectal muscle;
EUL – external urethral ligaments; PUL – pubourethral ligaments; ATFP – arcus tendineus fasciae pelvis; CL – cardinal ligaments; USL – uterosacral ligaments;
VVL – vesicovaginal ligaments; PB – perineal body; V – vagina; R – rectum; SR – baroreceptors at the level of Lieutaud's trigone

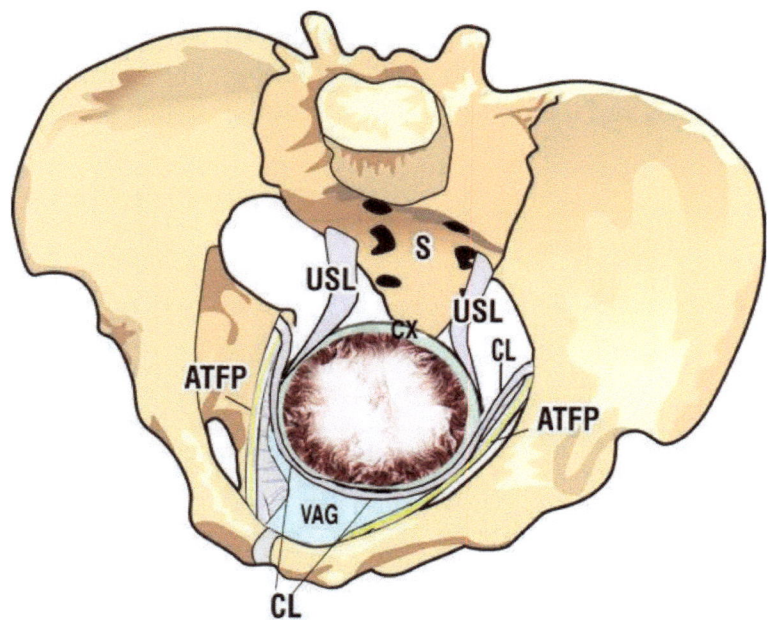

Fig. 4.15. Ligament damage during childbirth
(according to **Petros P., 2010**)
S – sacrum; USL – uterosacral ligaments;
CX – cervix; ATFP – arcus tendineus fasciae pelvis; CL – cardinal ligaments; VAG – vagina

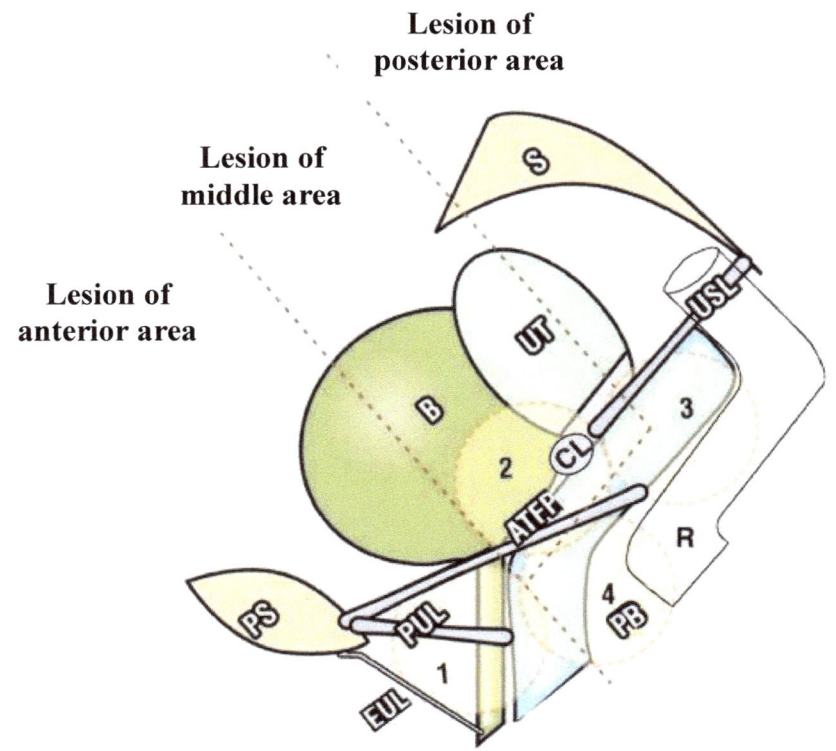

Fig. 4.16. Ligament damage at childbirth - saggital view
(according to **Petros P., 2010**)

PS – pubis; S – sacrum; USL – uterosacral ligaments; UT – uterus; ATFP – arcus tendineus fasciae pelvis; CL – cardinal ligaments; PUL – pubourethral ligaments; EUL – external urethral ligaments; PB – perineal body; B – bladder; R – rectum

This way the bladder wall is elongated with the consecutive stimulation of the baroreceptors at this level and the triggering of the *"imperiosity"* sensation at low urinary volumes, Fig. 4.14.

The main mechanism is the elongation of the ligaments and the fascias that have a role in the suspension of the pelvic organs beyond the limit of elastic resistance, with the consecutive disorganisation of the collagen fibers. Such an example is the passage of the fetus skull during childbirth, Fig. 4.15. In case of a full dilation, the maximum pressure exerted by the 10 cm of the movable fetal mass is on the insertion of the pubocervical fascia on the paracervix, uterosacral, and cardinal ligaments.

Each moment during childbirth can induce lesions at the level of some connective structures of the pelvis. Their extension, with the persistence of the fetal skull at a certain level, increases the risk of lesions to ligaments and fascias, not only by the prolonged mechanical elongation but also by vascular stasis and ischemic alteration of their structure.

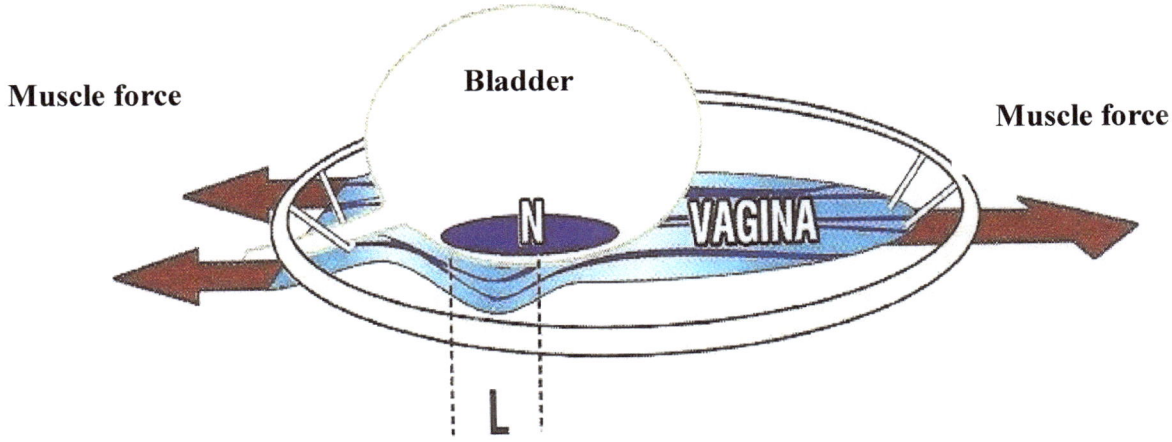

Fig. 4.17. Laxity of pubocervical fascia and disorder of muscle contraction
(according to **Petros P., 2010**)
L – length of defect, N – nerves endings

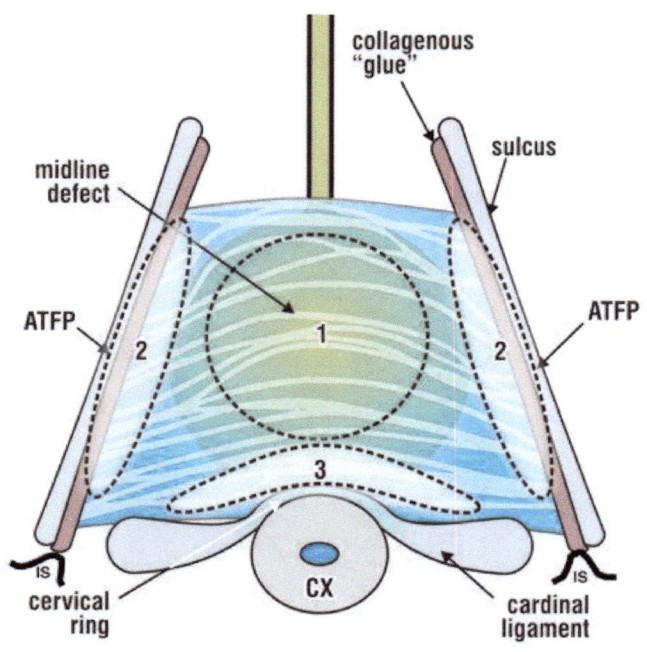

Fig. 4.18. **Areas prone to laxity of pubocervical fascia**
(according to **Petros P., 2010**)
ATFS – arcus tendineus fasciae pelvis

Some surfaces are numbered from 1 to 4 in fig. 4.16. They represent the positions of the fetal skull during the second stage of labour – the descent. The position in front of the second circle can induce the lesion of arcus tendineus fasciae pelvis, the cardinal ligaments and the anterior vaginal wall. The position of the third circle can induce the damage of the uterosacral ligaments and the posterior vaginal wall. The fourth circle can lead to the destruction of the perineal body and the rectovaginal fascia. The position in front of the first circle affects the pubourethral and external urethral ligaments, as well as the distal part of the vagina (**Petros P., 2010**).

4.4.2. Physiopathology of pelvic floor disorders
4.4.2.1. Mechanisms for the appearance of anterior prolapse *(cystocele)*

The pubocervical fascia is horizontally oriented, with an anterior insertion at the pubis level and the posterior one on the paracervix. It is laterally inserted on the ATFP. The bladder is sustained in a standing position by this fascia, which is made up of collagen fibers and some soft muscle fibers, and, which corresponds to the horizontal part of the vagina.

The damage of this structure is the cause for the appearance of anterior prolapse. The laxity of the connective tissue can lead to a dysfunction through the loss of resistance and excessive elasticity. Thus, the muscle force necessary for the tensioning of the vagina is greater, proportional with the magnitude of the defect, Fig. 4.17. (**Petros P., 2010; Swash M.,** *et al.*, **1985**).

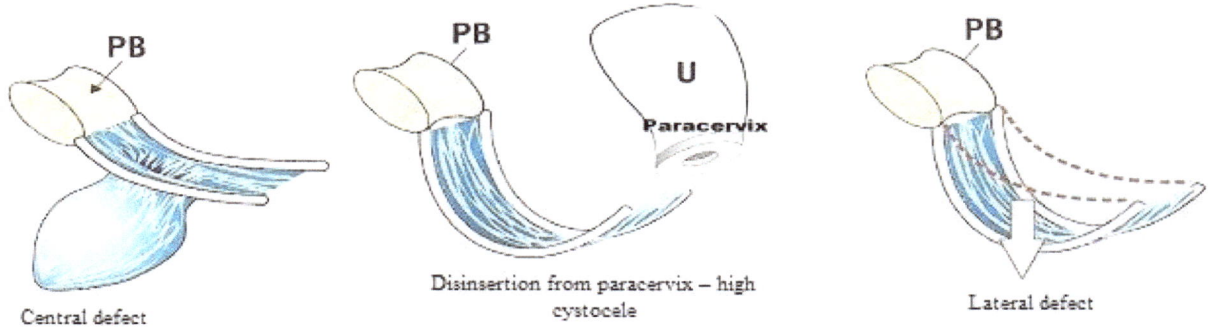

Fig. 4.19. Types of anterior prolapse
(according to **P. Petros, 2010**)
PB – pubis, U - uterus

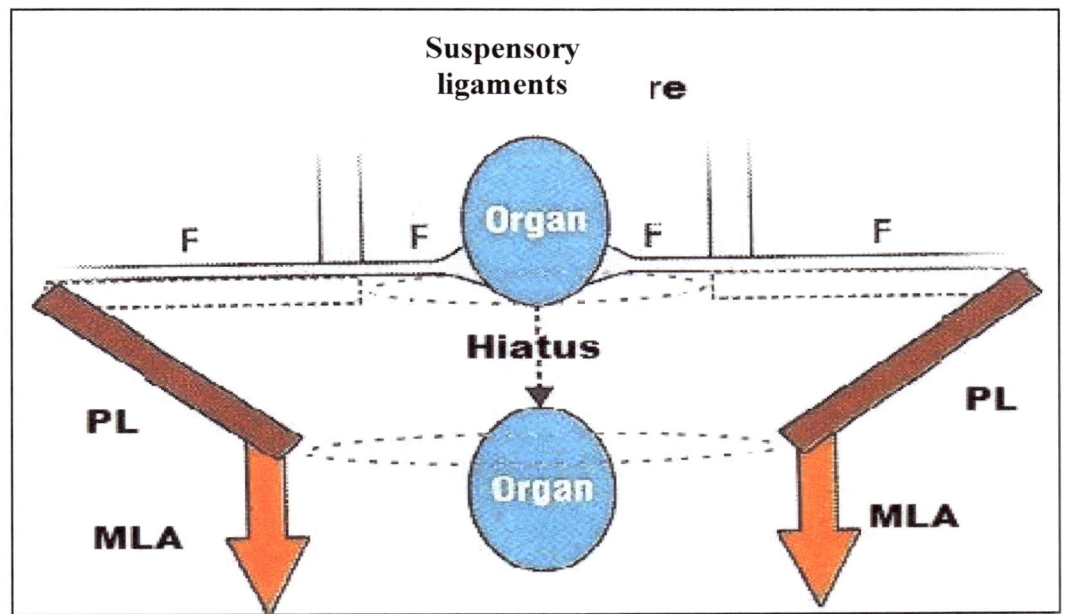

Fig. 4.20. Role of the levator hiatus in the occurrence of uterine prolapse
(according to **Petros P., 2010**)

More types of cystocele are described according to the part affected, Fig. 4.18.

Medial cystocele
Destruction of the median part of the pubocervical fascia, with the consecutive herniation of the bladder, which cambers the central area of the vagina.

Apical cystocele – disinsertion of the fascia from the paracervix. The bladder ruptures in the cranial side of the vagina and needs a more complex surgery. More often, it is also associated with a certain degree of uterine prolapse.

Lateral cystocele
It refers to the lateral disinsertion from the ATFP, Fig. 4.19 (**Petros P., 2010; Petros P., 2011c**).

4.4.2.2. Mechanisms for the appearance of uterine prolapse

From a biophysical point of view, the *levator hiatus*, which is located between the puborectal and pubococcygeus muscles, has an important role. It increases its diameter during Valsalva maneuver (**Dietz H.P. & Steensma A.B., 2005**). The connective tissue links the pelvic organs and the muscle sides of the hiatus, so that, their wombs is maintained in an approximately horizontal position. The size of the hiatus diameter determines an aspect of "*ditch*" through the descent of the muscle sides and is associated with a high risk of prolapse. This dynamics appears physiologically through the contraction of LAM, but the ligamentous apparatus maintains the pelvic floor. As the collagen and elastin fibers degrade and the connective tissue becomes more lax, the position of the prolabated pelvic organs, especially the uterus, becomes permanent, Fig. 4.20. (**Dietz H.P.**, *et al.* **2012**).

The second important factor that leads to the appearance of uterine prolapse is the angle of the vaginal axis with the horizontal. It has to be less than 45 degrees, so that, when the abdominal pressure rises, its vector result with the forces induced by the levator plate and the longitudinal anal muscle, would determine the posterior movement of the vagina and the compression on the rectum and on the levator plate. If the angle is greater than 45 degrees, the vectors result is oriented towards the levator hiatus and determines the utero-vaginal herniation in a telescoping way, Fig 4.21. (**Hsu Y.**, *et al.*, **2006**). The normal angulated position of the vagina is maintained by two essential structures: uterosacral and cardinal ligaments, Fig. 4.22., and their damage leads to the appearance of uterine prolapse. In major defects with complete uterine-vaginal prolapse, the connective tissue is affected at several levels, including the lateral anchoring through ATFP and the perineal body (Delancey levels II and III).

A particular case that is often confused with a form of prolapse is the "*hypertrophic elongation of the cervix*". Recent research has hypothesized that the pathophysiological changes underlying this entity are vascular (**Enache T,**, *et al.*, **2015**). The first step in the pathogenic chain is a posterior compartment defect that induces the appearance of a uterine prolapse.

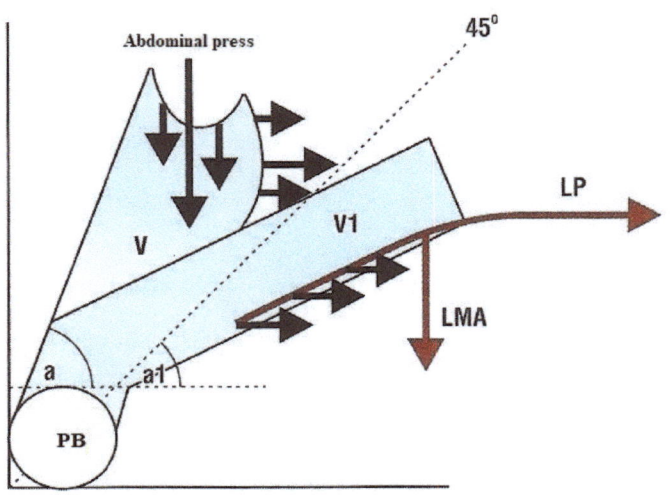

Fig. 4.21. Vaginal axis
(according to **Petros P., 2010**)
V1 – normal vaginal axis with a <45 degrees angle; V – vaginal axis predisposes to prolapse, the a >45 degrees angle

Pre and postoperatory ultrasound measurements revealed a statistically significant decrease in cervical length as well as a reduction of the resistivity index on both uterine arteries, in addition a reduction of resistance to blood flow (**Enache T**, *et al.*, **2016**). We can therefore infer that a degree of prolapse induces resistance to blood flow, perhaps through vascular obstruction. Being characterized by low pressure, the venous system is also influenced, thus resulting a venous stasis with consecutive edema. The edema seems to be responsible for increasing the size of the cervix. The studies conducted so far suggest that these modifications are transient, the blood flow resistance decreasing postoperatory.

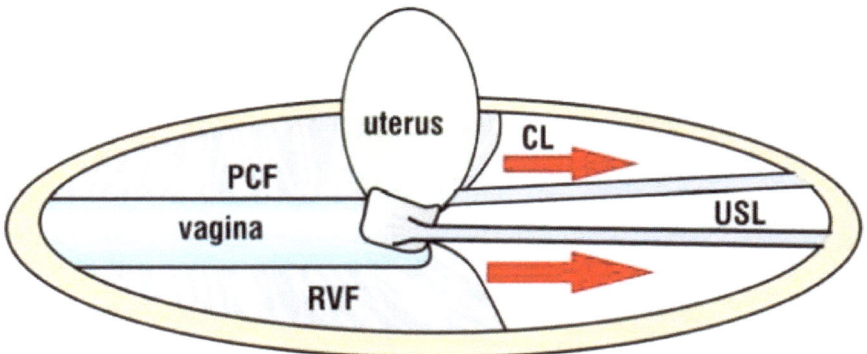

Fig. 4.22. The role of ligaments in the posterior anchoring of the uterus
(according to P. Petros, 2010)
USL – uterosacral ligaments, CL – cardinal ligaments, PCF – pubocervical fascia, RVF – rectovaginal fascia

We therefore consider that *"hypertrophic cervix elongation"* represents a reversible change associated with a degree of prolapse. This perspective involves a change in the surgical method, thus avoiding any cervical resection associated with any correction technique of pelvic floor disorders.

Moreover, the paracervix and rectovaginal fascia are also involved in this system, so, the defects occurring at this level can be associated with a degree of prolapse (**Petros P., 2010**).

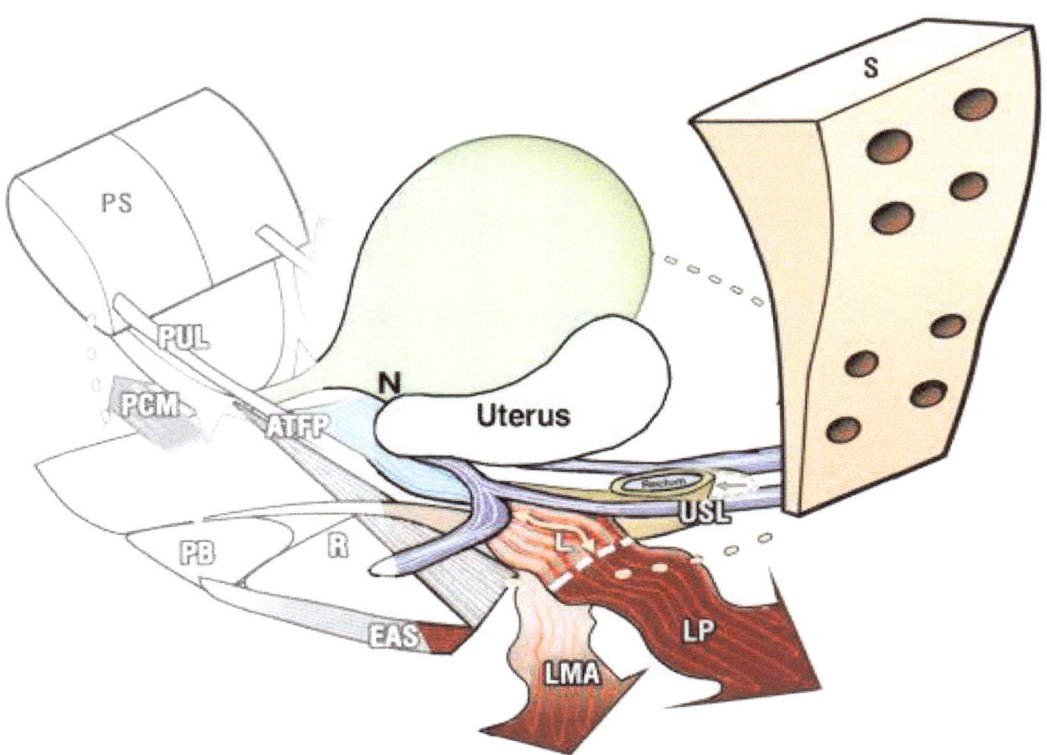

Fig. 4.23. Potential impact of uterosacral ligaments elongation according to Gordon's Law (according to **Petros P., 2010**)
PS – pubis; S – sacrum; N – nerve endings; PUL – pubourethral ligaments; PCM – pubocervical muscles; ATFP – arcus tendineus fascie pelvis; PB – perineal body; R – rectum; EAS – external anal sphincter; LAM – longitudinal anal muscle; USL – uterosacral ligaments; L – length of ligaments and muscles elongation

The functional impact can be deduced by applying the Gordon's Law to uterosacral ligament lesions, Fig. 4.23. Symptoms may include chronic pelvic pains, pollakiuria, and urinary urge, nocturia, bowel evacuation disorders, and anal incontinence. SUI may also occur to a very small extent.

4.4.2.3. Mechanisms for the appearance of vaginal vault prolapse and vaginal prolapse

The same ligament structures as in the uterus support are also involved in the support of posterior fornix: cardinal and uterosacral ligaments, paracervix, and, with a greater impact in this case, the rectovaginal fascia. The above-mentioned elements also contribute to supporting the vaginal vault after total hysterectomy; moreover, it is also attached to the pubocervical fascia. The degradation of uterosacral ligaments and rectovaginal fascia particularly may cause elitrocele and most often coexist with other defects and frequently associate rectocele or uterine prolapse, Fig 4.24 (**Davis K.** *and* **Kumar D., 2005**). We also reiterate the role of ligament ischemia due to the sectioning of the uterine arteries that normally vascularize these structures.

Because the uterus, which has a pivotal role in pelvic floor, does not exist anymore, a cystocele and a rectocele are usually associated in the case of vaginal vault prolapse. The prophylaxis of this type of postoperatory hernia is done through a solid anchoring of the vaginal bunt to the uterosacral and cardinal ligaments in the total hysterectomy, Fig 4.24.

4.4.2.4. Mechanisms for the appearance of posterior vaginal wall prolapse (rectocele)

The posterior vaginal wall prolapse, the rectocele, occurs as a result of damage to the rectovaginal fascia and the perineal body. The fascia can be damaged either by structural destruction of collagen fibers or by disintegration from the uterosacral ligaments or perineal body. Its disappearance as a mean of supporting the anterior rectal wall leads to the herniation of the rectum and the swell at the level of posterior vaginal mucosa. The detachment of the perineal body leads to the extension of the defect with the rectum prolapse to the level of the vaginal introit, Fig. 4.25 (**Abendstein B.,** *et al.,* **2008***a*; **Petros P., 2011***c*).

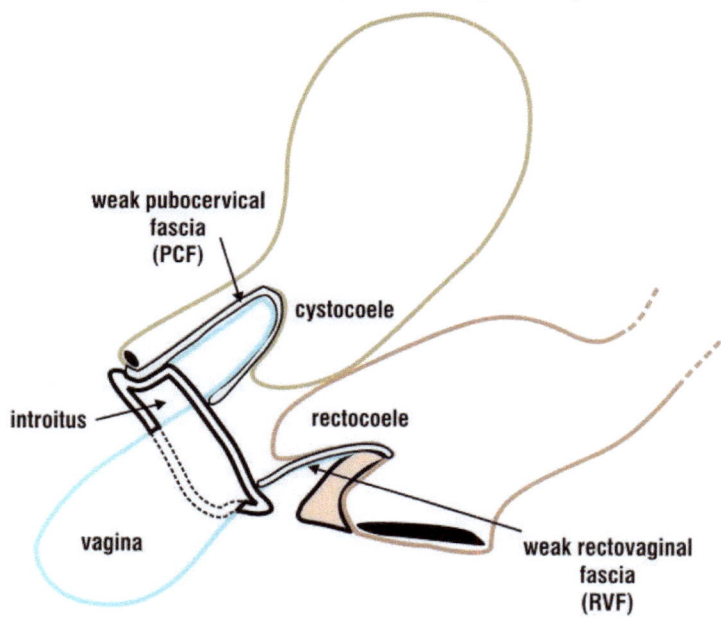

Fig. 4.24. Mechanism of occurrence of vaginal vault prolapse
(according to P. Petros, 2010)
USL – uterosacral ligaments, CL – cardinal ligaments, PCF – pubocervical fascia, RVF – rectovaginal fascia, EAS – external anal sphincter, LP – levator plate, RVF – rectovaginal fascia, PB – perineal body, A – anus

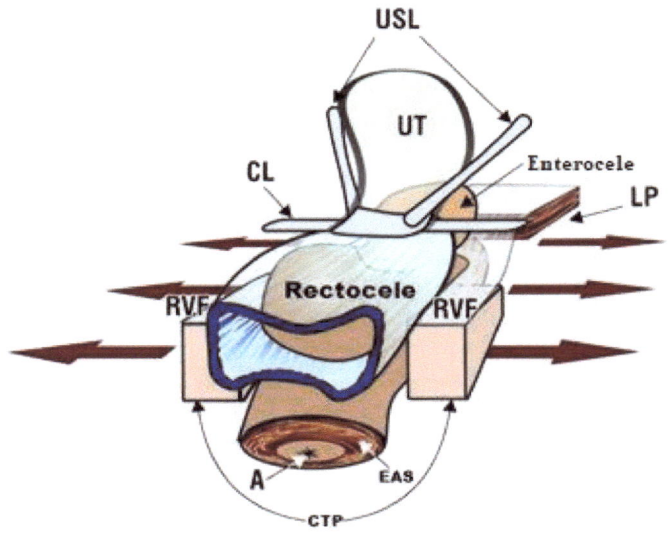

Fig. 4.25. Mechanism of occurrence of rectocele and enterocele
(according to **Petros P., 2010**)

4.4.3. Physiopathology of stress urinary incontinence

According to Integral Theory, stress urinary incontinence is the consequence of a ligament defect that has the pubourethral ligaments as a central element. Urinary retention is mainly the result of the angulation of the urethra, which is performed indirectly, through the vaginal wall.

The alteration of connective system, the diminution of elastin fibers in the absence of the estrogenic stimulus in menopause, as well as the atrophy specific to the aging process lead to the decrease in the force with which the pubococcygeus muscle participates in establishing the three active components that stabilize the perineum.

Thus, a vector imbalance occurs with the predominance of the posterior muscle component, represented by the levator plate and the longitudinal anal muscle, to the detriment of the anterior component, Fig. 4.26. The result is the posterior dragging of the vesical trigone with the opening of the evacuation tract and the decrease of flow resistance. The process is similar with what happens during micturition, which is however, a temporary controlled imbalance (**Petros P., 2011c; Strohbehn K.** *and* **DeLancey J.O.L., 1997**).

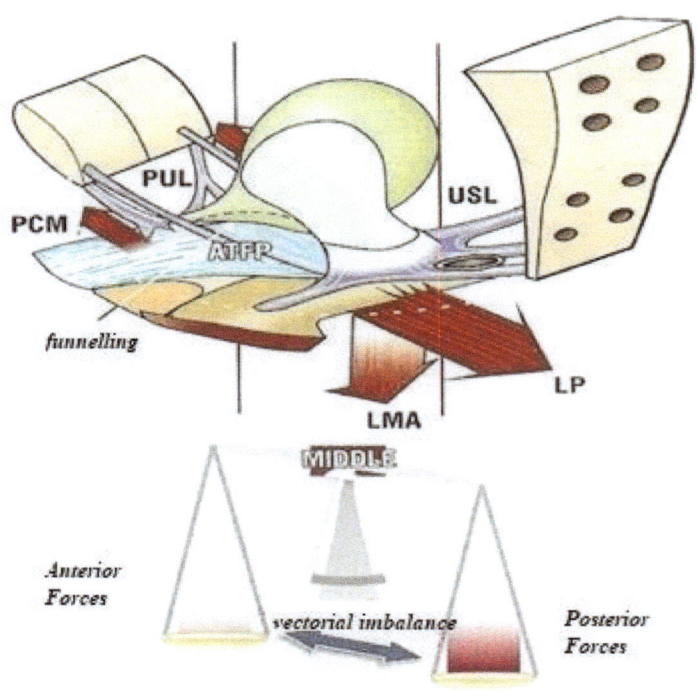

Fig. 4.26. Vector imbalance in the occurrence of effort urinary incontinence and fecal incontinence
(according to **Petros P., 2010**)
PCM – pubocervical muscle, LAM – longitudinal anal muscle, LP – levator plate, ATFS – arcus tendineus fasciae pelvis, PUL – pubourethral ligaments, USL – uterosacral ligaments

The mechanism through which the force of the pubocervical muscle is lower so that the predominant posterior vector could be understood by applying the Gordon's Law, Fig. 4.27. The laxity of pubourethral ligaments induces the elongation of the muscle fibers, over the "L" length, beyond the elastic resistance of sarcomeres, and with the consequent decrease of the developed force.

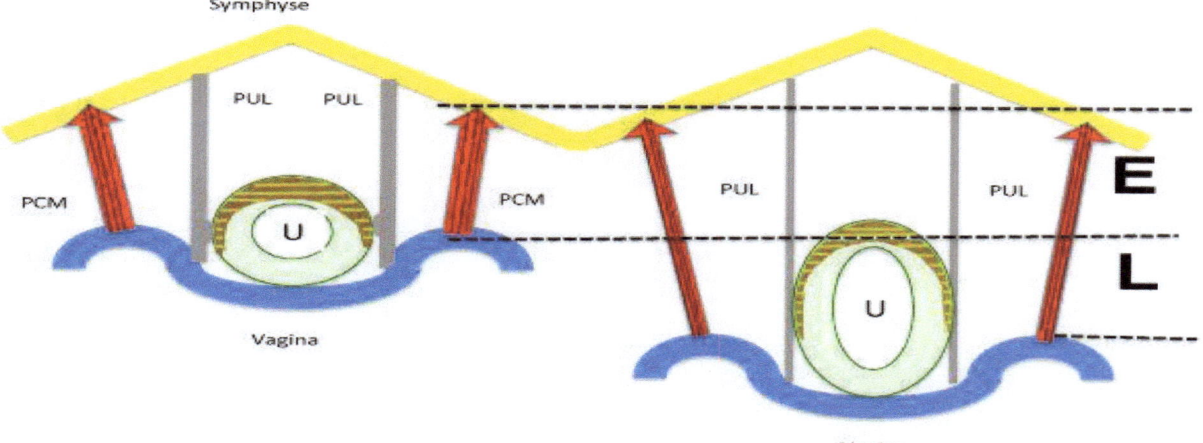

Fig. 4.27. Gordon's Law in SUI etiopathogeny
(according to **Petros P., 2010**) Left image – patient with continence
Right image – patient with SUI, PUL – pubourethral ligaments; PCM – pubocervical muscle; U – urethra; E – normal length of PUL; L – supplementary elongation of PUL

4.4.4. Physiopathology of anorectal dysfunction

Anorectal dysfunction means both digestive tract evacuation inability and low constipation, and rectal content continence and fecal incontinence. Pelvic floor disorders are not the only cause of fecal incontinence or rectal evacuation disorders, but are often associated with them. The mechanism through which it can occur is the impairment of the perineal body, the rectovaginal fascia, the uterosacral ligaments, or the pubourethral ligaments. The involvement of the latter occurs because the connective tissue is interconnected. The levator plate tensions the connective system, and, if the anterior anchoring through the pubourethral ligaments is deficient, then the vector deficit with the predominance of posterior forces appears, Fig. 4.26. Also, the affected uterosacral ligaments induce a downward oriented vector resultant. In both situations, no rectoanal angulation is obtained with a corresponding continence effect, Fig. 4.28 (**Huang W.C., et al., 2007**).

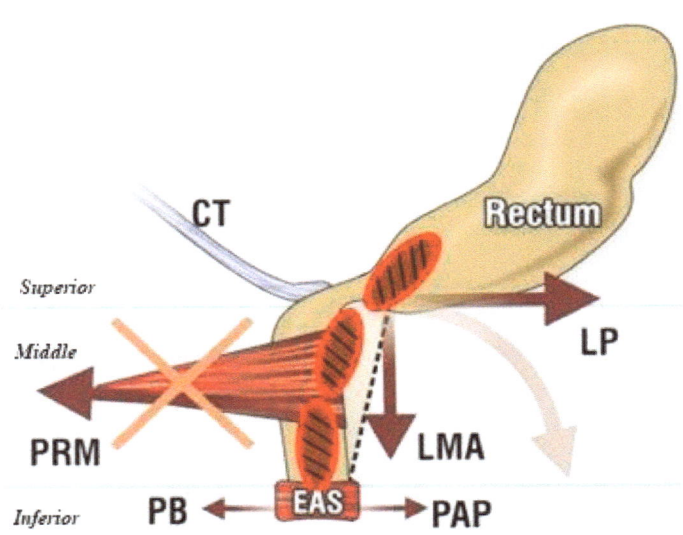

Fig. 4.28. Mechanisms of anorectal complex support – defecation
(according to **Petros P., 2010**)
CT – connective tissue of anchoring to the vagina and the uterosacral ligaments, LP – levator plate, LAM – longitudinal anal muscle, PRM – puborectal muscle, EAS – external anal sphincter, PB – perineal body, PAP – post-anal plate

The external anal sphincter (EAS) has an important role in anal continence through two mechanisms: the direct constrictor effect on the anal canal and the fact that it represents the lower anal insertion point of longitudinal anal muscle (LAM). EAS dysfunction leads to the LAM inactivation and thus no rectoanal angulation occurs anymore (**Petros P., 2010**; **Petros P., 2011***c*).

The alteration of the connective component can also lead to rectal evacuation disorders. The defect of the rectovaginal fascia leads to an anterior displacement of the anterior vaginal wall and thus can cancel the relaxation effect of the puborectal muscle.

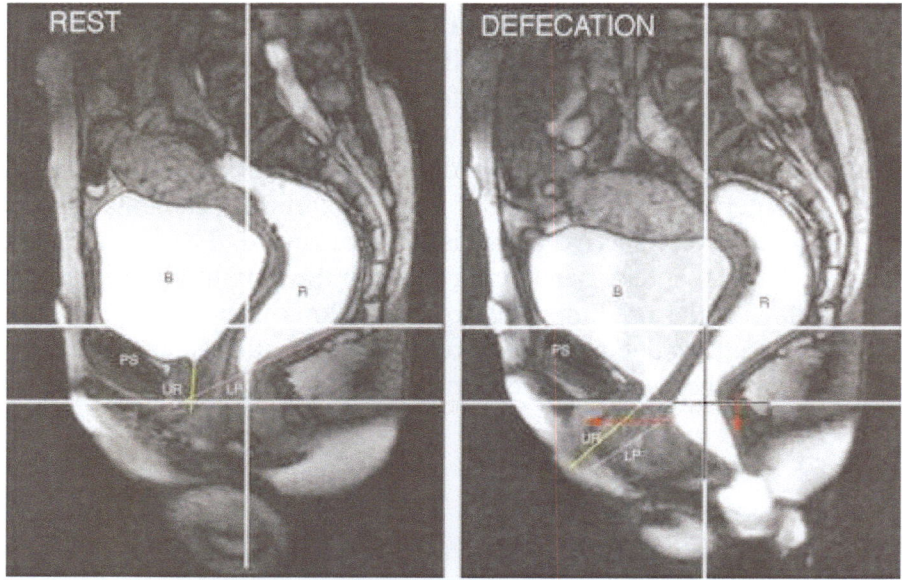

Fig. 4.29. MRI. Left: the female patient at rest. Right: the female patient during defecation (according to Petros P., 2010)
PS – pubis, B – bladder, R – rectum, UR - urethra, LP – levator plate

The radiological analysis of rectal retention and defecation in these patients highlighted some phenomena that may appear and may lead to the obstruction of the faeces. During defecation, both the urethra and the anterior rectal wall are pushed backward, altering the angle of the urethra with the horizontal from 92 to 40 degrees. The angulation of the levator plate modified from 28 degrees with the horizontal at rest to 38 degrees while defecating. However, the anorectal angle increased only a little, from 100 to 110 degrees, Fig. 4.29.

4.4.5. Physiopathology of rectal prolapse

The laxity of uterosacral ligaments and rectovaginal fascia can lead to poor anterior rectal wall anchoring in *rectal prolapse* (**Abendstein B., et al., 2008a**). The mechanism is represented by the absence of rectum stretching and, the anterior rectal wall tends to descend under the influence of the abdominal press. According to Poisseuille's law, an increase in resistance to flow, fecal bowl, on the rectal length unit with the consecutive increase of venous stasis and pulling of the rectal mucosa in caudal direction is achieved.

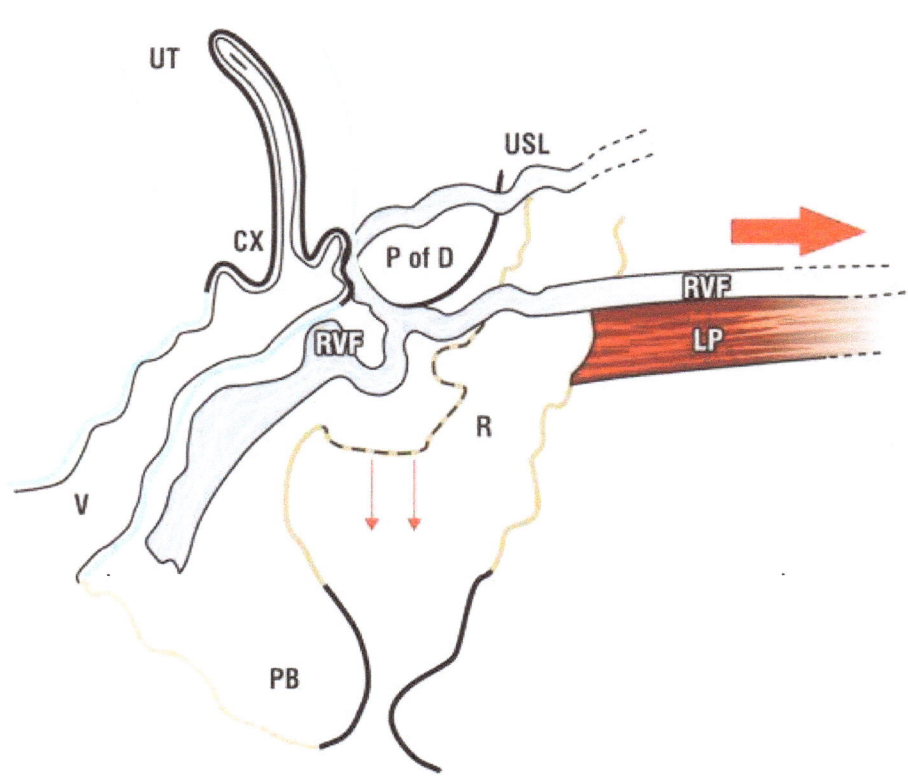

Figure 4.30. Physiopathology of rectal prolapse
(according to **Petros P., 2010**)
UT – uterus, PB – perineal body, CX – cervix, P of D – pouch of Douglas, V – vagina, USL – uterosacral ligaments, RVF – rectovaginal fascia, R – rectum, LP – levator plate

Rectal veins are low pressure veins located in the rectal wall. The laxity of uterosacral ligaments causes the breaking of the rectal wall due to its insufficient anchoring and thus induces the wrinkling of these veins with consecutive stasis. This is the mechanism, through which the pressure in the venous system increases and finally induces the occurrence of hemorrhoids, Fig. 4.30. The occurrence of hemorrhoids in the absence of rectal prolapse may have the same physiological mechanism, a stasis at the level of the pelvic circulation and implicitly rectal one, due to a pelvic floor disorder at the level of the posterior compartment (**Enache T., 2014**).

5. *Clinical and paraclinical diagnosis of pelvic floor disorders*

Diagnosis of perineal affections, though easy at first sight, implies some subtleties. Classically, the objective exam established both positive diagnosis and therapeutic conduct. According to the principles of the Integral Theory System and following a principle stated by Mircea Eliade that *"there are no illnesses, but only ill people"*, the anamnesis acquires a very important role. Each case must be evaluated according to the symptoms that bring the patient to the doctor and these should be correlated with the clinical signs observed during the examination. The observance of some pelvic floor disorders in asymptomatic patients does not necessarily require a surgical correction. Moreover, those symptoms that do not associate with an objective sign must be reassessed.

Generally, female patients go to the physician for a main symptom, and subsequently an entire series of signs and symptoms, which were tolerated without being attributed to a clear meaning, are discovered. Such an example is offered by Gold and Goeschen, who conducted a study on 198 patients who presented to the physician for pelvic pains. Applying the validated questionnaire of Integral Theory System, many other symptoms and various degrees of prolapse have emerged. Their graphic representation led to the figure below and the analogy with the iceberg Fig. 5.1.

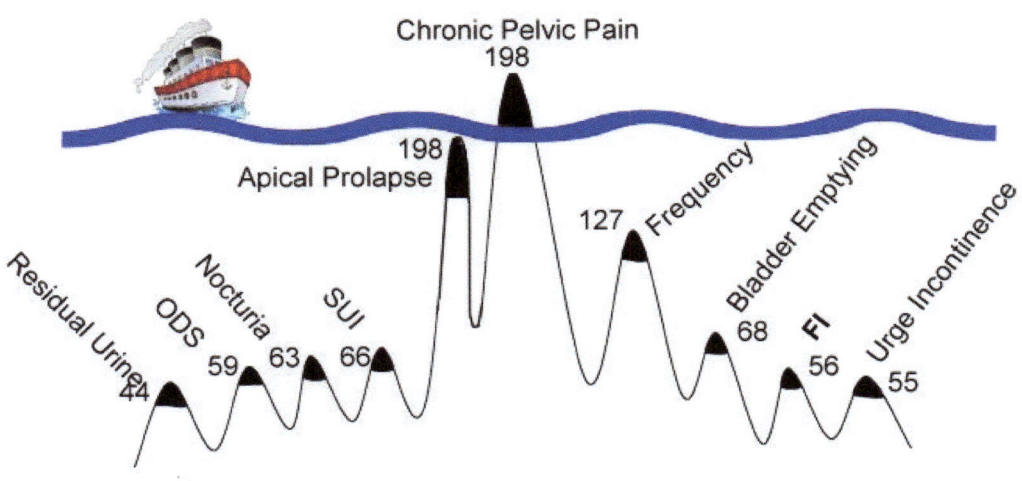

Fig. 5.1. The Pescatori Iceberg
(according to **Petros P., 2010**)

Initially, only one symptom is observed, but various symptoms and pelvic floor disorders that coexist can be observed below the level of waterline (the symptom that determines the female patient to go to the physician).

The imaging and urodynamic explorations have gained more and more importance over the last 20 years, providing additional therapeutic elements.

5.1. Semiology of pelvic floor disorders

The main method of diagnosing pelvic floor disorders anomalies is the clinical examination, which is fundamental for establishing the diagnosis and the therapeutic behavior.

5.1.1. Symptoms

The main symptom associated to pelvic floor disorders is stress urinary incontinence (SUI). However, a careful anamnesis signals a deeper influence of pelvic floor disorders on the function of the organs involved. Moreover, symptoms that are not classically associated with any perineal disorder, or which were treated exclusively medically until recently, are currently considered the consequence of this pathology, whose reevaluation may mean the extension of surgical indications (**Petros P., 2010**).

Symptomatology is very important in the diagnostic evaluation of the female patients with pelvic floor disorders. The suffering, of more or less importance, is the one that determines the presentation to the physician. Often, large anatomical defects are completely asymptomatic, and, in contrast, minimal anatomical defects can be symptomatic. This finding requires a reassessment of the therapeutic conduct, which must be centered on the patient and not necessarily on the objective examination. The ultimate goal of the surgical treatment should first be remission or at least the improvement of symptomatology and not only the strict correction of the anatomical defect (**Petros P., 2010**).

5.1.1.1. Stress urinary incontinence

SUI **(**Stress Urinary Incontinence**)** in women is clinically defined as the intermittent, sudden and involuntary loss of urine, resulting from a common physical effort such as coughing, sneezing, laughing or lifting a weight (**Abrams P.K.,** *et al.,* **2009**). The physiopathological mechanisms of appearance have been presented previously. SUI prevalence varies between 10 and 60%; almost half of the women at menopause can suffer from this pathology. Beyond the symptom itself, SUI determines a poor personal hygiene with important psychological and social consequences. Depending on the socio-cultural level of the female patient, this disorder is interpreted either as a disease, determining the patient's presentation to the physician, or as a natural evolution in senescence, thus, consequently minimized or as a shameful phenomenon, which must be overcome in silence.

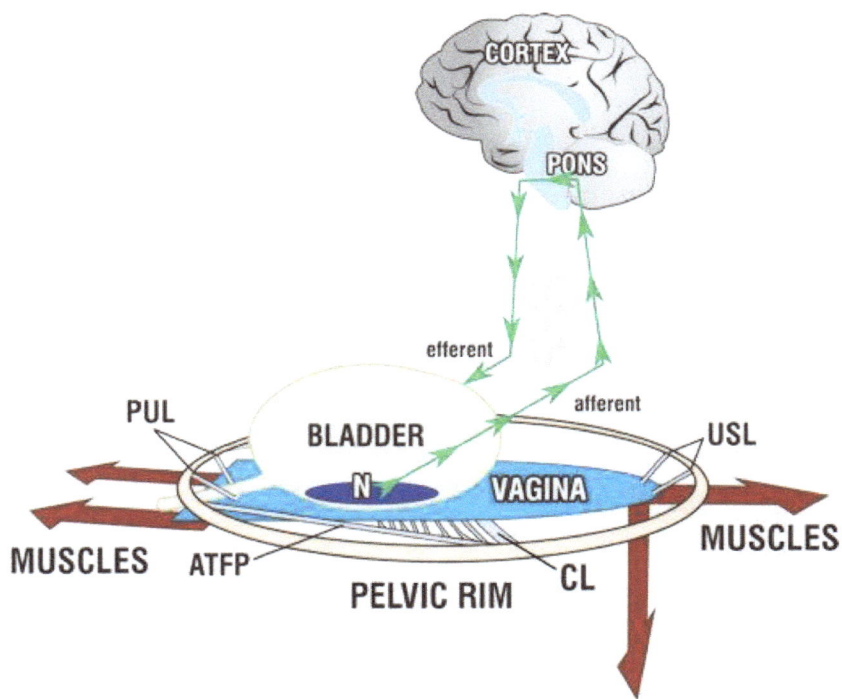

Fig. 5.2. Analogy with trampoline. Laxity of one of the suspensor ligaments induces the tensioning of the vaginal membrane, with a consecutive elongation and premature release of nervous impulses
(according to **Petros P., 2010**)
ATFP – arcus tendineus fasciae pelvis, PUL – pubourethral ligaments, USL – uterosacral ligaments, N – nerves

The patients feel stigmatized, most often isolate themselves from society, and delay the treatment due to shame.

The differential diagnosis is made with the continuous loss of urine as it occurs in urinary fistulae, multiple sclerosis, or other neurological disorders (**Petros P., 2010**).

5.1.1.2. Urinary urge and urge urinary incontinence

In 2002, ICS (International Continence Society) defined the urinary urge as the "*sudden and imperious sensation of urinating, which cannot be delayed*" (**Rosier P.F. & Bosch J.R., 2002**). Urgency urinary incontinence can appear to the extent that conditions do not allow it and the patient cannot urinate, which is characterized by the involuntary loss of urine that was preceded by urinary urge. Traditionally, this is a condition that benefits from drugs treatment, unlike SUI, which can be treated surgically. Urinary urge most often appears secondary to an intrinsic or extrinsic bladder disease, or an infection or a malignant disorder. However, this can also be a consequence of pelvic floor disorders. Usually, when such a cause is found, the urge is also associated with other anatomical symptoms and defects.

The mechanism is represented by the early stimulation of baroreceptors that determine afferent nervous impulses and premature triggering of the micturition sensation. The peripheral neurological mechanism is realized by a musculo-elastic complex that contains baroreceptors.

They are sensitive to pressure variations in the bladder wall. The bladder wall is the starting point of the reflex arc that controls the micturition. Lieutaud's trigone has an important role, with an intimate relationship between the vagina and the bladder. This elastic structure can be compared with a trampoline Fig. 5.2. (**Adekanmi O.A., et al., 2003**). Ligament laxity causes a compensatory muscular contraction to maintain the pelvic floor, inducing a further elongation of the vaginal membrane. The tension present in the vaginal wall is transmitted to the Lieutaud's trigone and thus the sensitivity of baroreceptors is affected. This way, the alteration of the connective component or a nervous hypersensitivity may induce the onset of excessive impulses and the premature activation of micturition reflex at low urinary volumes (**Petros P., 2010**).

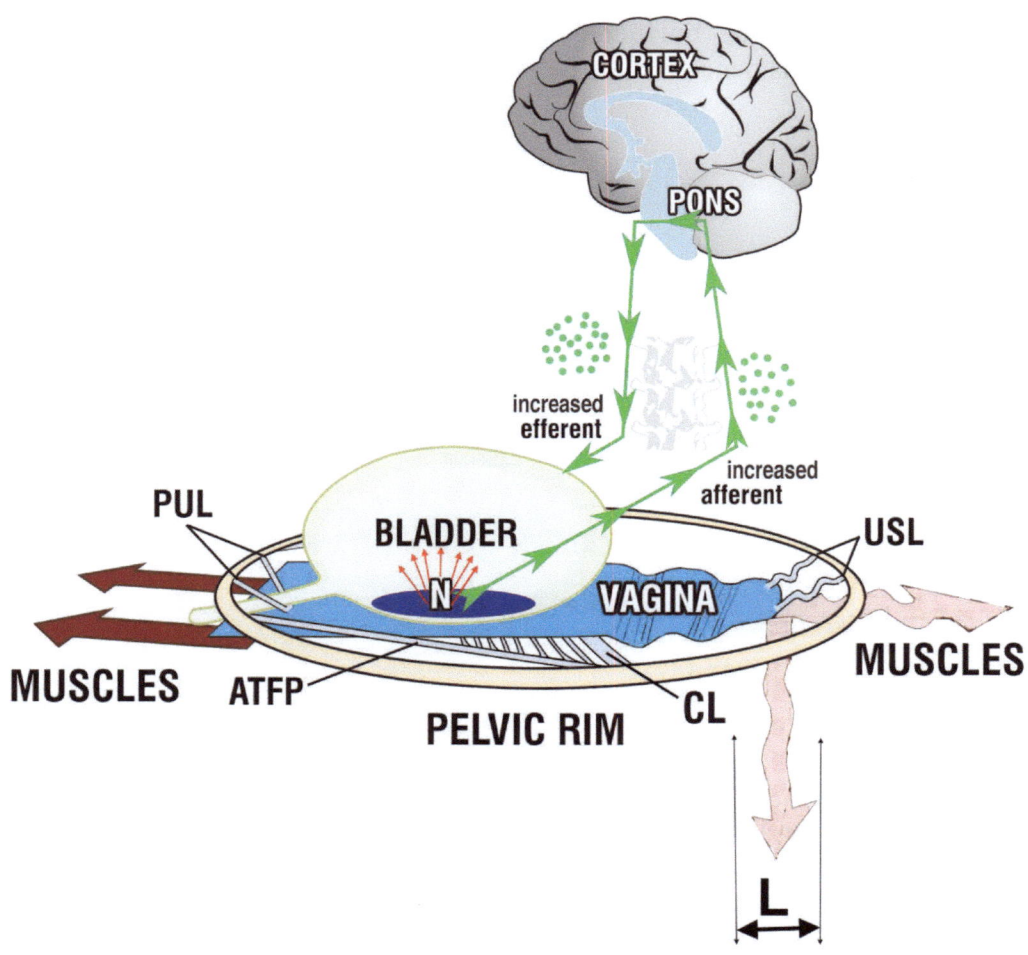

Fig. 5.3. Urinary urge. Gordon's Law
(according to **Petros P., 2010**)

USL – uterosacral ligaments; CL – cardinal ligaments; PUL – pubourethral ligaments; ATFP – arcus tendineus fasciae pelvis; increased afferent; increased efferent; pelvic rim; bladder; muscles; widening of some structures denotes ligament elongation and decrease of muscle strength; N – nerve endings; L – length of uterosacral ligaments elongation

In the context of pubourethral ligaments damage, through the predominance of posterior vector component, the vagina is no longer sufficiently tensioned. The consequence is a relative deficiency in the support of Lieutaud's trigone, with its elongation being transmitted to the trigone baroreceptors and thus triggering early nerve impulses (**Petros P., 2010**). Insofar the uterosacral ligaments are affected, their elongation induces the proper stretching of the muscle fibers that provide the posterior vector component and according to Gordon's Law, the strength developed decreases significantly. Thus, the vaginal membrane can no longer be tense and cannot support the Lieutaud's trigone, which is relaxed, thereby causing the premature stimulation of the nervous receptors Fig. 5.3.

These changes occur more frequently after the age of 70 and are probably secondary to ligament apparatus atrophy and loss of elasticity of the vagina. These symptoms can also be encountered in female patients who underwent surgery with alloplastic material, which causes recurring scars at the level of Lieutaud's trigone Fig. 5.4. The interpretation of these biophysical observations is that virtually any ligament defect, irrespective of the affected compartment can induce urinary urge.

Hyperstimulation of baroreceptors to small vesical volumes is perceived at the cortical level as urinary urge, an event that occurs in healthy female patients when the bladder is full. Efferent impulses induce an increase of posterior muscle tone to achieve bladder continence. Insofar as the urethral support apparatus is affected, a vector imbalance appears which is similar to the one of SUI and consequently involuntary leakage of urine occurs. This phenomenon is known as "*urgency urinary incontinence*".

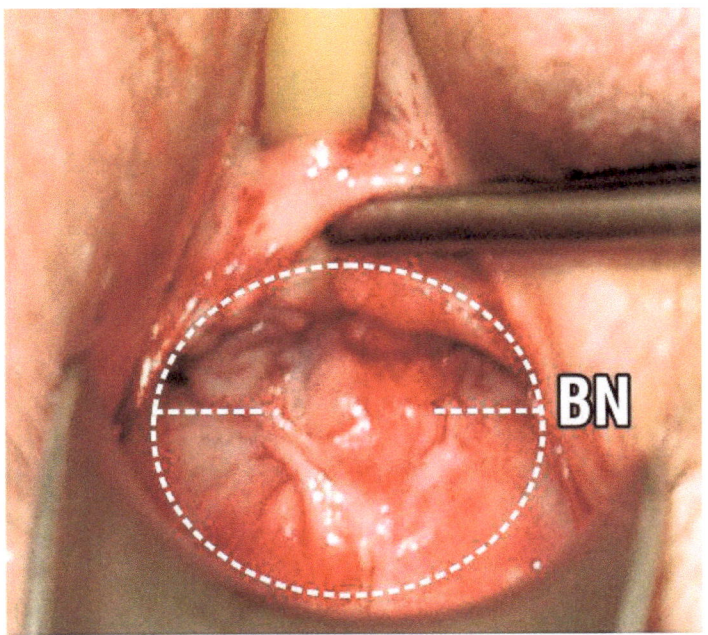

Fig. 5.4. Extensive scar at the level of bladder neck in a female patient with urinary urge
(according to **Petros P., 2010**)
BN – bladder neck

    This symptom can be relieved through the maneuver of gently palpating the anterior vaginal wall, thus achieving the diagnosis of pelvic floor disorder that induced the urge. The explanation is given by the reduction of tension at the level of Lieutaud's trigone Fig. 5.5. (**Bartolo D.C.C.** & **Macdonald A.D.H., 2002**).

Detrusor contraction

    This reflex triggered by various factors is subcortical, and the cortex tends to counteract the micturition reflex by an additional contraction of pelvic muscles. Handwashing in healthy patients (**Petros PE.P.** & **Ulmsten U., 1993**) can trigger overactive contractions. E. Mayer suspects as a mechanism of appearance the suppression of cortical means of micturition inhibition (**Mayer E.A., 2006**).

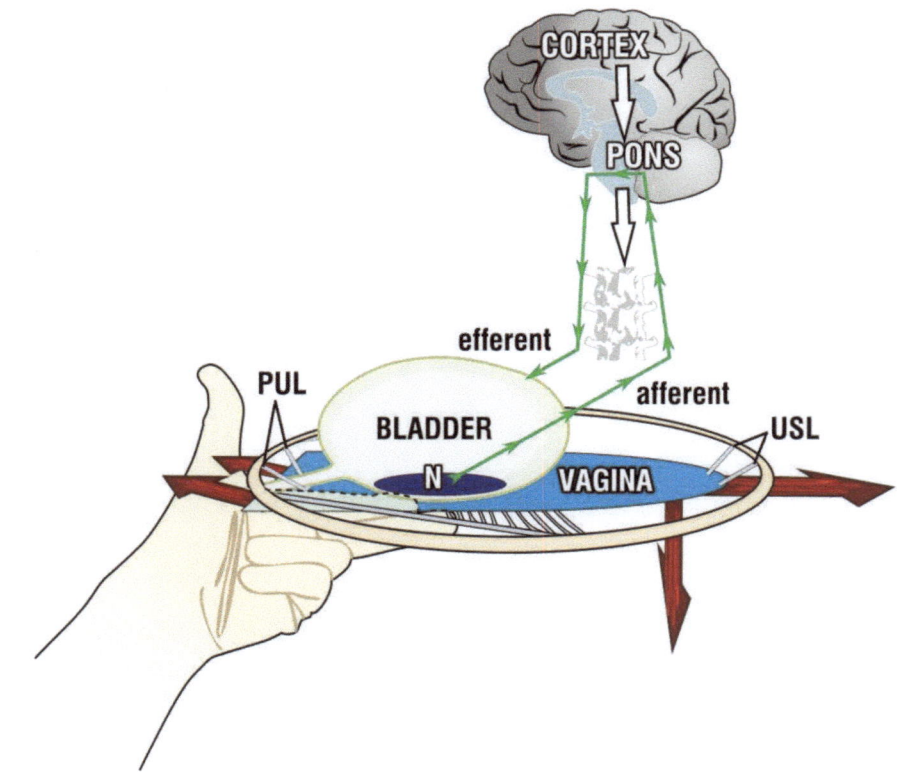

Fig. 5.5. **Diagnosis of pelvic floor disorders involved in the occurrence of urinary urge**
(according to **Petros P.P., 2010**)
USL – uterosacral ligaments; PUL – pubourethral ligaments; increased afferent; increased efferent; bladder;
N – nerve endings

5.1.1.3. Pollakiuria

Pollakiuria is defined as an increase in micturition frequency at over 8 times per day. Usually, small urine volumes are evacuated, but in extreme forms, it seriously affects the quality of life. Classically, this is the consequence of bladder inflammations (infections, bladder tuberculosis, and interstitial cystitis), bladder tumors with reduced bladder volume or affections that determine the narrowing of the urethra – urethritis, rare in women. Besides the elimination of these causes, if they exist, the classical therapeutic conduct is exclusively based on drugs (**Tiny A.**, *et al.*, **2011**).

In the context of pelvic floor disorders, pollakiuria is a rather common symptom and the mechanism of appearance is similar to that of urinary urge, and, most often, the two occur simultaneously. In the case of urinary urge, the frequency of small volume of urine micturitions increases significantly to eliminate the entire quantity of urine accumulated continuously in the bladder for a 24 hours period (**Goeschen K., 2007**).

5.1.1.4. Nocturia

Nocturia is the urge to urinate at night, each micturition being preceded and followed by sleep (**Rosier P.F.** & **Bosch J.R., 2002**). This symptom has a pathological significance when it occurs at least twice during the night. Until the advent of the Integral Theory System, nocturia was not associated with pelvic floor disorders. The main traditional recognized causes are the following: ingestion of large quantities of liquids in the evening, caffeine, pregnancy, and diseases of urinary apparatus, diabetes, and cardiac insufficiency (**Lee Y.-S.**, *et al.*, **2010**).

Nocturia also occurs in the context of a pelvic floor defect, more exactly through the damage of uterosacral ligaments. In clinostatic position, the bladder is supported in about 2/3 of its surface by the posterior vaginal compartment, anchored by uterosacral ligaments. Under the influence of gravity, as the bladder fills with urine, it tensions to the posterior vaginal wall.

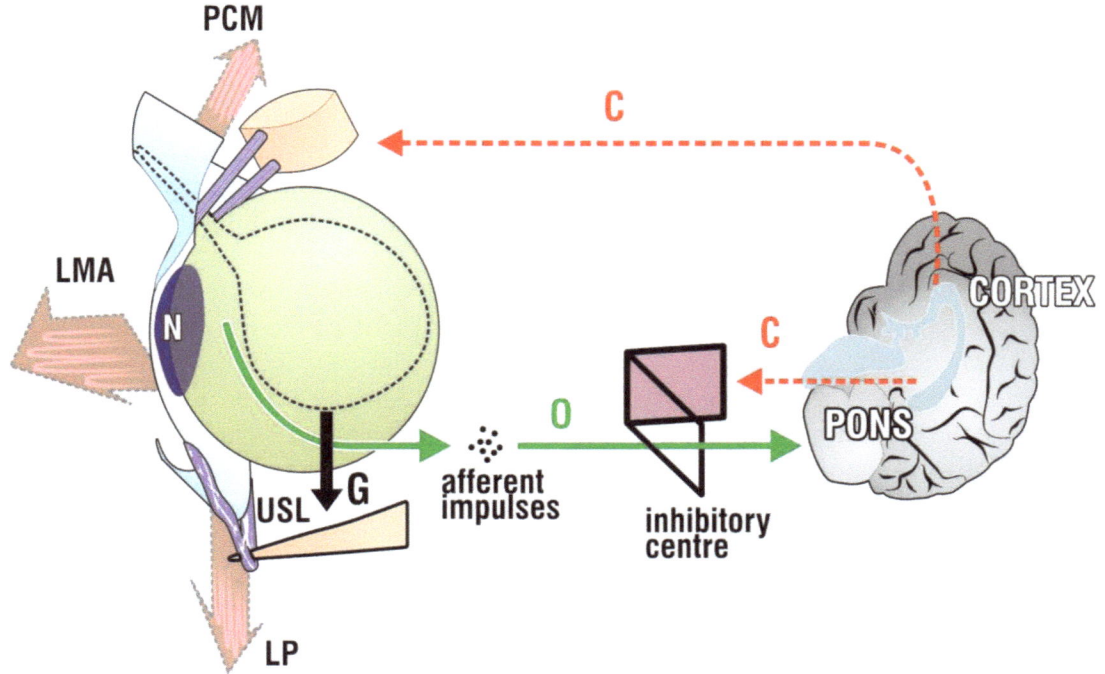

Fig. 5.6. **Mechanism of occurrence of nocturia**
(according to **Petros P.E.P., 2010**)
USL – uterosacral ligaments; LP – levator plate; L M A– longitudinal anal muscle; PCM – pubocervical muscle; C – closing reflex

If the uterosacral ligaments are firm, they support the bladder base. However, if the ligaments are affected, the posterior third of the vagina is no longer properly anchored, the vagina tends to elongate further, thus tensioning the bladder wall at the level of Lieutaud's trigone with a premature stimulation of the baroreceptors at this level and precocious triggering of urinary reflex even at a low urinary volume. The afferent impulses reach the cortical level and awake the patient to urinate. Sometimes, especially when the elasticity is low, with senescence, the activation of the micturition reflex can lead to the loss of small quantities of urine in bed, Fig. 5.6. (**Petros P., 2010**).

Urinary urge, pollakiuria and nocturia present a common physiopathological mechanism, so they most *often* coexist (**Petros P. & Ulmsten U., 1993**), forming the *posterior vaginal fornix syndrome*.

5.1.1.5. Bladder voiding disorders

This type of dysfunction is defined as the difficulty of bladder emptying. The pathophysiological mechanism of occurrence is an increased resistance to urinary flow during micturition.

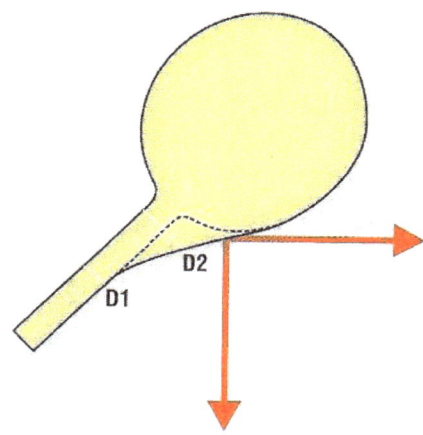

Fig. 5.7. **The physical origin of bladder voiding disorders – Poiseuille's Law: D2 is twice higher than D1**
(according to **Petros P.E.P., 2010**)

According to Poiseuille's Law, the diameter at the level of the bladder neck (D2) is twice higher than the one at the caudal level of the urethra (D1), which mathematically translates by a 16-plication decrease in flux resistance (two to four).

Considering that D2 is lower, a significant increase of resistance to urinary flow appears, Fig. 5.7. **(Petros P., 2010)**.

By affecting the pubocervical fascia, cystocele can prevent the tensioning of the vagina by the posterior vector component. This way, the posterior bladder pulling is disrupted and the bladder neck does not open properly anymore.

On the other hand, a voluminous cystocele causes voiding disorders by angulation of the urethra and lowering the bladder's lower point below the plane of the urethra during micturition **(Petros P., 1997)**.

Voiding disorders may also occur in the case of damage to the uterosacral ligaments. They represent the anchoring point of the inferior vector component (longitudinal anal muscle – LAM), so that this component is inactivated. Consequently, the evacuation tract does not open properly anymore and the detrusor pressure must overcome a higher resistance to the flow, Fig 5.8.

The main clinical manifestation is the prolongation of the micturition.

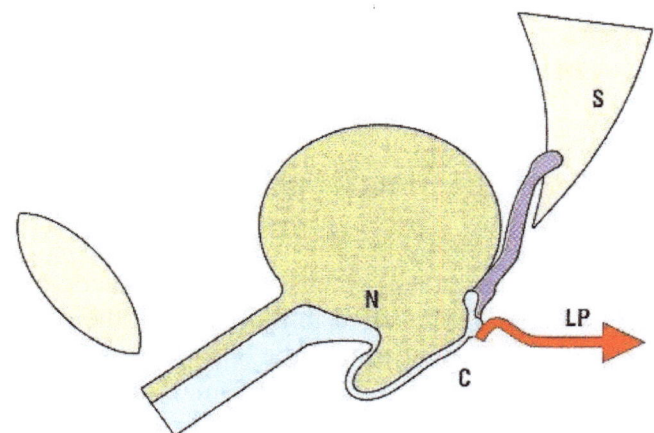

Fig. 5.8. Obstruction of the bladder voiding with the presence of cystocele
(according to **Petros P.E.P., 2010**)
S – sacrum, N – afferent nerve endings, c – cystocele, LP – levator plate

Although Petros admits a maximum of 60 seconds for a normal micturition, there is no accepted standard. Most frequently, the female patient mentions the increase in the time needed to empty the bladder content compared to the previous one. Moreover, there is also a post-micturition residue, which translates into a feeling of incomplete bladder voiding. Physiologically, the bladder should be emptied completely at each micturition, so the residue should not exist. However, clinically, a post-micturition physiological residue is admitted, but regarding the volume, no conclusion has been reached. Petros admits a residual volume of up to 30 ml, while several studies **(Kelly C.E., 2004)** mention it as a residue that exceeds 100 ml.

The symptoms associated with voiding disorders include the urge of urination (forcing), prolonged urinary jet, incomplete urinary voiding. The most common complication of voiding disorders is urinary infection due to urinary stasis. Thus, specific symptoms may be added to those already existing, such as polaki-dysuria, etc.

5.1.1.6. Fecal incontinence

Fecal incontinence is the patient's impossibility to control fecal continence and is manifested by involuntary loss of gas or faeces. Depending on the severity of the symptomatology, initially the capacity of liquid stool continence is lost, then even the solid one. This affects between 10 and 20% of the female patients at menopause and the psychological consequences are major **(Petros P. & Swash M., 2008)**.

5.1.1.7. Constipation

Constipation is a disorder of the digestive system characterized by the delay of the stool for over 3 days. In case of pelvic floor disorders, constipation is *obstructive* and most frequently associated with the rectocele.

Depending on its localization, there is a defect of the uterosacral and cardinal ligaments or a defect of the rectovaginal fascia or perineal body. Regardless of the localization of the damaged area, the consequence is a prolapse of the anterior rectal wall. Constipation occurs when the anatomical defect is important, with anterior rectal sacculation. This results in a stasis of the faecal bowel at the level of the hernia sac. Typically, defecation can still be achieved as the patient reduces the rectocele by pressing the posterior vaginal wall with the finger (**Bartolo D.C.C. & Macdonald A.D.H., 2002**).

5.1.1.8. Vaginal discomfort and other symptoms associated with pelvic organs prolapse

In case of important anatomical defects with large anomalies such as large cystocele; advanced uterine prolapse; etc., the prolapsed organ induces some symptoms by its own presence (**Butrick C.W.**, *et al.*, **2009**).

In less advanced stages, a discomfort or a sensation of foreign body can appear intravaginally (**Kato T.**, *et al.*, **2002**) with a more abundant leukorrhea accompanied by burns and pruritus. A certain degree of inconvenience to orthostatism and walking is associated in female patients in whom uterine prolapse or anterior or posterior vaginal mucosa determine the exteriorization of the defect by vaginal introduction. The most important defects are encumbered in comparison with the noisy symptoms due to the involvement of adjacent organs and specific lesions. The most common are the decubitus lesions, which can sometimes have a hypertrophic vegetative aspect due to superinfection. A biopsy may be indicated for a correct differential diagnosis, Fig. 5.9.

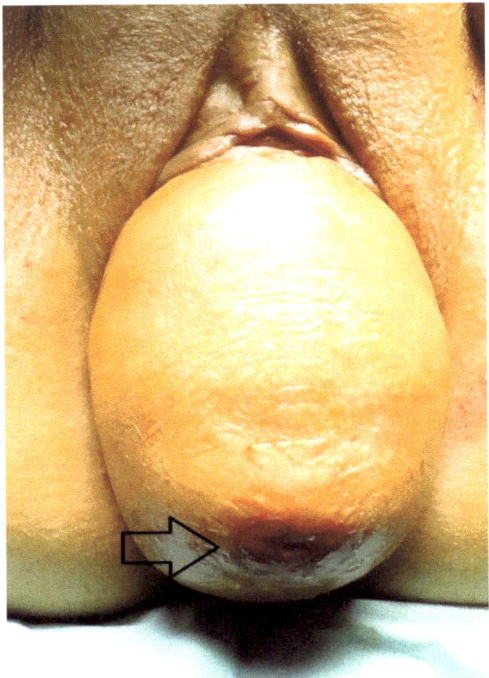

Fig. 5.9. Decubitus lesion associated to a 4th degree prolapse
(according to **Enache T., 2014**)

5.1.1.9. Pelvic pain and dyspareunia

In the woman's body, pelvis represents a very vulnerable place for a major pathology, often invalid, particularly pain, bladder and intestinal disorders and dyspareunia. Dysmenorrhea, uterine fibroids, menstrual disorders, persistent uterine retroversion, endometriosis, pelvic inflammatory disease, ovarian tumors, vaginal or uterine prolapse, are all involved in the etiopathogeny of pelvic pain. These pains are characterized as persistent upper abdominal floor or as low sacral pain.

However, most aspects of chronic pelvic pain syndrome (CPPS) are considered of unknown origin, classified as "neurological", or in German literature as "*pelvipathia vegetativa*", "*spastic parametropathy*", "*spasmophilia genitalis*", "*plexalgia hypogastrica*", "*pelvic neuralgia*" or "*cervical syndrome*" (**Zetkin M. & Schaldach H., 2005**). Pelvic pain can be caused by disorders of blood circulation in the pelvis, as for example in functional hyperemia forms during menstruation or due to inflammation. In literature, venous congestion due to varicose vein dilations of the pelvic veins, "*pelvic congestion syndrome*", has been well known for many years.

Several decades ago, Heinrich Martius published in German literature the fact that in approximately 30% of the cases, the posterior irradiated pains are caused by pelvic organs suspension and supporting ligaments affection (**Martius H., 1946**). The two "*recto-uterine ligaments*", which are connected with the sacrum through paraproctium and which are generally known as "*uterosacral ligament plication*" or "*uterosacral ligaments*" (USL), are located at the center of numerous pathophysiological pathways. Unfortunately, the concepts of Martius remained totally unknown in the Anglo-Saxon literature.

In 1993, Petros and Ulmsten described the CPPS independently as being caused by lax uterosacral ligaments as part of the "*posterior fornix syndrome*" (**Petros P. & Ulmsten U., 1993**), along with other pelvic symptoms: nocturia, urinary urge, voiding disorders. They reported a significant rate of healing of CPPS and of other posterior fornix symptoms following the correction of uterosacral ligaments (**Petros P. & Ulmsten U., 1993**).

Petros made the classical description of this type of pain in 1996.

"In its acute manifestation, the pain is invariably severe, frequently unilateral, located at the level of the right or left iliac fossa, usually improved by dorsal decubitus, frequently relieved by the insertion of a pessary, reproducible at the palpation of the cervix or its posterior displacement while the patient lies in dorsal decubitus position. Although chronic pain varies considerably in intensity, there have been cases of deep dyspareunia that occurs only in deep penetration or in specific positions. Frequently, the female patient complains of a constant pain in the lower abdominal floor the day after sexual intercourse. Half of the female patients have complained of low sacrum pain, which was also surgically treated. Six female patients, two of whom had a nulliparous pregnancy, were included in the study" (**Petros P., 1996**).

In 2008, Abendstein et al. expanded the concept of posterior fornix syndrome through their report regarding the "*obstructed defecation syndrome*" (ODS), severe sacral and abdominal CPPS and non sphincter faecal incontinence with a posterior intra-vaginal mesh (PIVS) (**Abendstein B., et al., 2008**). These papers have led to a diagnostic algorithm that immediately separates CPPS of uterosacral origin from other forms such as endometriosis, the key element being that in the uterosacral origin one, other posterior compartment symptoms appear invariably, Fig. 5.10.

The posterior vector component of the levator plate (LP) and the longitudinal anal muscle tension the cardinal ligaments (CL) and the uterosacral ligaments (USL) during urethral and anorectal closure, stretching the pubocervical fascia (PCF) and thus stimulating the nerve endings inducing afferent impulses. The lax ligaments cause the decrease of the muscular force and the appearance of symptoms and signs. The intensity of a symptom can be more frequently linked to the affection of a particular ligament, for example, SUI is related to pubourethral ligaments injury, nocturia, and pain being most often associated with USL. The structures highlighted with the red border are surgically reconstitutable with polypropylene meshes. The importance of strictly stressing the damaged structures and their reconstruction is highlighted once again.

So far, the discussion regarding the importance of the suspension and support system of pelvic organs is still unknown in the Anglo-Saxon and international literature. The Expert

Committees from ICS (International Continence Society) and the European Association of Urology do not mention the role of USL laxity as a major cause of CPPS (**Abrams P.**, *et al.,* **2002**; **Fall M.**, *et al.,* **2010**).

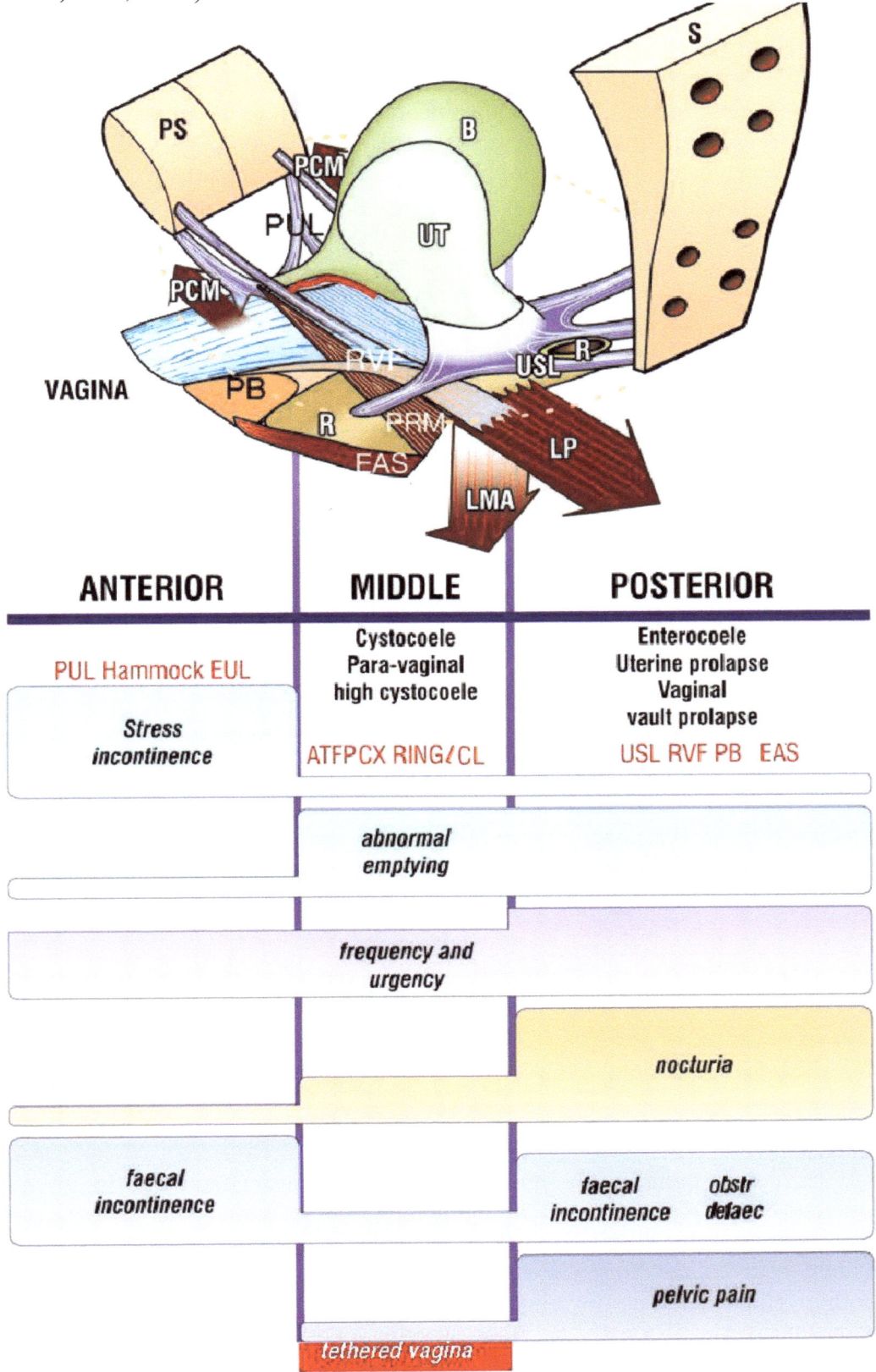

Fig. 5.10. Diagnostic algorithm

Also, neither the recent article on CPPS does not mention the right posterior ligament defect as a possible cause (**Evans S.F., 2012**). Important articles published in 1993, 1996, 2001, 2010 and 2012 that focus heavily on this subject, are still being ignored (Petros P. *&* Ulmsten

U., 1993; Petros P., 1996; Farnsworth B.N., 2011; Petros P. **& Richardson P.A., 2010**; **Forgács S.,** *et al.,* **2012**).

There are two defining aspects in the case of pelvic pain and dyspareunia.

The first aspect is given by the importance of the posterior pelvic support and suspension system in CPPS induction.

The second aspect is defined by the therapeutic possibilities of curing these symptoms.

a) Anatomy of posterior support system

USL has a major role in the anatomy of the posterior compartment. Its importance has started to be known and emphasized since the beginning of the 18th century. The early 20th century marked several observations that changed the perception regarding USL. Symington (**Symington J., 1914**) noted the topographic report regarding *"plexus pelvicus"*. Balisdell (**Blaisdell F.E., 1917**) demonstrated the presence of the muscle tissue in the USL structure. Martius (**Martius H., 1938**) highlighted the painful contraction of these muscle fibers, Fig. 5.11. The figure shows that the parametrium fibrous tissue mainly has a posterior orientation to the iliosacral region, connecting and suspending the cervix to the posterior side of the pelvis.

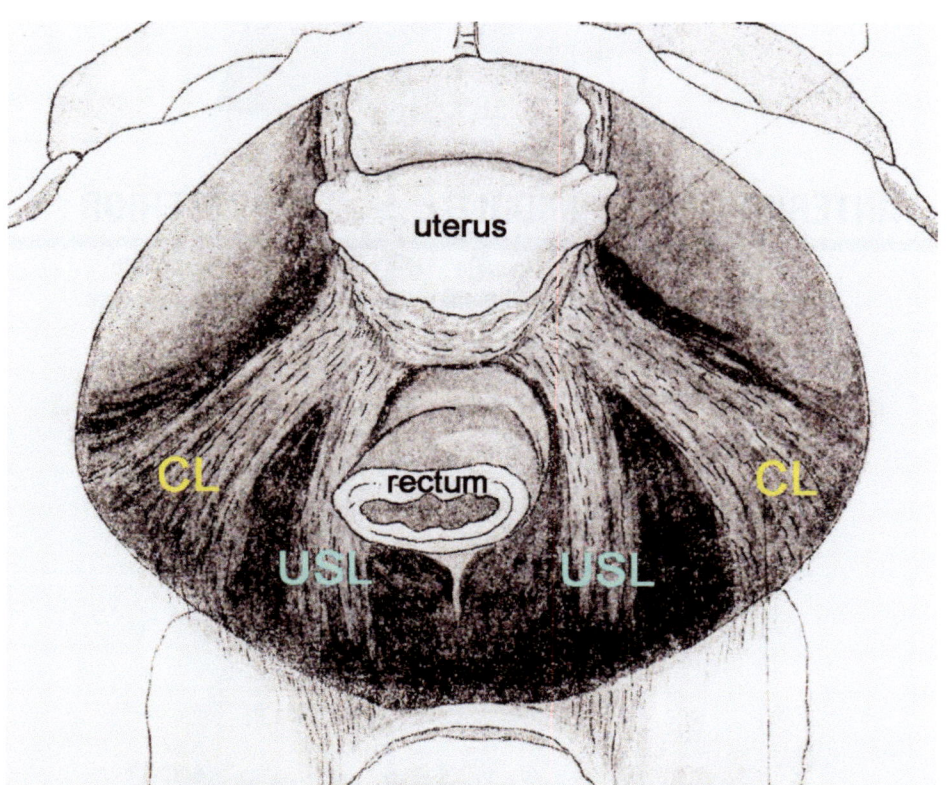

Fig. 5.11. Parameter. Highlighting the posterior anchoring of the cervix
(according to **Martius H. 1938**)
USL – uterosacral ligaments; CL – cardinal ligaments

In 1996, Petros performed a prospective study to understand this issue and to find treatment methods (**Petros P., 1996**), including female patients with an unknown pelvic pain and with laxity of the posterior vaginal fornix. The histological examination of USL was part of this study and demonstrated the presence of soft muscle tissue, collagen, and elastin and nerve endings, both myelinated and non-myelinated in all samples. USL nerve fibers were classified as visceral parasympathetic fibers. In his view, visceral innervation incorporating T12-L1 fibers offers an adequate explanation for the distribution of pain in the lower abdomen, especially in the area innervated by the ilioinguinal nerve. The author assumed that the lax and weakened USL stretching under the influence of gravity could stimulate the nerve endings in these tissues and cause pain.

Even today, there are still different views on the importance of the posterior suspension of pelvic organs. For example, in his book published in 2008, Fritsch mentioned only one recto uterine ligament as a plication stretching from the rectum to the uterus. This ligament forms the cranial limit of "pouch of *Douglas*". For the author, there is no evidence of the existence of a structure linking the sacrum to the rectum or uterus (**Fritsch H., 2008**).

Petros and Goeschen underlined in their treatises that the USL originate from the S2-4 sacral vertebrae and attach behind the cervical ring, Fig. 5.29 (**Petros P., 2010**; **Goeschen K. & Petros P., 2008**).

USL fixes the vaginal fornix in its place. Age or births in the medical history of the patient that induce a loss of collagen/ elasticity lead to uterine prolapse due to USL elongation. The descending branches of uterine arteries replace the blood supply of the proximal parts of USL, so that hysterectomy can cause atrophy and weakening of USL by removing the main source of vascularization. The nerves of the USL are sensitive to tension. This aspect is easily highlighted in patients by using the posterior valve of a bivalve speculum. Discrete support relieves pain. The pulling of the cervix will exacerbate the symptoms (**Wu Q., *et al.*, 2013**).

In 2012, Forgács and colleagues highlighted the „*ligamentum recto-uterinum*" in all dissections of female bodies examined (**Forgács S., *et al.*, 2012**). They detected a connection between the lateral side of the rectum and the cervical ring and also between the connective tissue of the paraproctium and the adjacent area of the sacrum. Considering these, they concluded that the term "*uterosacral ligament*" is correct. Moreover, they also histologically examined two 1 cm long sections of the anterior and posterior ligaments. Both specimens obtained contained firm fibrous connective tissue, typical of a ligament, vessels, and smooth muscle fibers disposed along the ligaments.

b) Pain transmission ways

Time limited pain caused by tension, compression, contraction, or spasm is a physiological phenomenon very often met in women during childbirth. These pains are predominantly mechanical and are thus comparable to situations that besides pregnancy induce similar pressures on pelvic floor. In this context, the following issues are very important.

i) How does pain actually occur at birth?

ii) What nerve tract is the pain transmitted to the central nervous system?

iii) Do similar pains occurring in non-pregnant women have the same source and identical ways of transmission?

Birth pain consists of the following:
- labor pain due to contraction or uterine spasm
- pain induced by continuous cervical dilation and
- pain caused by the tensioning and stretching of the pelvic floor as a result of fetal skull descending.

In the first period of birth, pain is secondary to uterine contraction and is transmitted via the Frankenhäuser ganglion, Fig. 5.15., lower hypogastric plexus, sympathetic fibers of the hypogastric nerve to the posterior roots of the spinal cord at T11 – T12 level, Fig. 5.12 and 5.13. Pains resulting from cervical dilation are predominantly transmitted through parasympathetic fibers of the lower hypogastric plexus to S2-S4 sacral roots.

The fetal skull that descends via the pudendal nerve and the plexus sacralis to the same S2 – S4 area, Fig. 5.12, causes pains during the second period of birth.

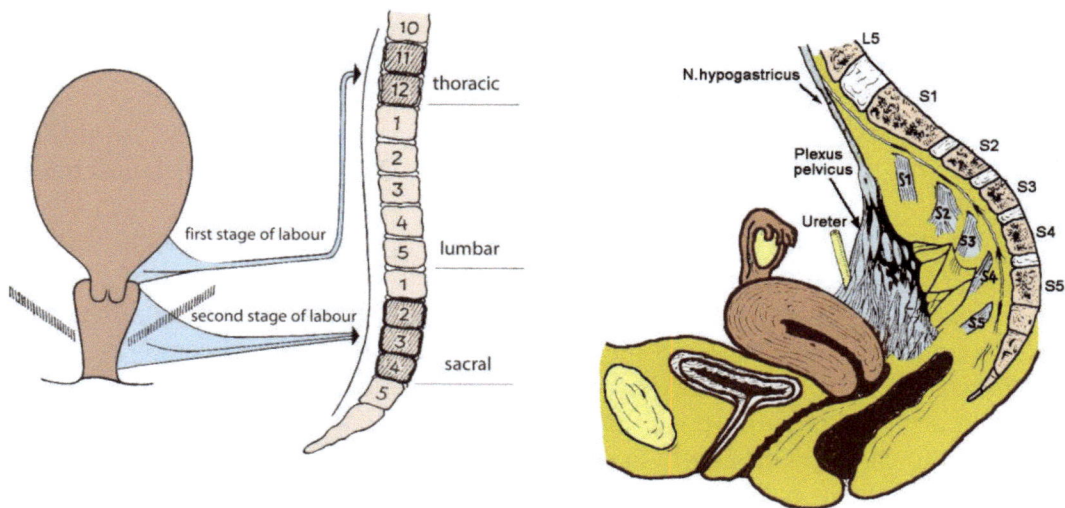

Fig. 5.12. Schematic diagram of uterine visceral innervation

Fig. 5.13. Schematic diagram of pain transmission during labor

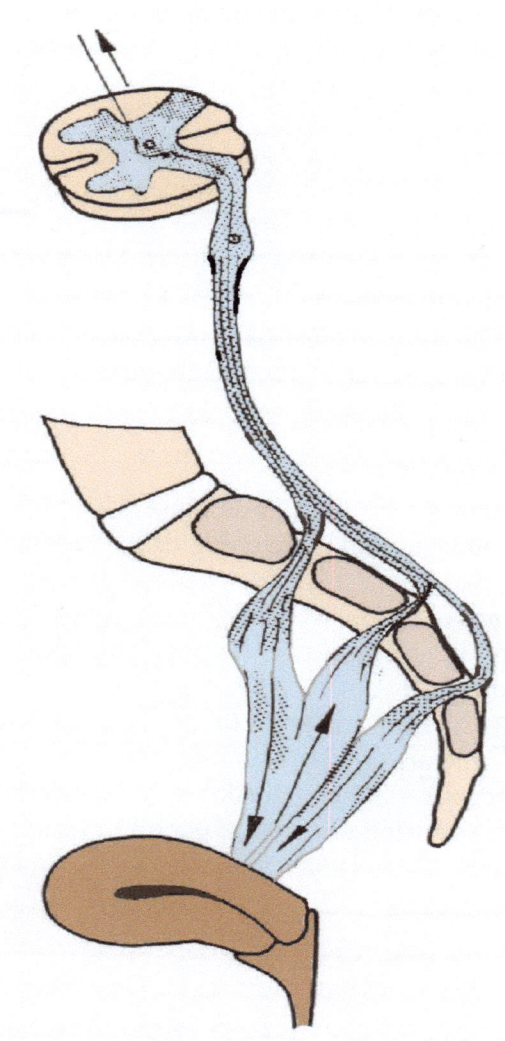

Fig. 5.14. The mechanical origin of posterior irradiated gynecological pain and cerebrospinal transmission

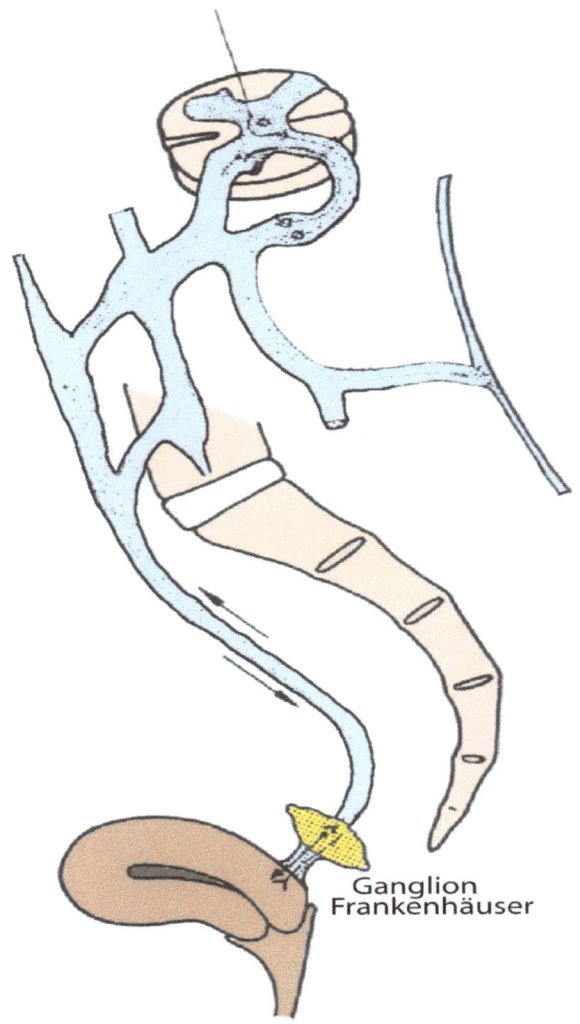

Fig. 5.15. The visceral origin of posterior irradiated gynecological pain

Over the past two decades, epidural anesthesia has become the most common procedure for stopping pelvic pain, while during previous years, Frankenhäuser ganglion was the preferred spot for paracervical block. When performed by professionals, both methods are very efficient for pain relief (**Roemer H., 1967**).

In 1946, Martius (**Martius H., 1946**) mentioned two ways of transmitting the lumbosacral pain in non-pregnant women. The first goes directly to the central nervous system via the somatic afferent fibers and the stimuli are the mechanical irradiation of free nerve endings Fig. 5.14. The second way, in case of pathological visceral irradiation, the primary visceral afferent stimuli are directed to the spinal cord and can be taken over by the somatic afferent fibers and interpreted at the cerebral level as coming from somatic areas served by them.

The projection of pain is thus present at the level of the lumbosacral region, the anterior and lateral abdominal wall, the inguinal region, and the thigh root Fig. 5.16.

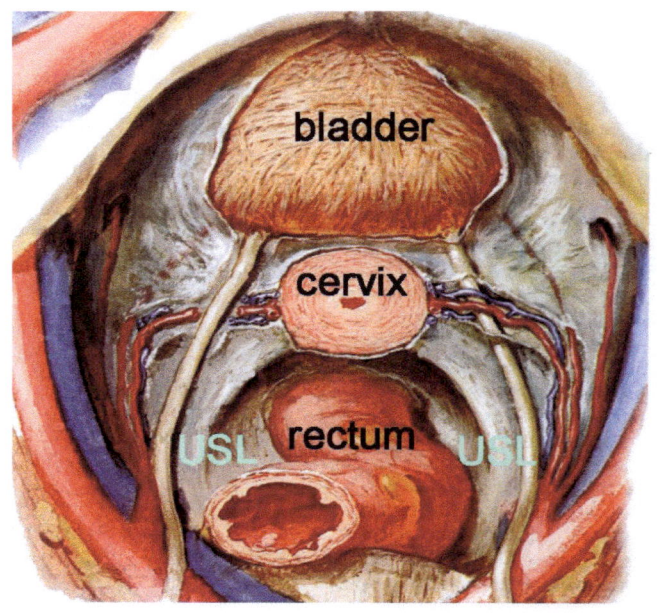 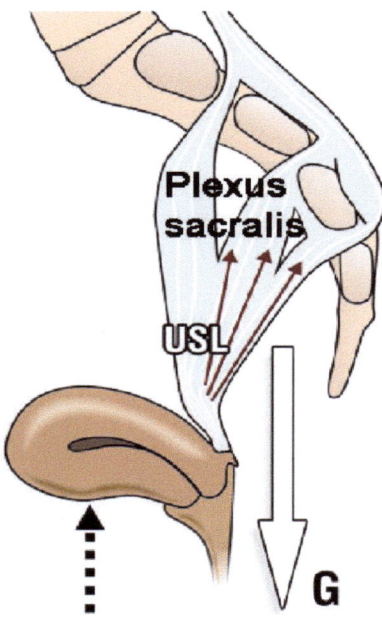

Fig. 5.16. Schematic diagram of pelvis in woman
USL – uterosacral ligaments

Fig. 5.17. In the case of lax USL or an inadequate support of the pelvic floor (the dotted black arrow)

The most common and most important is the shorter, directly cerebrospinal way.

The vertical position of the human being imposes a serious tension on the suspension and support system of the uterus, especially because the pelvis in women extends particularly posteriorly, Fig. 5.11, 5.16. and 5.17., where it can be observed that gravity (G) pulls the uterus caudally, tensioning the plexus sacralis.

There are many somatosensory receptors on the pelvic wall, which can cause lumbosacral pain by traction of the support apparatus. Symptomatology includes lower abdominal and deep sacral pains. It is not surprising that both concepts, the pains associated to pregnancy or not, are compatible. Regardless of the pregnancy stage, it is very likely that the pelvic pain caused by tension, compression, contraction, or spasm of the pelvic organs appears and is transmitted in the same way, given the nervous transmission ways that will not change after birth.

c) Possible causes of lumbosacral pains

This subchapter deals with the importance of the posterior sustaining and supporting system of the vagina, uterus, bladder, and rectum. The goal is not to list all the possibilities that determine pelvic pain. This would lead to a monotonous listing of almost all entities of gynecological pathology. Our discussion is limited to uterus and posterior vaginal wall as shown in Fig. 5.10., cardinal and uterosacral ligaments, perineal body, and rectovaginal fascia. Because USL incorporates connective tissue, collagen, elastin and also nerves, smooth muscles and vessels, the question that arises is what mechanical or pathophysiological alteration can cause the chronic pelvic pain.

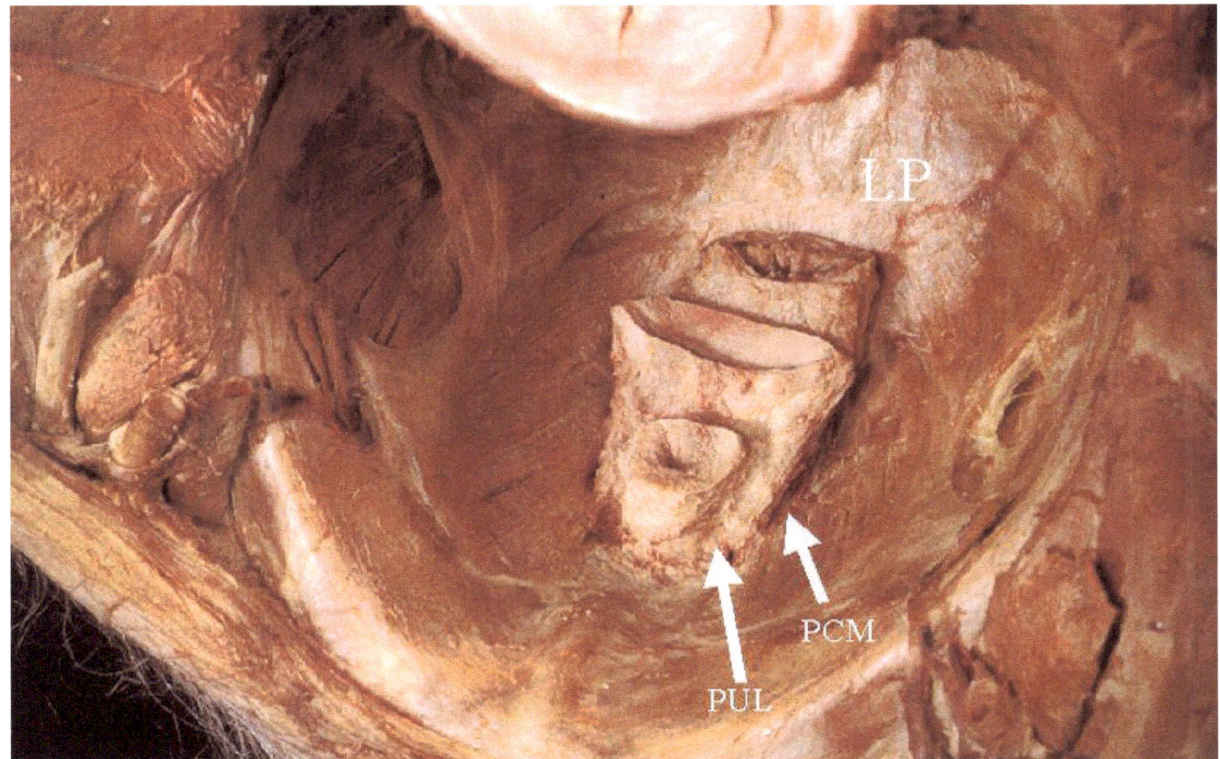

Fig. 5.18. Interconnection of pelvic organs with the levator ani muscle through connective tissue
Corpse specimen – cranial view from front to back: urethra, vagina, and rectum
PUL – pubourethral ligaments; PCM – pubococcygeus muscle; LP – levator plate

i) Pain as a result of spastic contractions and colics of USL

A long time ago, it has been hypothesized that smooth muscle fibers inside the USL can induce painful spastic contractions. These colic pains are located especially on the left side of the pelvis associated with spastic constipation. For this clinical case, Martius created in 1938 the term "*parametropatia spastica sinistra cum obstipationem*" and indicated the link between spasm and pain in the area of the posterior suspension system (**Martius H., 1936**). A frequent finding in these cases is the irradiation of severe pain at the sacral level while touching the posterior vaginal fornix during the gynecological examination. Pain is particularly accentuated at the insertion points of the USL. Pain intensity increases exponentially if the cervix is mobilized laterally or especially anteriorly. Posterior irradiated pains may occur during deep sexual penetration.

This situation has been and is still confused, being interpreted as adnexitis, parametritis, or proctitis. Proctitis is often taken into account because pain accentuates at defecation. And yet, this is not the result of inflammation. It is caused exclusively by the condensed faecal bowel that passes and tensions the USL.

ii) Pain induced by irritation of Frankenhäuser ganglion

The Frankenhäuser ganglion, the cervico-uterine ganglion, or the so-called "*pelvic brain*" is located bilaterally paracervical and paravaginal in the posterior fornix (**Frankenhäuser F., 1867**; **Robinson B., 1997**) Fig. 5.15. It is located in the connective tissue of the parameter, at the conjunction of the two halves of the uterine cervix and approximately 2.5 cm lateral to it. Topographically, it is located at the base of the broad ligament and at the distal end of the lower hypogastric plexus. The Frankenhäuser ganglion is practically located at the junction between the cervix and the posterior vaginal fornix and has deep and extensive connections with the uterus, vagina, rectum, urethra, and bladder. The distension and contraction of the pelvic organs, with consequent changes in the positions of the organs, somehow alter their anatomical relations with the ganglion.

During parturition, labor is initiated by mobilizing the presentation distally with the mechanical consequences of irritation, pressure, and ganglion stimulation. The more this movement in the distal sense is broader, the more the mechanical irritation is more intense on the Frankenhäuser ganglion, and secondary, many nerve endings are stimulated.

This explains the growing pain during labor.

Very experienced obstetricians know Frankenhäuser ganglion especially because of the paracervical block. Injecting the local anesthetic into the paracervical area blocks the nerve endings of the presacral nerve and plexus sacralis.

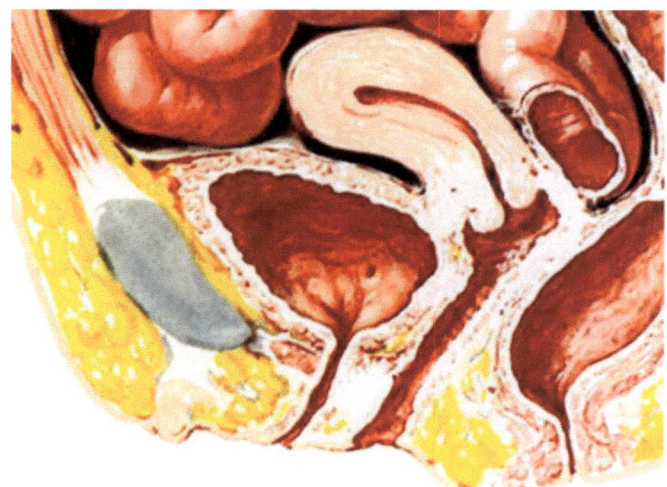

Fig. 5.19. Normal anatomy
A stable support of the pelvic floor is necessary for the normal uterine position

Immediately after the injection, patients experience pain relief. Pain determined by dilation of the uterine inferior segment as well as pain generated by the enormous stretch of the uterus support system during delivery is no longer present as long as the anesthetic is active.

Considerations regarding the source of pain can be made outside pregnancy.

Located in the parameter, Frankenhäuser ganglion is subjected to permanent stimulation if the uterus or vagina is descended. This way, pains of increased intensity, similar to those in labor, can result.

The mechanical support of the uterus and vagina restored by the correction of the support and suspension structures should stop the permanent ganglionar stimulation. In these patients, remission should be definitive in the absence of relapses.

iii) Pain generated by non-physiological tension exerted on the plexus sacralis

This pain can be caused by defects of the support ligaments or of the perineal muscles.

Defects of support ligaments

The lumbosacral area in woman provides an extensive support and suspension apparatus for pelvic organs, which is deeply connected with the posterior pelvic bone periosteum, skeletal muscles, and sensory receptors of somatic nervous system.

It is logical that a support defect of pelvic organs leads to an increased tension on the plexus sacralis with the effect of severe pain occurrence at this level, Fig. 5.18.

There are two simple mechanical reasons that the pelvic organs change their physiological position, causing the tensioning of the support and suspension system.

1) Because of the bipedal position of the human being, pelvic organs are exposed to gravity. Thus, pelvic organs are predestined to descend.

2) The fixation of the genitals must be flexible so that the huge modifications of the uterus position during pregnancy are possible.

Therefore, in recent years, it has become well known that pelvic pain is mainly linked to vaginal or uterine prolapse caused by defects of support structures. As a result, even patients with minor prolapse may present major symptoms, because the downward force applied on the plexus sacralis Fig. 5.17 generates these pains. Martius has made observations about the intensity of the symptoms and the extent of the prolapse in 1946 (**Martius H., 1946**).

Defects of perineal muscles

As mentioned earlier, in women, the pelvis content is not only suspended but it is also supported from the base. The perineal muscles contain three layers of muscles one on top of the other, just like the roof tiles. The striped muscles alone cannot provide the permanent tonus necessary to support these organs. It is obvious, as shown in 5.10., that the three directions of muscular forces, shown by the arrows in the figure, which tension and support the pelvic organs, are vectorally opposed to the suspension ligaments. A weakened ligament will induce a reduced muscle force. Thus, the whole system is interconnected and ultimately relies on firm suspension ligaments. For this reason, the elastic system of viscerally innervated musculoskeletal tissue must be intact. It is the so-called fiber-musculo-ligament system or the endopelvic fascia in Fig. 5.10. This system is connected with striated muscle fibers, sealing the interstices and working unitarily, Fig. 5.18.

The pelvis has two functions.

The first function is the inferior delineation of the abdominal cavity.

The second function is to ensure the evacuation of some intra-abdominal organs, Fig. 5.19.

The fact that the voiding of the bladder, rectum and uterus correspond to the gravitational direction due to the bipedal posture and require a perfect coordination of the fiber-musculo-ligament system, especially since this system should also function after birth. A decline in the pelvic floor followed by a descending of the pelvic organs inevitably determines a tension on the support ligaments, Fig. 5.20. This phenomenon can induce pain, primarily caused by a pelvic floor deficiency. Although support ligaments are secondary tensioned, they result in pain in the lumbosacral area.

Predominantly, these pains can be treated by repairing the pelvic floor defect, which restores the physiological position of the affected organs by the disappearance of the ligament tension. As long as the ligaments are weak, their simple plication will not work. The surgical augmentation of ligaments must follow the principle of neo-ligaments (**Petros P.,** *et al.,* **1990; Abendstein B.,** *et al.,* **2008; Farnsworth B.N., 2001**, Petros P. & Richardson P.A., 2010; **Goeschen K.** & Petros P., 2008).

Chronic severe sacral pain may be the result of previous pathological processes in the parametric region. Martius made this statement (**Martius H., 1946**).

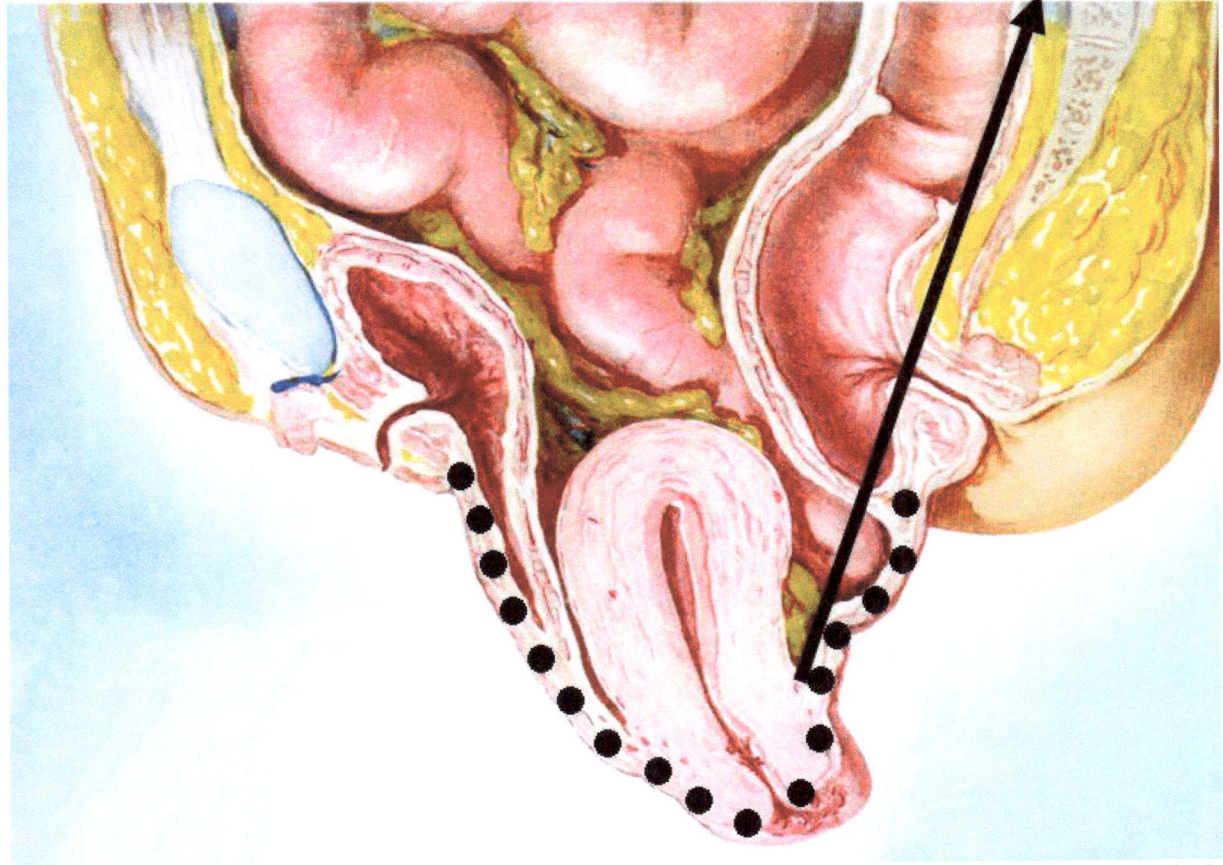

Fig. 5.20. Elitrocele. Injured pelvic floor (black dotted line) **cannot support the pelvic organs, causing prolapse, raised tension of support ligaments** (black arrow) **and pain**

In the case of a pelvic floor defect or a pathological suspension of the uterus, posterior irradiated pain of increased intensity may occur if the uterus is firmly attached to the pelvic wall by parametric scar tissue Fig. 5.21.

Deficiency of support mechanisms leads to an increased pulling of suspension mechanisms, even in female patients with minor prolapse. According to Sellheim, this situation is called "*suspension agony*" in ancient literature (**Sellheim H., 1926**).

iv) Pain induced by overload of uterosacral ligaments (USL)

Regarding USL, Petros published the following hypothesis for the pathogenesis of chronic sacral pain.

"*Pelvic pain associated with USL laxity is characterized by chronic abdominal pain in the lower compartment, (often unilateral), deep dyspareunia and often low sacral pain. Sometimes, it can be severe enough for the patient so that she is determined to urgently see the physician.*" (**Petros P., 1996**).

The nerve fibers present at the level of USL are visceral parasympathetic. The visceral innervation incorporating fibers with integration into T12-L1 adequately explains the irradiation of pain in the lower abdomen, especially in the area of the ilioinguinal nerve. It has been hypothesized that the tension followed by the elongation of lax ligaments due to the gravity can stimulate the respective nerve fibers and cause pain, Fig. 5.22a) and b), where an analogy between the USL and a telephone cable is made.

This pain is often relieved in decubitus position, and, is usually part of the "*posterior fornix syndrome*" (**Petros P., Ulmsten U., 1993**), which also includes urinary urge, nocturia, and more recently, faecal incontinence, bladder and rectum voiding disorders (**Abendstein B.**, *et al.*, **2008**). Pain in CPPS may appear even in the context of a small degree of prolapse. This pain can be reproduced and "*simulated*" by the digital tensioning of USL. It is assumed that pain relief after surgical treatment with intravaginal posterior mesh is linked to the mechanical support and tension release of USL mechanical support and, consequently, to S2-S4 unmyelinated fibers that pass through these ligaments. Mounting a pessary can have effect through the same mechanic support mechanism for ligaments that induce relief of nerve endings.

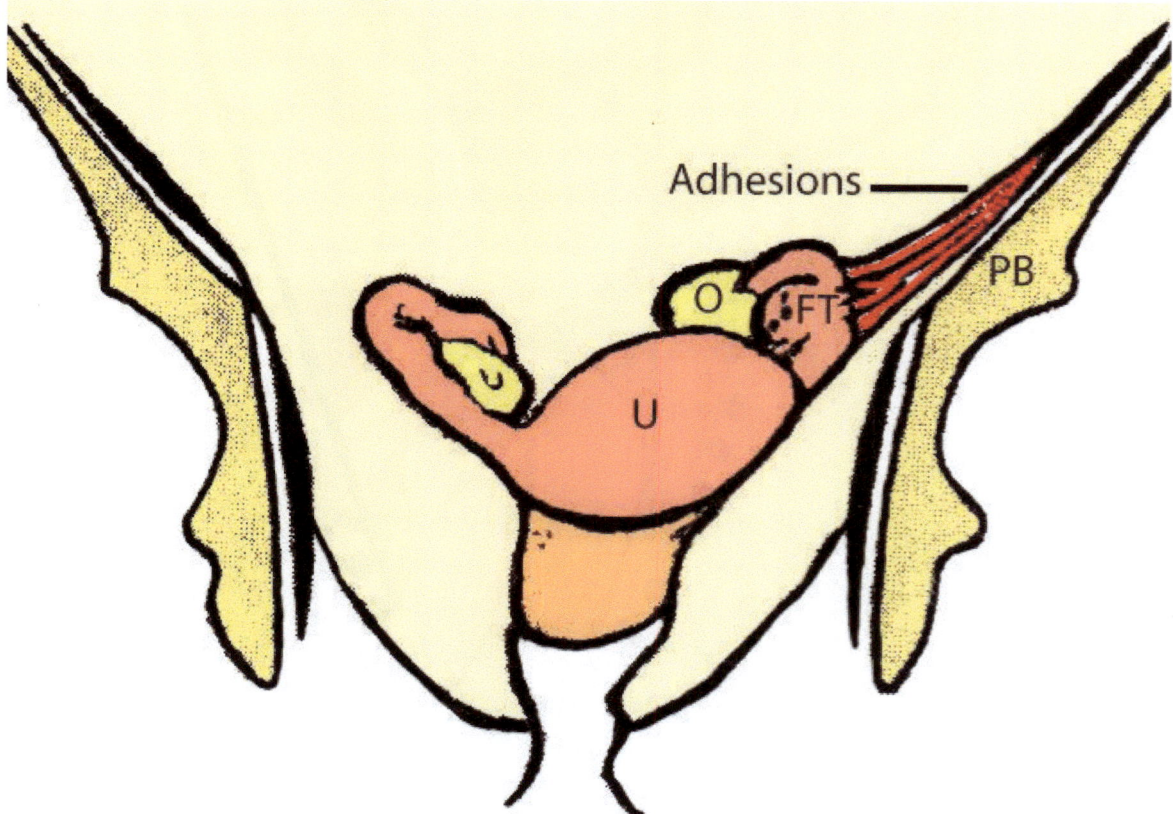

Fig. 5.21. "*Suspension agony*" caused by pulling on parametrial scar tissue
U-uterus; O-ovary; FT- fallopian tube; PB – perineal body

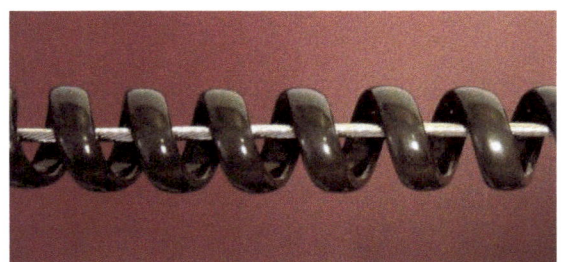

Fig. 5.22*a)* **USL with firm elastic connective tissue (spiral black cable) prevent the elongation of nervous fibers inside**

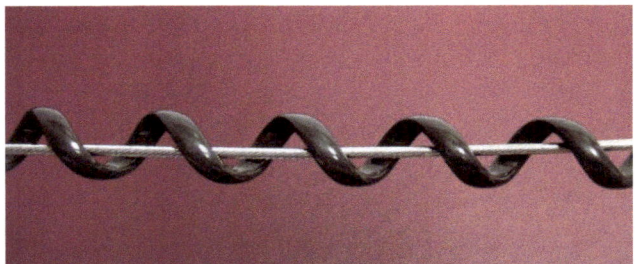

Fig. 5.22*b)* **Lax USL cannot stop the tension of nervous fibers inside**

v) Pain induced by vascular disorders

"*Pelvic Venous Congestive Syndrome*" (PVCS) is characterized by chronic pain affecting 13-40% of women and is due to lower pelvic varicose veins. PVCS generates chronic pain, as well as the feeling of tension in the lower abdomen and/ or the pelvis.

Varicose veins usually appear in the lower limbs, where the venous valves are deficient, or where there is a downstream obstruction. In these cases, the venous blood flow is reversed and no longer circulates to the heart, causing stasis and pain.

The same mechanism is also present in the appearance of PVCS.

PVCS appears most frequently in young women who gave birth. During pregnancy, the pregnant uterus can compress the pelvic veins. This may affect the valves of the veins. After birth, the connective tissue in women is lax and the support system is overloaded. This leads to the lowering of pelvic organs with circulatory obstructive effect followed by the dilation and swelling of the venous walls. Pain increases in orthostatism, during or after sexual intercourse and is usually relieved by the decubitus position. Transvaginal ultrasound is very useful in determining abnormally dilated veins. However, in dorsal decubitus position, it may be difficult to demonstrate the presence of dilated pelvic veins because the hydrostatic pressure is low and the vein diameter seems normal. Considering this, the ultrasound examination should be performed in orthostatism.

From the point of view of Petros (**Petros P.** *&* **Ulmsten U., 1993**), pelvic congestion is secondary to ligament laxity and may occur even in nulliparous or independently of pregnancy, in the following conditions: normally, cardinal and uterosacral ligaments support the uterus, possibly the contraction of pelvic floor muscles also participate. It is assumed that due to ligament laxity, gravitational force can induce the "wrinkling" of the pelvic veins in these tissues, thus obstructing the flow and generating congestion.

d) Painful symptoms

Women with pelvic organs support or suspension deficiencies most often present after a long-suffering period, often accompanied by failed treatment attempts. Pain can be so severe that these patients may experience psychiatric disorders. Some even mentioned suicide attempts. Invariably, laparoscopy is negative in these cases, which induces the idea to the physicians that the pathologic substrate is psychogenic (**Petros P.** *&* **Ulmsten U., 1993**). This is a great tragedy, as pain can be significantly improved or even healed.

Pain can occur in the following forms:
- persistent abdominal pain in the lower part of the body, often unilateral;
- low sacral pain;

- dyspareunia and postcoital pain;
- asthenia;
- irritability.

Pain gets worse during the day and improves in decubitus position. It can be reproduced while palpating the cervix and the posterior fornix.

Chronic pains can induce asthenia and irritability (**Petros P. & Ulmsten U., 1993**), the decrease of libido and the appearance of marital stress with depression, all of which, in another context, can be interpreted as psychological associations or even considered psychosomatic causes. According to Martius, these pains can be induced by shifting the cervix anteriorly or laterally during the gynecological examination (**Martius H., 1946**).

In this context, Petros (**Petros P. & Ulmsten U., 1993**) revealed that the deficiency of the non-myelinated nerve endings support connective tissue, whose trajectory is along the uterosacral ligaments, could be the cause of lower abdominal or sacral pains. The pressure exerted on these nerves can induce deep dyspareunia.

The lower abdominal and sacral pains can be reproduced by touching the posterior fornix or with a clip. This has been described as *"painful excitation"* or *"cervical pain"* or *"vaginal pain"*. As already mentioned above, pelvic pain is often part of *"posterior fornix syndrome"*, which includes urinary urge, pollakiuria, nocturia, bladder, and rectal voiding disorders. Pain can even appear in patients with a low degree of prolapse.

In 1938, Martius (**Martius H., 1938**) considered that these symptoms to be related to somatic problems rather than local causes, mechanical stimuli amplifying the tension in the parametric tissue. In a high percentage, this mechanical, local irritation originates in a defect of pelvic organs support or suspension system.

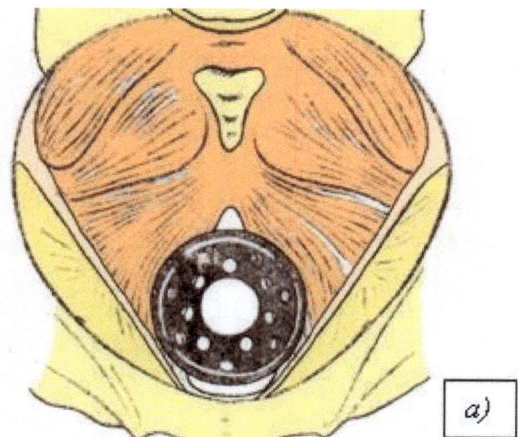

Fig. 5.23*b*) Schatz pessary in correct position

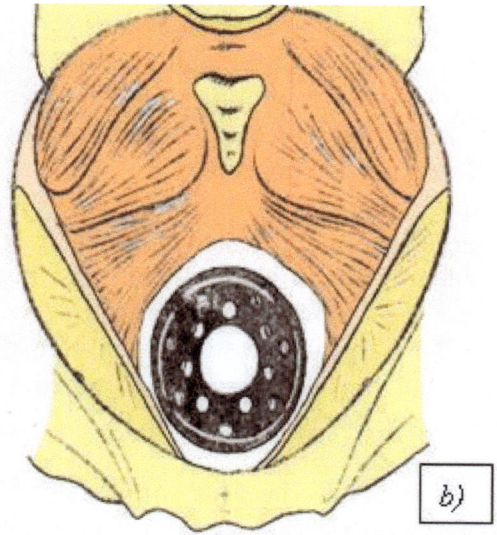

Fig. 5.23*b*) Schatz pessary that does not function properly because of enlarged levator hiatus

In his view, the treatment by introducing a pessary is not a good idea, as it is only a palliative and not an etiopathogenic treatment. On the contrary, the pessary treatment can even worsen the situation by the appearance of ulcerations and/ or inflammation. The device will stand in position only if the levator hiatus is smaller than the circumference of the ring. If the hiatus is too large, or if the support area of levator ani muscles is weakened, the pelvic organs together with the pessary will fall, Fig. 5.23*a)* and *b)*. Thus, the insertion of a pessary must be only temporary, since it can induce many problems for the patients.

In this view, Martius noted in his 1936 surgical treaty that "*this problem can be solved by a surgery capable of restoring natural anatomy*" (**Martius H., 1936**). He further underlined that "*a narrowing of the vagina by the so-called anterior or posterior colporrhaphy is not enough, because the support ability of the vagina is inadequate*". Unfortunately, this so-called widespread prolapse surgery is net effective for anatomical repair, but encourages surgeons to use it because the name seems convincing.

In 1993, in collaboration with Ulmsten, Petros (**Petros P. & Ulmsten U., 1993**) described pain as part of "*posterior fornix syndrome*", with symptoms that include pelvic pains, nocturia, urge, pollakiuria, and voiding disorders. In 1996, when still not knowing Martius' research from German literature, Petros (**Petros P. & Ulmsten U., 1993**) justified Martius' statements through scientific research. He published his results on the relationship between pelvic pains of unknown origin and the laxity of posterior vaginal fornix in a prospective study. In a 3 months review, 85% of the patients were cured, and at 12 months, 70%. Petros' conclusion was that non-organic pelvic pain was attributed to psychological factors. He suggested that this could be a lower abdominal pain with T12-L1 parasympathetic integration, probably due to the gravitational force that induces painful stimuli in the nerves that are not supported by lax uterosacral ligaments.

He concluded that the laxity of the posterior ligaments of the vagina should be excluded primarily in patients with discomfort or pelvic pains and the ones undergoing psychiatric care. A pessary can be useful before surgery as a diagnosis method in pain relief, "*simulated surgery*", by offering a mechanical support to ligaments, thus for nerve endings at this level. Another more recent diagnosis test is the soft introduction of a posterior vaginal valve (**Wu Q., et al., 2013**). A personal communication between Gunnemann and Petros offers as a diagnosis method the introduction of a large buffer at the level of the posterior fornix. Due to the decrease in the healing rate by a simple plication surgery over time (**Petros P., 1996**), Petros developed the posterior mesh surgery Fig. 5.24., for the reinforcement of injured uterosacral (**Petros P., 2001***b*; **Petros P., 1997**) and cardinal (**Petros P. & Richardson P.A., 2010**) ligaments.

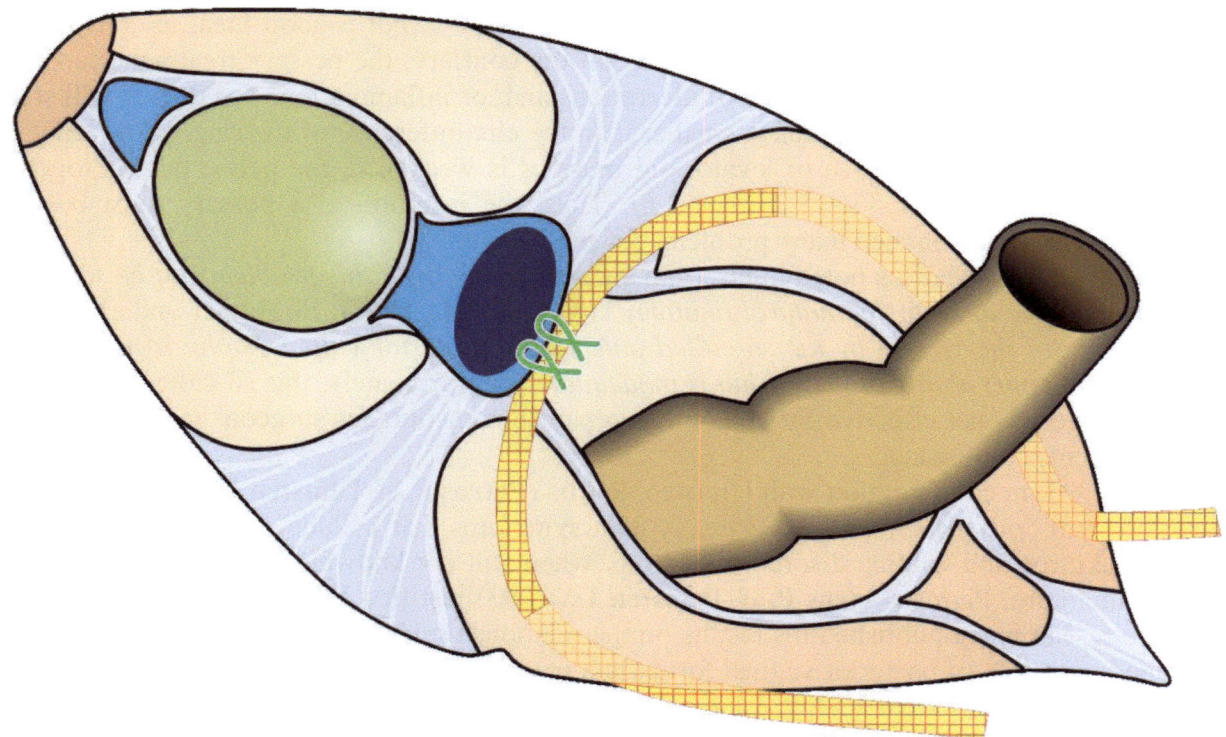

Fig. 5.24. Posterior intravaginal mesh placed along the uterosacral ligaments (USL)

Figures 5.25*a), b),c),* and *d)* demonstrate the physiological reconstruction of the anatomy before and immediately after the reinforcement of uterosacral and cardinal ligaments, according to Petros. The captured laparoscopic images show a sufficient support of newly created ligaments (according to **Enache T., 2014**). Keeping the uterus in a natural position prevents pulling on the lumboplexus sacralis and pain.

At the same time, Petros' persuasive data (**Petros P., Ulmsten U., 1993**) are validated by many surgeons. In 2002, Farnsworth had already published a 78% pain relief rate after the surgical treatment of vaginal vault prolapse after hysterectomy. Since then, many studies have confirmed these results (**Petros P.** *&* **Richardson P.A., 2010**; **Goeschen & Gent H-J., 2004; Goeschen K., 2015; Gold D.M.** *&* **Goeschen K., 2016; Caliskan A.,** *et al.,* **2015; Wagenlehner F., 2014; Markovsky O., 2014; Petros P., 2014; Müller-Funogea A., 2014).**

The healing rates of chronic pains vary between 62 and 83%.

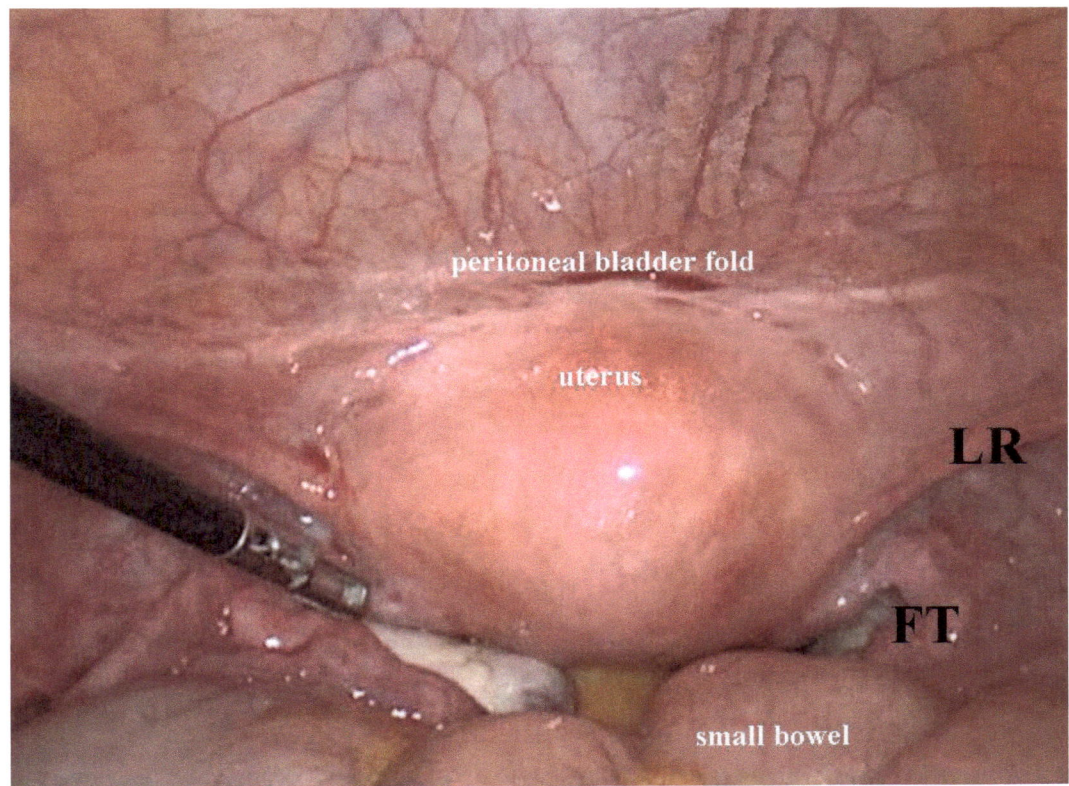

Fig. 5.25*a*) Uterus in descending position

The round ligaments are lax (RL) and the fallopian tubes are deep inside the pouch of Douglas.

Another therapeutic option for pelvic pains is surgery of nerve pathways interruption such as: laparoscopic uterine nerve ablation and presacral neurectomy, hysterectomy with or without adnexectomy (**Stones W.,** *et al.,* **2007**) or neuromodulation, following which patients reported an improvement of painful symptoms by 40%, 15 months after surgery (**Zabihi N.,** *et al.,* **2008**). But according to Daniels, laparoscopic destruction of the nervous tissue is not more effective than a diagnostic laparoscopy (**Daniels J.,** *et al.,***2009**).

In PVCS patients, pelvic embolization proved to be a safe procedure with a relief of painful symptoms and varicose dilations. Up to 80% of the patients achieved an improvement by using this method 2 weeks after the procedure was performed (**Ignacio E.A.,** *et al.,* **2008**; **Ganesh A.,** *et al.,* **2007**). However, this treatment does not eliminate the cause of venous dilations.

The problem of congestion and pain will recur if the hypothesis is correct: cardinal and uterosacral ligaments, potentiated by the contraction of the pelvic floor muscles, normally support the uterus. Petros (**Petros P., Ulmsten U., 1993**) has hypothesized that where the support ligaments are lax, the gravitational force acting on the uterus induces congestion by wrinkling the pelvic veins in these tissues and the obstruction of the venous flow. The same laxity could be an important cause of hemorrhoids (**Paradisi G.** *&* **Petros P., 2010**). The collapse of the anterior rectal wall to the rectal lumen could disturb the venous return, leading to venous distension and increase of pressure in the local venous system, which can cause pains and bleedings.

This theory provides an explanation for the fact that PVCS and hemorrhoids appear not only in women who gave birth but also in nulliparous. Therefore, PVCS and hemorrhoids are not only secondary to births but also due to the congenital tissue laxity. Often, pains, PVCS, and hemorrhoidal diseases disappear after a correction on DeLancey's three levels of support (**Paradisi G.** *&* **Petros P., 2010**)

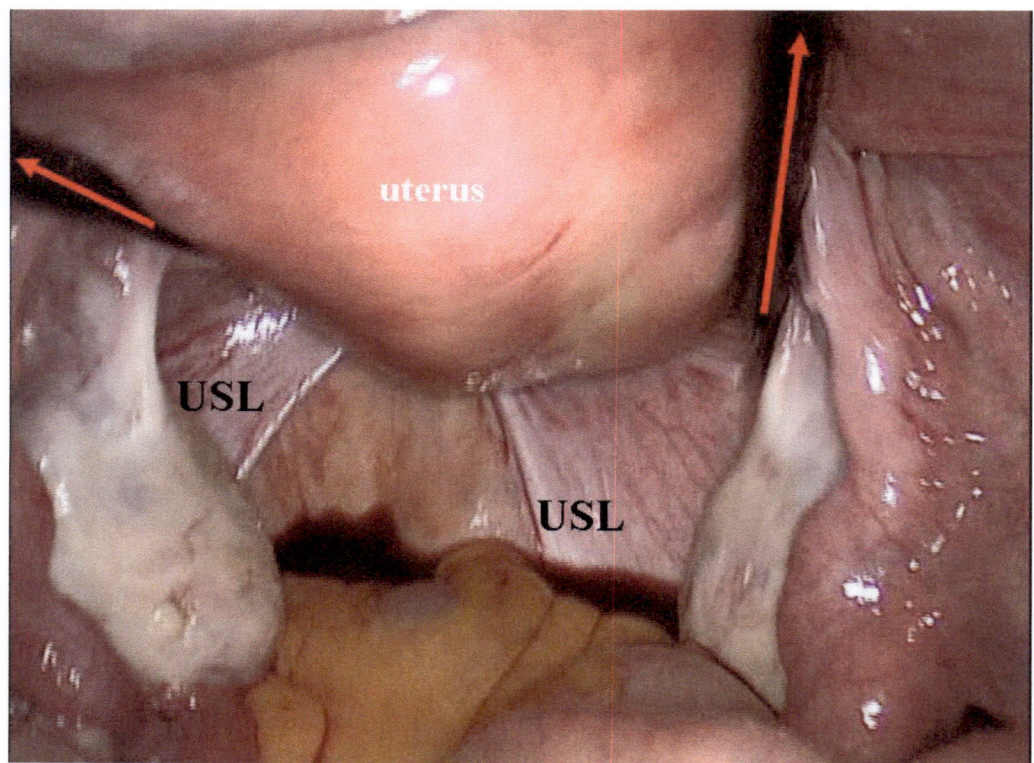

Fig. 5.25b) Anteversion and uterus lifting (red arrows) **tension elongated USL**

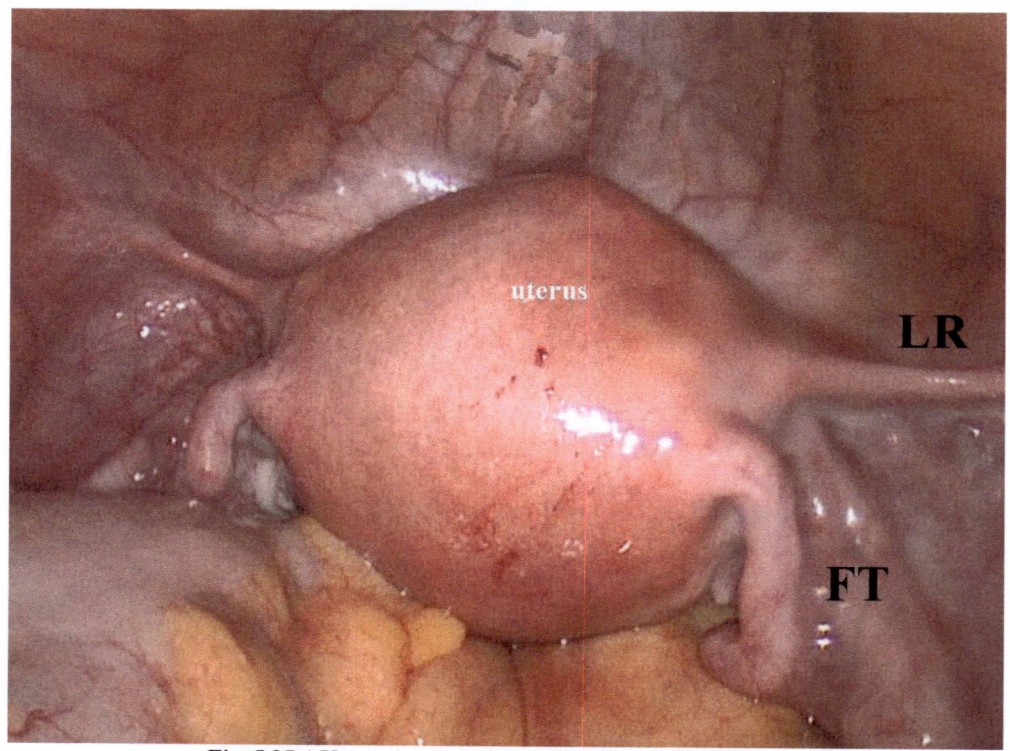

Fig. 5.25c) Uterus in normal position after vaginal surgery
Posterior mesh with sacrospinous fixation. Normal shape fallopian tubes and LR are far from the pouch of Douglas

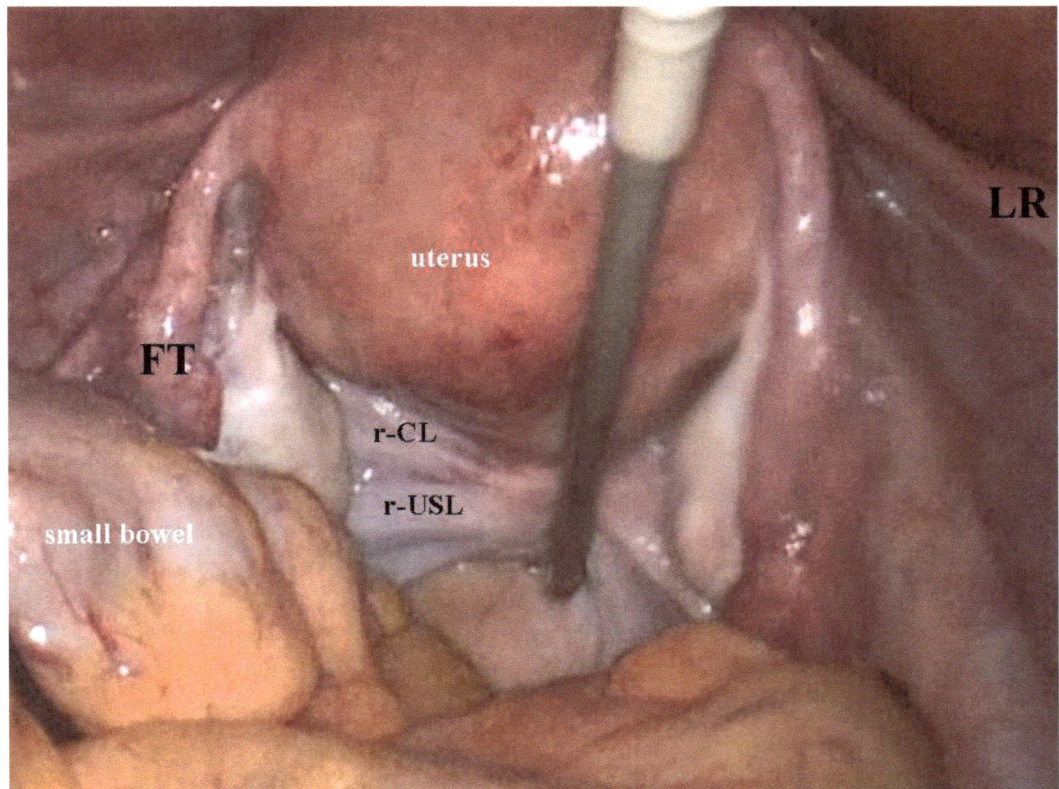

Fig. 5.25*d)* USL and cardinal ligaments (CL) rebuilt (r-USL and r-CL) in a bilateral physiological position efficiently support the uterus

Based on 1200 patients examined, Forgács (**Forgács S.,** *et al.,* **2012**) recently admitted that the muscle fibers located in the (sacrogenital plication) plica rectouterina have a colic contractile activity and thus can cause a visceral pain in the inferior pelvis in women. By laser stimulation of certain points in skin and vagina, it was able to stop or reduce pain in approximately 80% of the patients. On the other hand, if anatomical changes are the cause of pain, this method does not provide a lasting response.

From this point of view, CPPS is even a major public health problem, not only individual (**Abrams P.,** *et al.,* **2002**; **Fall M.,** *et al.,* **2010**). Laparoscopic inspection often does not reveal obvious causes of pain (**Petros P., Ulmsten U., 1993**), which leads to the symptomatology due to psychological reasons. Moderate and chronic pain affects 19% of the adult women in Europe, seriously affecting the quality of life with impact on the work capacity (**Breivik H.,** *et al.,* **2006**). Although it has been well known for several years that CPPS is caused in 30% of the cases by defects of the pelvic organs support ligaments (**Martius H., 1946**), experts and expert committees state that the pathogenesis of chronic pelvic pain is little understood (**Abrams P.,** *et al.,* **2002**, **Evans S.F., 2012**). In a 1996 study, the direct medical costs estimated for patients with CPPS, treated ambulatory in the U.S.A. were of 881.5 million dollars/ year. Moreover, 15% reported wage losses by not presenting to work and 45% reported low productivity (**Mathias S.D.,** *et al.,* **1996**). Considering all these, it is very important to cure those patients.

With regard to anatomical changes in the pelvic organs support or suspension system, there are 5 different reasons for inducing persistent pelvic pain and low sacral pain. All five possibilities lead to the conclusion that either the nerve endings or the muscle fibers in the uterosacral ligaments are tense, causing pulling on the plexus sacralis or Frankenhäuser ganglion, or pelvic veins dilations generate pressure on adjacent areas.

However, as mentioned earlier, pelvic congestion may be secondary to ligaments defects (**Petros P., Ulmsten U., 1993**).

From the therapeutic point of view, these patients can be divided into three groups.

i) Patients with intact pelvic floor but with damage to support ligaments. In these cases, the uterus, vagina, rectum, and bladder lose their physiological positions, causing a tension in the nerve fibers from the structure of the uterosacral ligaments or on the lumbosacralis plexus.

ii) Patients with lesions of the hard pelvic floor with unharmed ligaments. This situation leads to an insufficient support of the intestinal tract, followed by a lowering of the pelvic organs generating painful pulling on the sacrospinous plexus. These pains may occur even if the support system is efficient, because gravity tracts caudally insufficiently anchored pelvic organs, generating tension on the uterosacral ligaments and thus the lumbosacralis plexus.

iii) Patients with a combination of the two mentioned above.

This differentiation is not only of scientific interest, but has important therapeutical consequences and provides explanations for different success rates of vaginal or abdominal surgical methods in literature. Many surgeons are in favor the abdominal approach to restore the anatomy or to cure the lumbosacral pains, either by laparoscopy (**Bojahr B., et al., 2012; Ganatra A.M., et al., 2009; Agarwala N., et al., 2007; Sundaram C.P., et al., 2004; Ross J.W. & Preston M., 2005; Higgs P.J., et al., 2005**) or by laparotomy (**Nygaard I.E., et al., 2004; Baessler K., Schuessler B. & 2001; Maher C.F., et al., 2004; Maher C.F., et al., 2010**). The success rate, defined by the lack of postoperatory apical prolapse varies between 78 and 100%, and when defined as the lack of postoperatory prolapse varies between 58 and 100% (**Burrows L.J., et al., 2004**). Taking into account Cochrane analyses (**Maher C.F., et al., 2010**) and a recent review article (**Elterman D. & Chughtai B., 2013**), we came to the following conclusion: *„Abdominal sacrocolpopexy is the standard sacrocolpopexy for vaginal vault prolapse and is superior to vaginal sacrocolpopexy with less recurrences of prolapse and a lower rate of dyspareunia. Laparoscopic sacrocolpopexy increases the results of the gold standard, abdominal sacrocolpopexy with a minimum morbidity rate".*

Since there is a weak correlation between prolapse extension before and after sacrocolpopexy and pelvic symptoms (**Petros P. & Ulmsten U., 1993; Mouritsen L. & Larsen J.P., 2003; Burrows L.J., et al., 2004**), Bojahr and col. (**Bojahr B., et al., 2012**) conducted ca cohort retrospective study of 300 patients in order to evaluate subjective results after laparoscopic sacrocolpopexy. The subjective success of prolapse surgery was determined by the absence of symptoms. The study showed a "*significant postoperatory reduction of almost all the studies assessed*". However, the persistence of sacral pains was 82.9%. This means that the success rate was only 17%. In addition, 40% of the patients requiring a pessary postoperatory, needed it after the surgical treatment too, and 22.4% needed an additional prolapse procedure during the medium follow-up period of 24.5 months.

In contrast to abdominal surgery, several recent studies present superior results after vaginal sacrocolpopexy with regard to sacral pain and other symptoms. The healing rates for lumbosacral pain after posterior vaginal mesh (**Petros P., 2001a; Petros P., 2001b**) vary between 62 and 83% (**Farnsworth B.N., 2001; Petros P. & Richardson P.A., 2010; Goeschen K. & Gent H-J., 2004; Goeschen K., 2015; Gold D.M. & Goeschen K., 2016; Caliskan A., et al., 2015; Wagenlehner F., 2014; Markovsky O., 2014; Petros P., 2014; Müller-Funogea A., 2014**). Data from many studies demonstrate a high rate of healing of CPPS, which leads to the conclusion that abdominal surgery obviously can no longer be accepted as gold standard, if we include the symptoms in the assessment criteria (**Farnsworth B.N., 2001; Petros P. & Richardson P.A., 2010; Goeschen K. & Gent H-J., 2004; Goeschen K., 2015; Gold D.M. & Goeschen K., 2016; Caliskan A., et al., 2015; Wagenlehner F., 2014; Markovsky O., 2014; Petros P., 2014; Müller-Funogea A., 2014**).

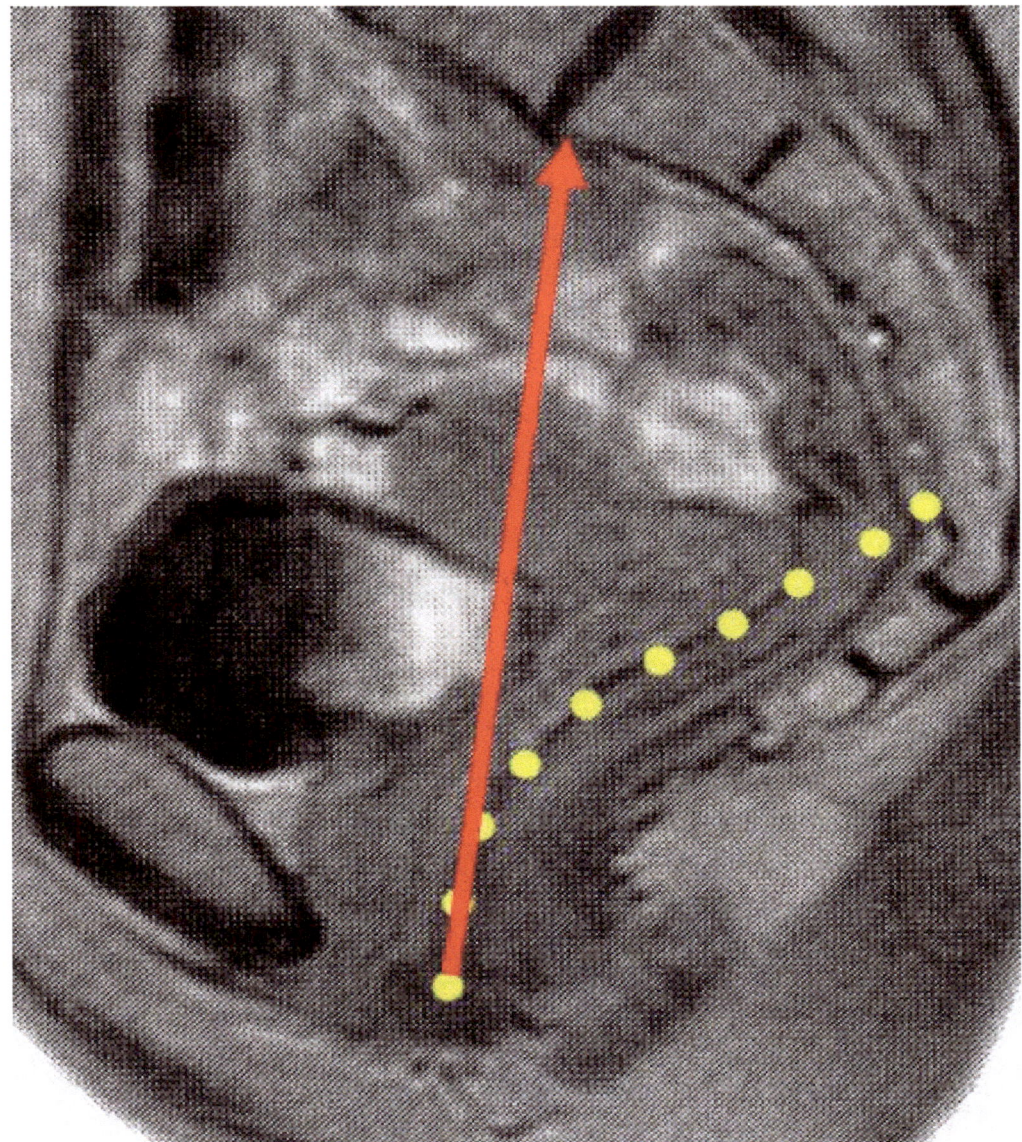

Fig. 5.26. Saggital MRI image of the pelvis in women in orthostatism
Yellow dotted line – normal vaginal axis the shape of a banana posteriorly oriented
Red arrow – vaginal axis nonphysiologically oriented upwards after laparoscopy/ laparotomy sacrocolpopexy

Is there any contradiction between the adequate restoration of the vaginal apex anatomy and the failure to treat accompanying symptoms?

From the point of view of an engineer, architect or surgeon, the optimal results in terms of symptomatology and anatomy can be achieved through a rigorous reconstruction of the anatomy, the way it is done "*in vivo*". In 150 AD, Galen had also specified that the normal function of the organs follow the reconstruction of form and structure.

Out of these observations, there are three possibilities.

i) If the entire support system is deficient, it may be sufficient to repair only injured ligaments.

ii) In case of damage to the pelvic floor, this problem should be solved by restoring the base so as to support the pelvic organs and the intestines.

iii) If both structures are affected, both must be restored. Taking into account these aspects, the following question arises.

"*What kind of approach, surgical, abdominal, or vaginal, offers the best results with regard to the three different situations?*"

Case 1 – Patients whose uterosacral and/ or cardinal ligaments are exclusively injured and responsible for pelvic pain.

This problem can be solved both abdominal and vaginal. However, the abdominal approach, as it is performed today, does not recreate the natural axis of the vagina due to the fixation of the mesh in the promontorium sacrum, Fig. 5.26, 5.27. and 5.28.

Thus, this process induces a vaginal axis oriented abnormally vertically. Physiologically, the uterosacral ligaments originate at S2-S4 sacral vertebrae, Fig. 5.27., at a significant distance from the promontorium sacrum.

In contrast, new vaginal techniques such as the *"posterior vaginal mesh"* or *"tissue fixation system"* (TFS) (**Petros P. & Richardson P.A., 2010**) are capable of placing neoligaments in the exact position as the natural ligaments, Fig. 5.24., 5.25., 5.29., 5.30. and 5.31*a)* and *b)*.

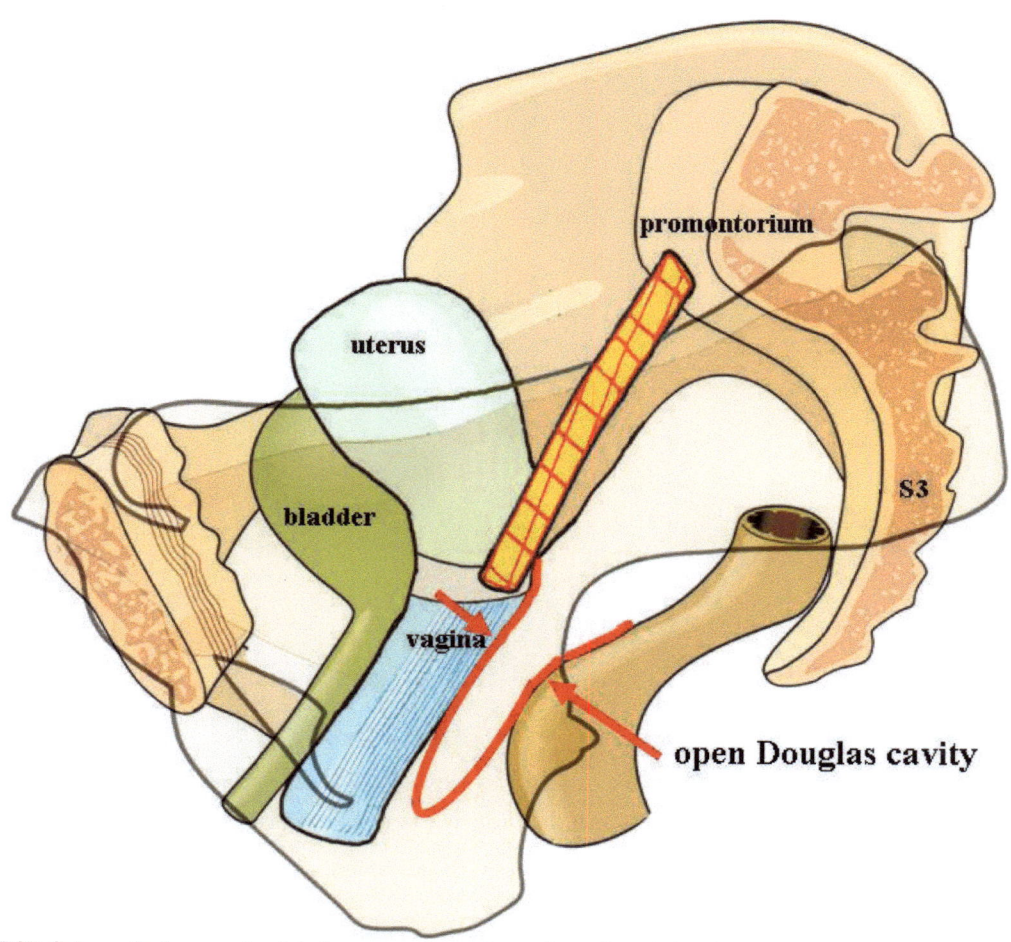

Fig. 5.27. Schematic image of pelvis in women in orthostatism after abdominal sacrocolpopexy – sagittal view
Fixing the vaginal apex and the cervix with mesh in promontorium sacrum pulls the uterus anteriorly and opens the pouch of Douglas

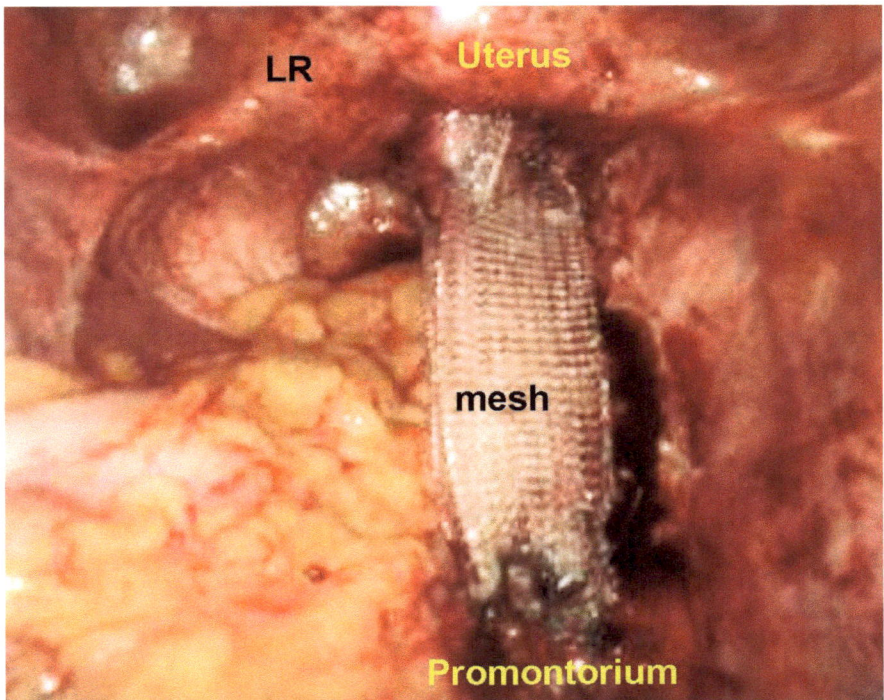

Fig. 5.28. Laparoscopic fixation of the uterus in promontorium sacrum with polypropylene mesh
In contrast to the vaginal fixation illustrated in Fig. 5.24., this procedure does not reconstruct either the vaginal axis or the physiological disposition of the USL or CL

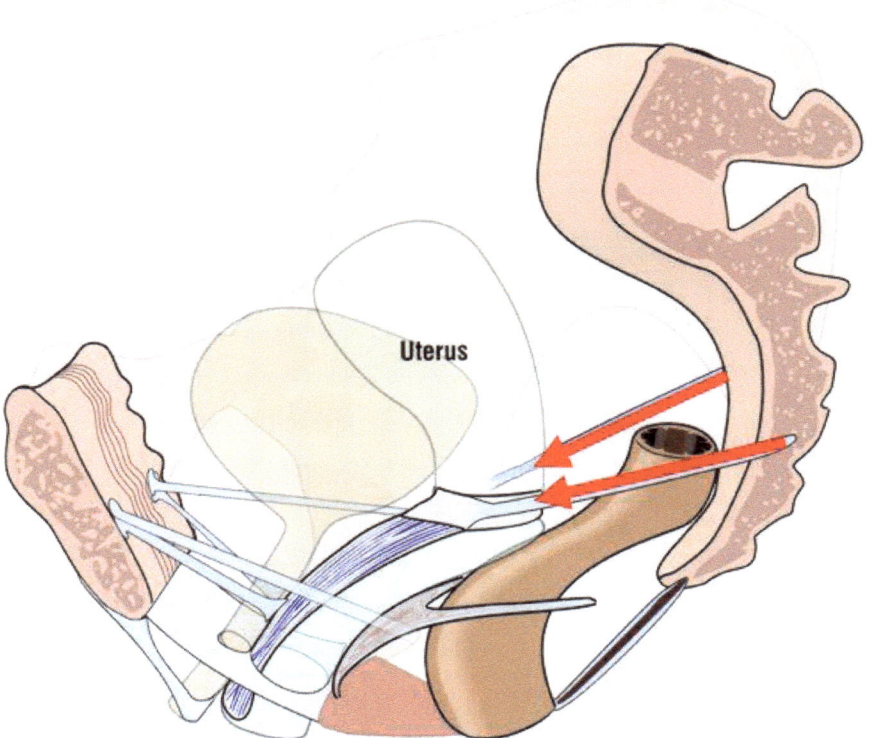

Fig. 5.29. Vaginal axis abnormally vertically oriented
USL (red arrows) appear at the S2-S4 sacral vertebrae and are inserted in the paracervix posteriorly

A vertical vagina after abdominal sacrocolpopexy is non-physiological and can generate three problems.

i) The more the vagina and the pelvic organs are in an upright position, the more they are exposed to the effect of gravity and are predestined to descend Fig. 5.32.

ii) The more the vagina and pelvic organs are in an upright position, the greater the posterior space, favoring the appearance of elitrocele, Fig. 5.25. and Fig. 5.33.

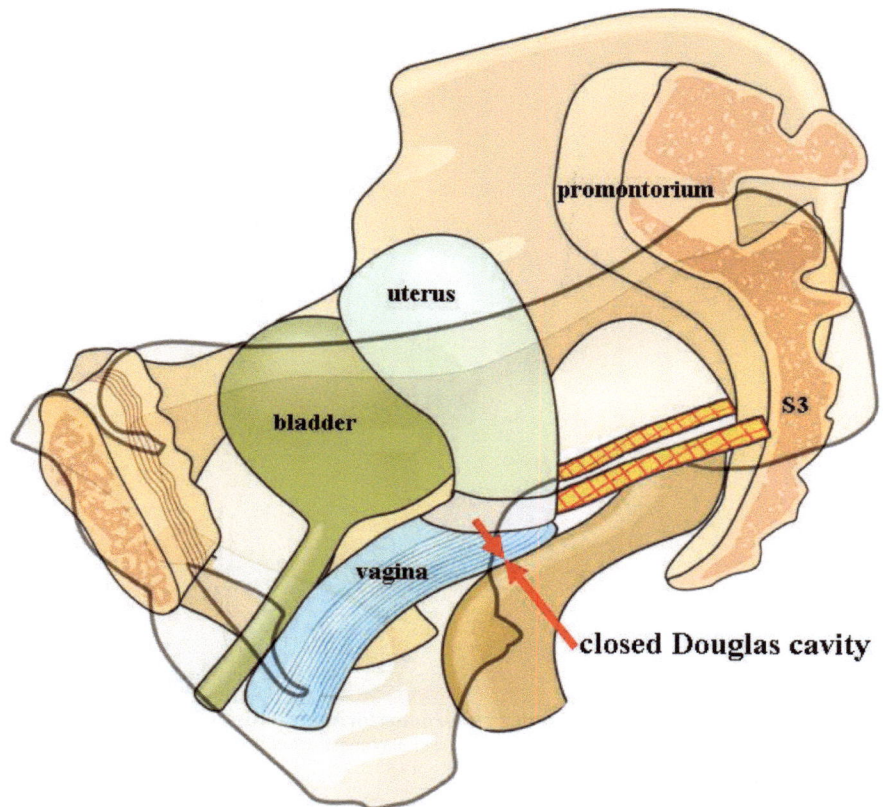

Fig. 5.30. Description of the pelvis of woman in orthostatism after vaginal sacrocolpopexy
Saggital section: fixation with mesh of the vaginal apex and the cervix at S3 vertebra creates a normal vaginal axis, keeping the pouch of Douglas closed

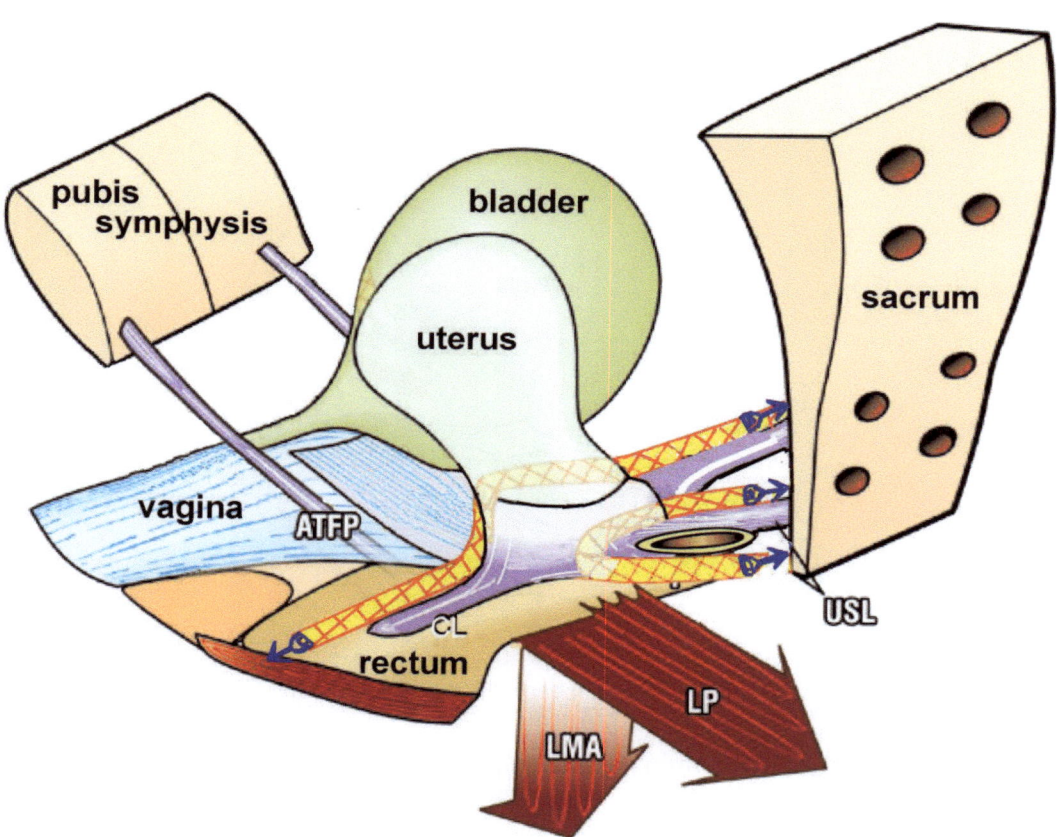

Fig. 5.31.*a)* Physiological reconstruction of vaginal shape and axis, after the insertion of artificial ligaments along the exact path of USL and CL
ATFP – arcus tendineus fasciae pelvis, LP – levator plate, LAM – longitudinal anal muscle

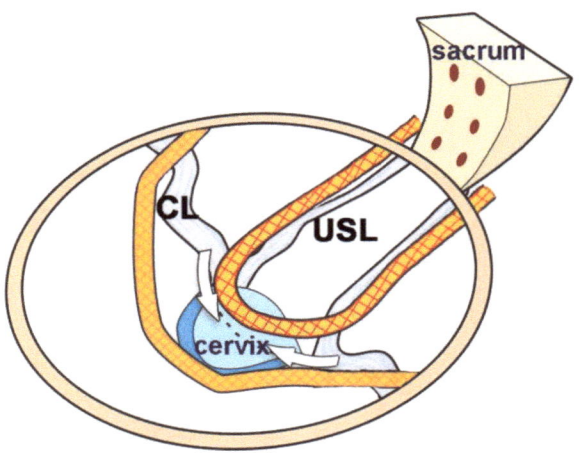

Fig. 5.31._b)_ **Physiological reconstruction of vaginal shape and axis, after the insertion of artificial ligaments along the exact path of USL and CL**
ATFP – arcus tendineus fasciae pelvis, LP – levator plate, LAM –longitudinal anal muscle

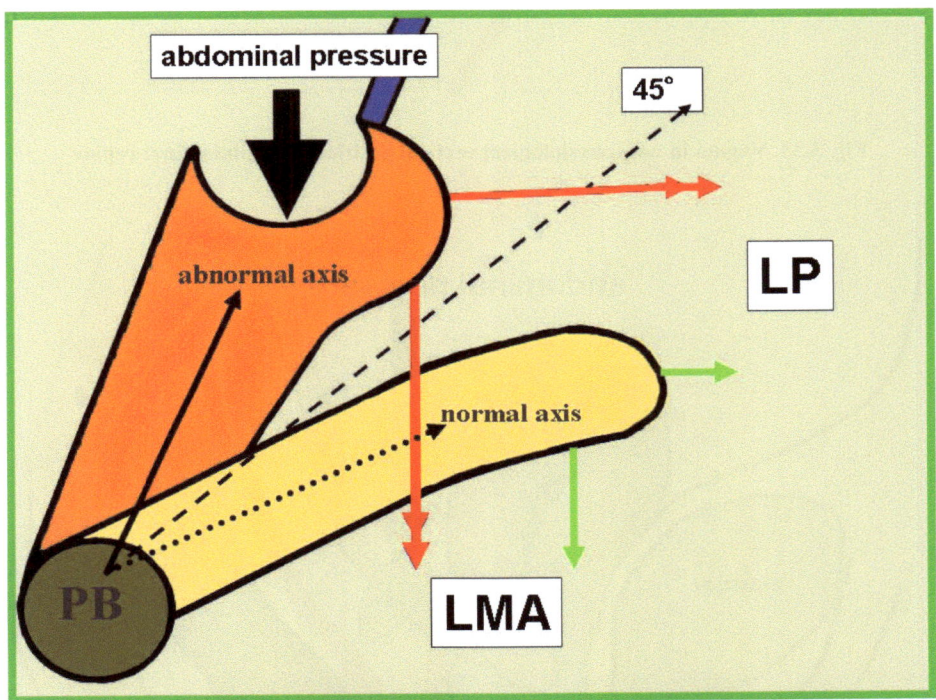

Fig. 5.32. Abnormal vertical axis due to fixation on promontorium sacrum (blue line)
In case of a vertically oriented vagina with an angle of > 45 degrees, the abdominal press, posterior pulling exerted by the LP and the posterior force of LMA accelerate the appearance of prolapse, elitrocele, or rectocele. PB – perineal body

Unsupported and posteriorly open space allows the abdominal press and gravitational force (dark blue arrow) to press the pouch of Douglas, causing prolapse of vaginal vault, elitrocele/ rectocele and even rectal prolapse.

iii) The more the vagina and the pelvic organs are in an upright position, the less the levator plate and the longitudinal anal muscle that opens and closes the bladder and the rectum will compress the vagina posteriorly Fig. 5.32.

The more the vaginal axis after laparoscopy/ laparotomy will be upright, the more the relapse or the "*de novo*" appearance of prolapse is more likely than the vaginal approach Fig. 5.26., 5.27. and 5.33.

It is expected compared to the vaginal approach. Furthermore, the unsupported posterior space allows the abdominal press and gravity to tension Frankenhäuser ganglion caudally, Fig. 5.34. Mechanical irritation of Frankenhäuser ganglion stimulates a high amount of nerve fibers generating pain due to pressure and tension.

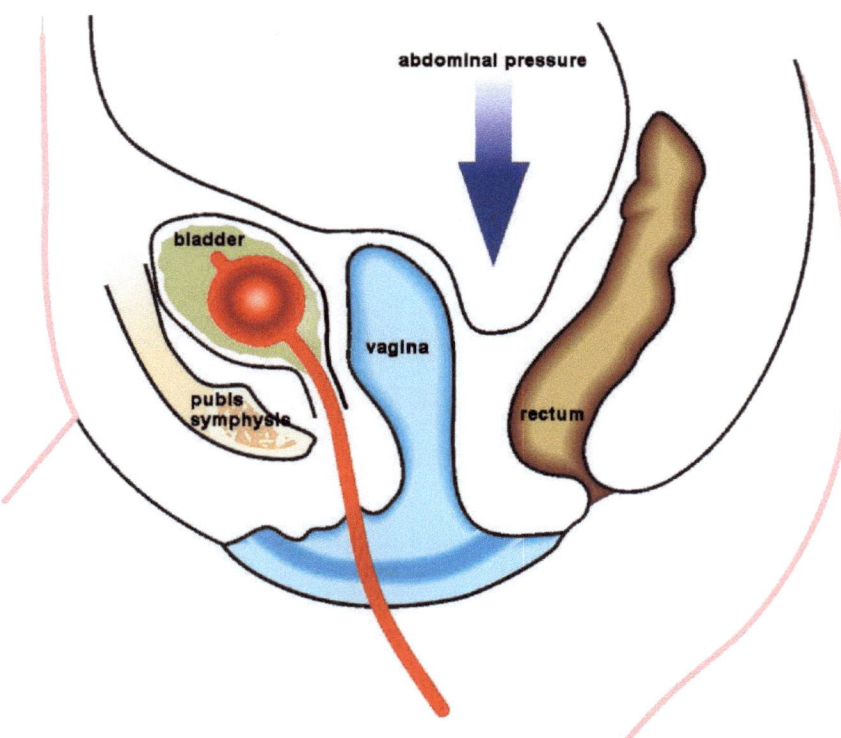

Fig. 5.33. Vagina in non-physiological vertical position after abdominal repair

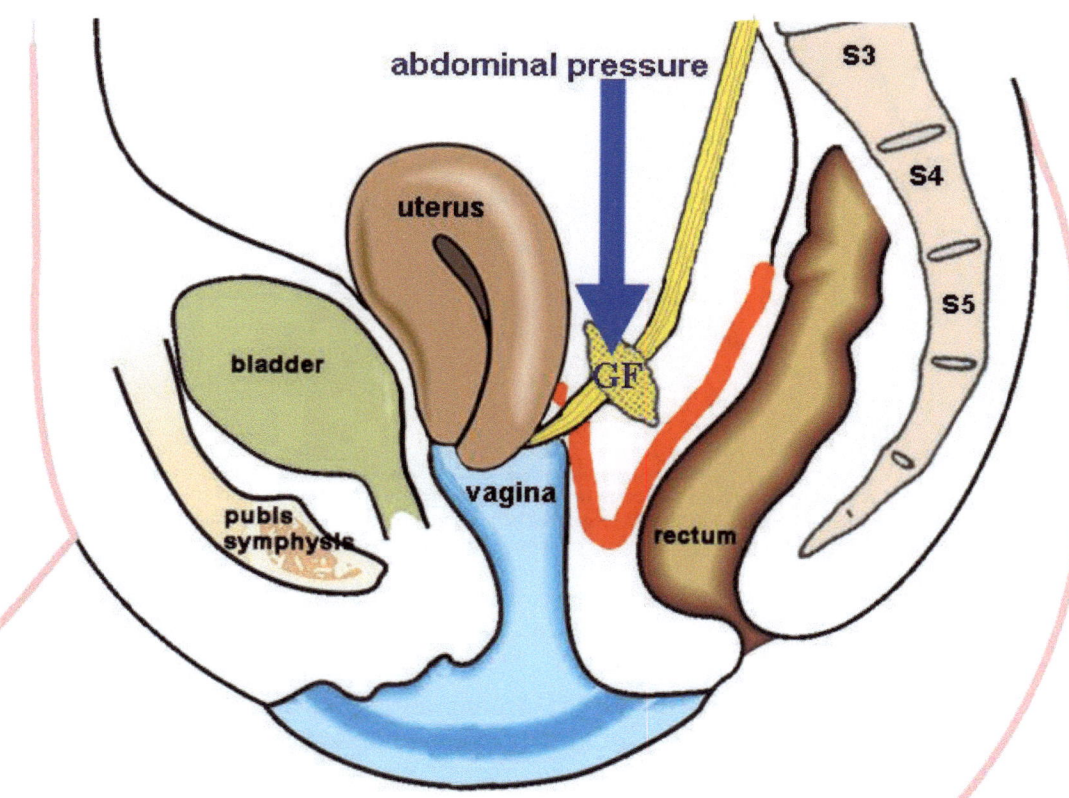

Fig. 5.34. Vagina in non-physiological vertical position after abdominal repair
Intra-abdominal pressure (dark blue arrow) and gravitational force tension the unsupported Frankenhäuser ganglion (FG, yellow) by caudal pulling, generating pain

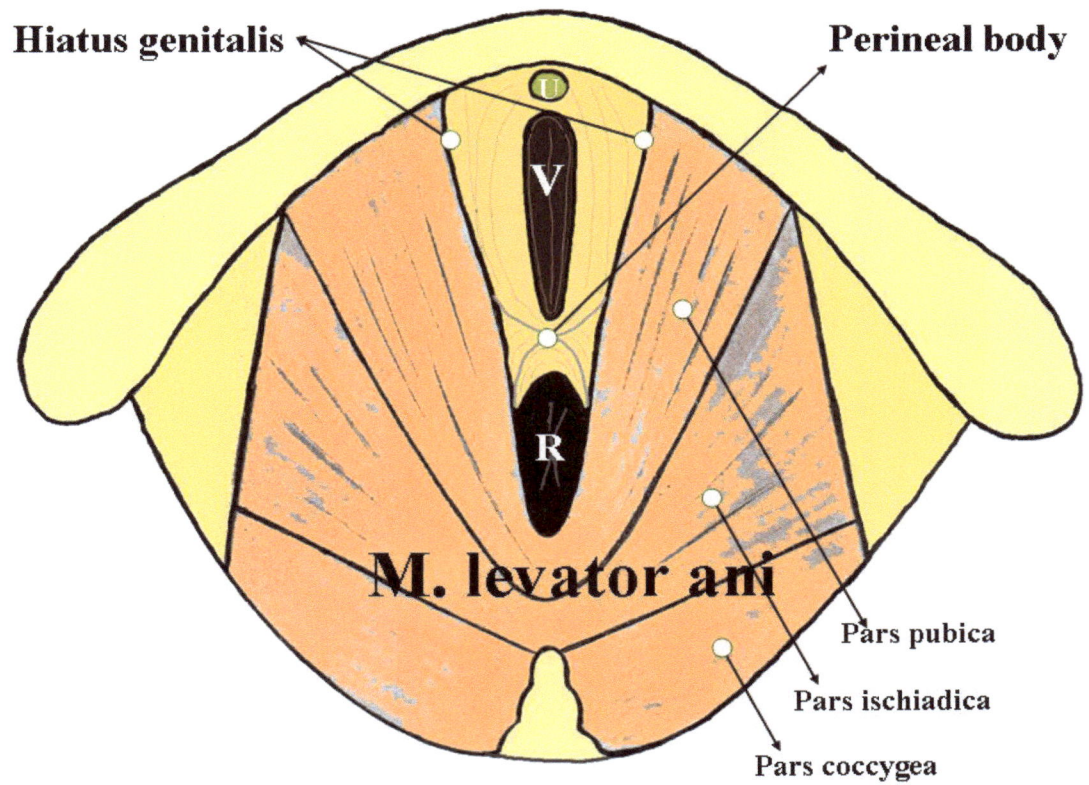

Fig. 5.35. Stabile and firm levator hiatus protected by the vigorous pubocervical muscle

This means that if Frankenhäuser ganglion is not caudally supported, the abdominal press can cause pain by pulling it lower, even if there is no traction on the plexus sacralis. This explains why in case of a new elitrocele, due to vaginal axis modification, the reconstruction of uterine suspension is not always efficient in pain relief.

Case 2 – Patients with pains and lesion of pelvic floor muscles, but with unharmed ligament anchoring.

These first need the reconstruction of the base, presented in Fig. 5.20.

In healthy women, the pelvic floor is stable and firm, due to the three muscle layers closely interconnected with the endopelvic fascia Fig. 5.18. The strongest muscle layer is made up of levator ani muscle and coccygeus muscle. The first one consists of two components:
- pars pubica;
- pars iliaca, Fig. 5.35.

As for patients with prolapse, pars pubica is the most affected.

„Levator crus", medial parts of levator ani muscle, are located close to the median line and define the urogenital hiatus, urinary tract, vagina, and rectum. Urogenital hiatus has a triangular shape with the wider part on the pubic symphysis. A stable and narrow urogenital hiatus is necessary to prevent the descent of pelvic organs. In case of uterine prolapse, the urogenital hiatus is dilated. This may be the consequence of lesions of the levator ani insertions and/ or of the perineal body, Fig. 5.36.

In many cases, "levator crura" moved laterally, opening wide the hiatus during the increase of abdominal pressure. This problem can be solved by a surgery that restores the natural anatomy of the area Fig. 5.37.

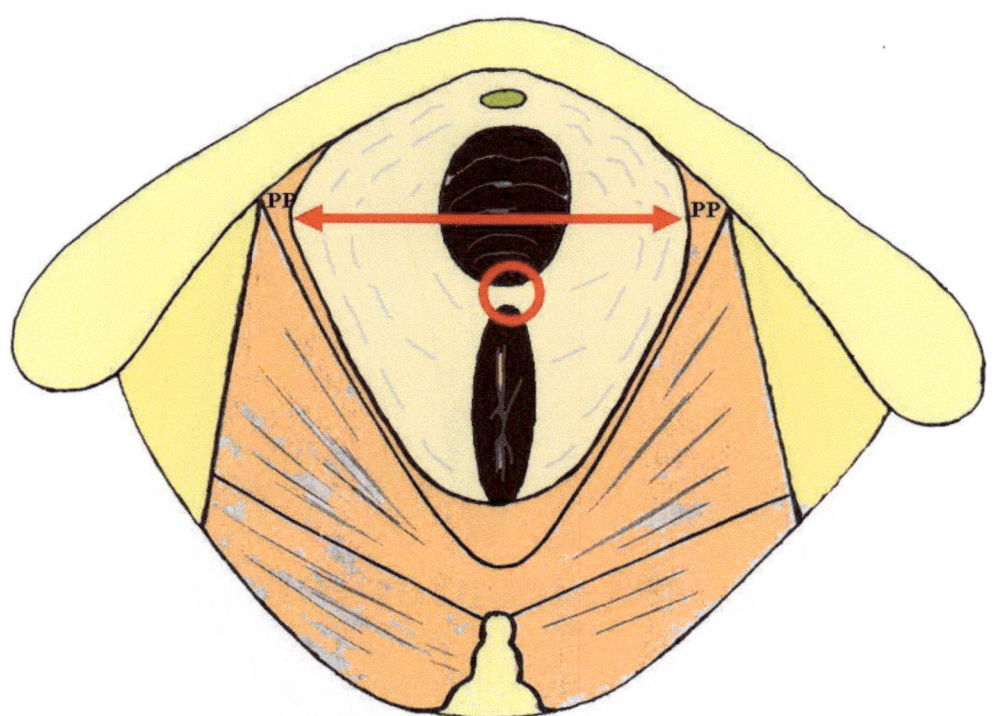

Fig. 5.36. Widened levator hiatus (red arrow) **caused by lesion of levator ani muscle and endopelvic fascia**
The levator ani muscle edges are thinned and laterally displaced. The perineal body is deficient (red circle)

It is logical and has been recognized for several decades that abdominal surgeries do not provide access to the important area of the hiatus (**Martius H., 1936**). However, vaginal surgeries can be efficient only if both urogenital hiatus and perineal body can be efficient. The narrowing of the vagina through the so-called "anterior and posterior colporrhaphy" is not efficient because the vaginal support capacity is inadequate. Besides, Martius has already mentioned the role of the suture of levator ani muscle in reducing the urogenital hiatus (**Martius H., 1936**), Fig. 5.37.

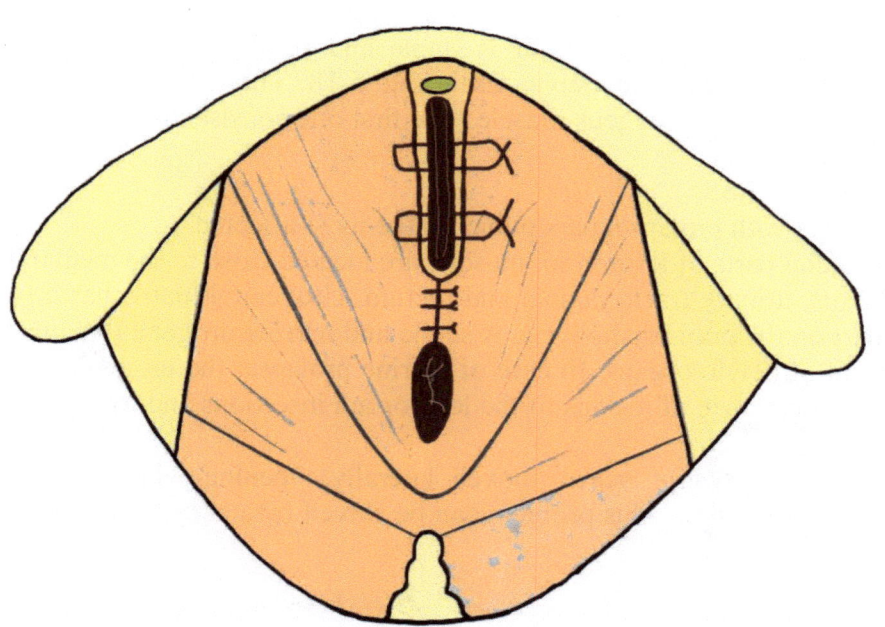

Fig. 5.37. Levator hiatus after levator ani muscle edges and the perineal body reconstruction

Still, the suture of the hiatus will inevitably induce pain and tension on the structures, which can be torn out, as met in perineal body native tissue repair. The reunion of dehiscence muscles is accomplished through the TFS technique, which uses an adjustable mesh.

Pain is minimal and the tissues are simply placed in the original position by the mesh, which, over time, contains fibrous tissue to form a new central tendon, Fig. 5.31.

Case 3 – Patients with a combination of the two types of defects

An isolated ligated defect is excluded because the affected connective tissue is responsible for the appearance of prolapse and the pelvic floor disorder. In most cases, a descent of the pelvic organs is the consequence of both mechanisms, connective and muscular.

A new level of understanding appeared in 1992, when DeLancey, relying on corpse dissections, demonstrated the importance of connective tissue structures for organs support, describing three levels of vaginal support (**De Lancey JOL., 1992**), Fig. 5.38.

Level 1 – Superior fixation – uterosacral-cardinal ligament complex.

Level 2 – Lateral fixation – superolateral insertion points of anterior wall, rectovaginal fascia.

Level 3 – Distal fixation – perineal body, perineal membrane.

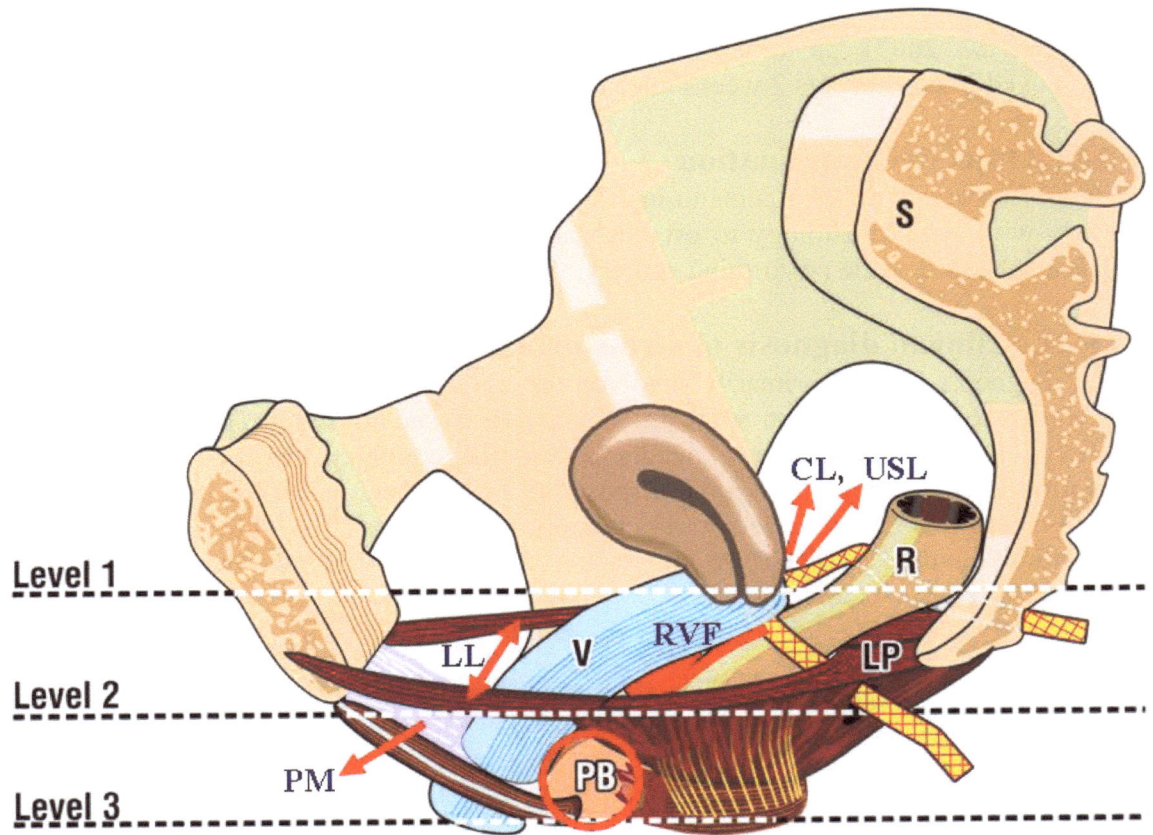

Fig. 5.38. Three-levels repair
Level 1 – cardinal ligaments (CL) and uterosacral ligaments (USL)
Level 2 – rectovaginal fascia (RVF) and levator limits (LL)
Level 3 – perineal body (PB) and of perineal membrane (PM)

Petros created a new vaginal surgical technique for pelvic floor disorders, based on the Integral Theory (**Petros P. & Ulmsten U., 1993**), which deals with prolapsed symptoms and organs as being both determined by lax suspensory ligaments: pubourethral, cardinal, arcus tendineus fasciae pelvis (ATFP), uterosacral and perineal body. Applying the neoligaments principle used in TVT (**Petros P. & Ulmsten U., 1993**), healing rates that have never occurred until then, have been reported (**Petros P., 2010**, **Goeschen K. & Gent H-J., 2004; Goeschen K., 2015**; **Gold D.M. & Goeschen K., 2016; Caliskan A.,** *et al.,* **2015; Wagenlehner F., 2014**; **Markovsky O., 2014**; **Petros P., 2014**; **Müller-Funogea A., 2014**). He accurately rebuilt the three levels, fig. 5.38., as it follows:

- insertion of a non-tensioned mesh to create artificial ligaments: pubourethral, uterosacral and cardinal, a level 1 repair;

- reinforcement of rectovaginal fascia and the narrowing of genital hiatus, a level 2 repair;

- restoring the perineal body and the perineal membrane, a level 3 repair.

Following the principles of Integral Theory (**Petros P. & Ulmsten U., 1993**), the symptoms due to prolapse are mainly due to the laxity of the pelvic connective tissue. Thus, an isolated defect of support ligaments is almost excluded. In most cases, the entire support system will be affected. In most patients with pelvic floor disorders, a repair at all three levels is necessary for the reconstruction of natural anatomy and the healing of symptoms.

Considering all these, there is a narrow path for the abdominal approach. Laparotomy and laparoscopy only allows the ascension of structures from level 1, such as the vaginal apex or the uterus and can suture the anterior vaginal wall disinsertion from the ATFP level. However, these procedures do not reconstruct the physiological anatomy. Therefore, it is not surprising that the abdominal approach offers healing rates of symptoms inferior to vaginal procedures (**Bojahr B., et al., 2012**).

Patients with persistent pelvic pains after a satisfactory pelvic floor correction should be examined to see if a spastic parameter or a pelvic congestion secondary to varicose dilations is responsible for symptomatology. According to Ignacio (**Ignacio E.A., et al., 2008**) and Ganesh (**Ganesh A., et al., 2007**), up to 80% of the patients with pelvic pains caused by varicose dilations achieved improvements 2 weeks after embolization.

5.1.2. Objective examination

The objective examination aims to highlight the anatomical defects and to correlate them appropriately with symptomatology to establish adequate therapeutic conduct. Often, the final diagnosis is established while performing surgery, the patient being under anesthesia.

5.1.2.1. **Clinical diagnosis of stress urinary incontinence** *(SUI)*

The diagnosis of SUI primarily involves the objectification of urine loss. The patient sitting in a gynecological position with full bladder, is asked to cough (**Falconer C., et al., 1996**). An involuntary urine leakage occurs during the coughing effort. This maneuver is repeated with a forceps, which is laterally disposed to the urethra, and, if the urine leakage does not repeat, it means that there is a defect of pubourethral ligaments (PUL) Fig. 5.39. As far as the external urethral ligaments (EUL) are affected, a bloating of urethral mucosa is also noted, (**Petros P., 2010**), Fig. 5.40. and 5.41.

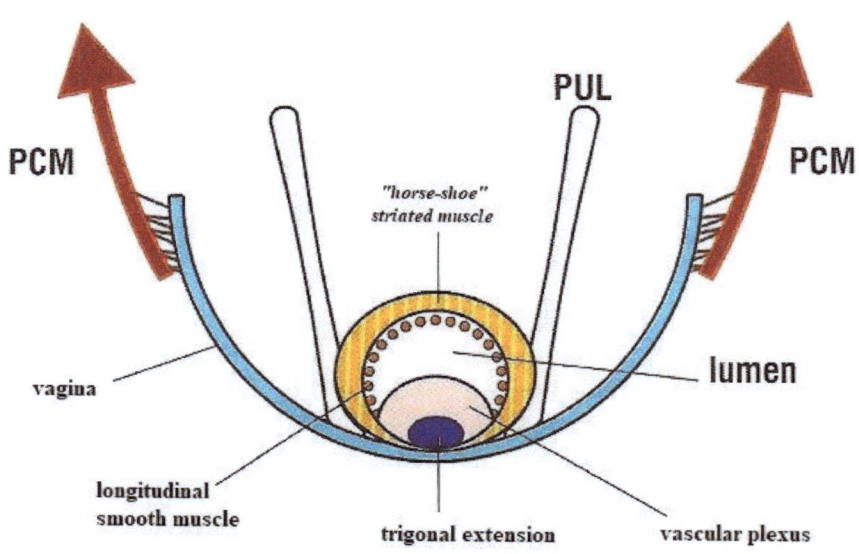

Fig. 5.39. **Urethral occlusion, saggital section**
(according to **Petros P.E.P., 2010**)
PCM – pubocervical muscle. PUL – pubourethral ligaments

One of the diagnostic tests of SUI is Petros' simulated surgery, (**Petros P., 2010**), which consists in positioning a forceps at the level of a unilateral pubourethral ligament, lifting the tissue without compressing the urethra, and observing the SUI disappearance following the maneuver Fig. 5.42.

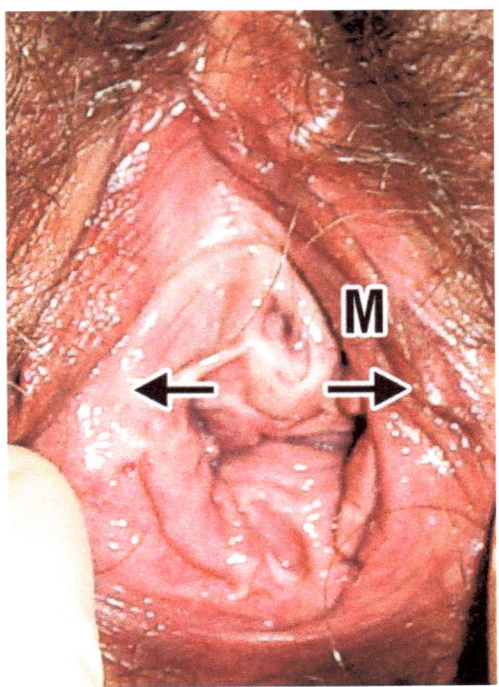

Fig. 5.40. Normal urinary meatus
(according to **Petros P.E.P., 2010**)

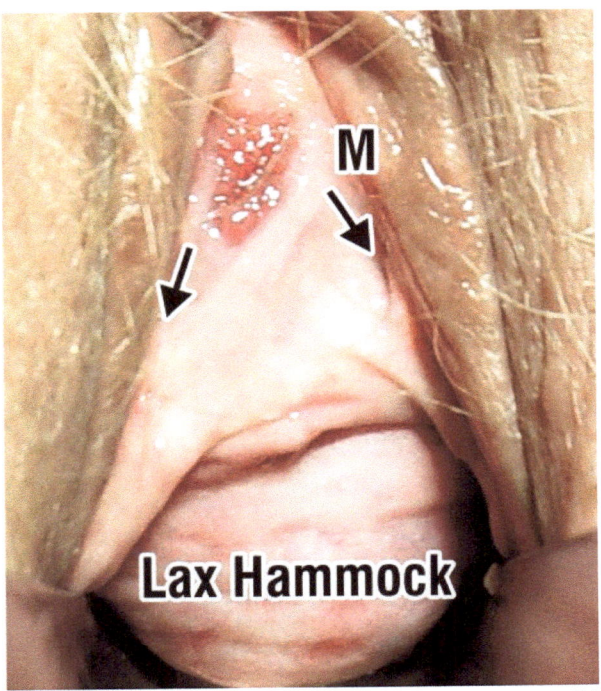

Fig. 5.41. External urethral ligaments and hammock. Elongated urethral meatus (M) with urethral mucosa bloating
(according to **Petros P.E.P., 2010**)

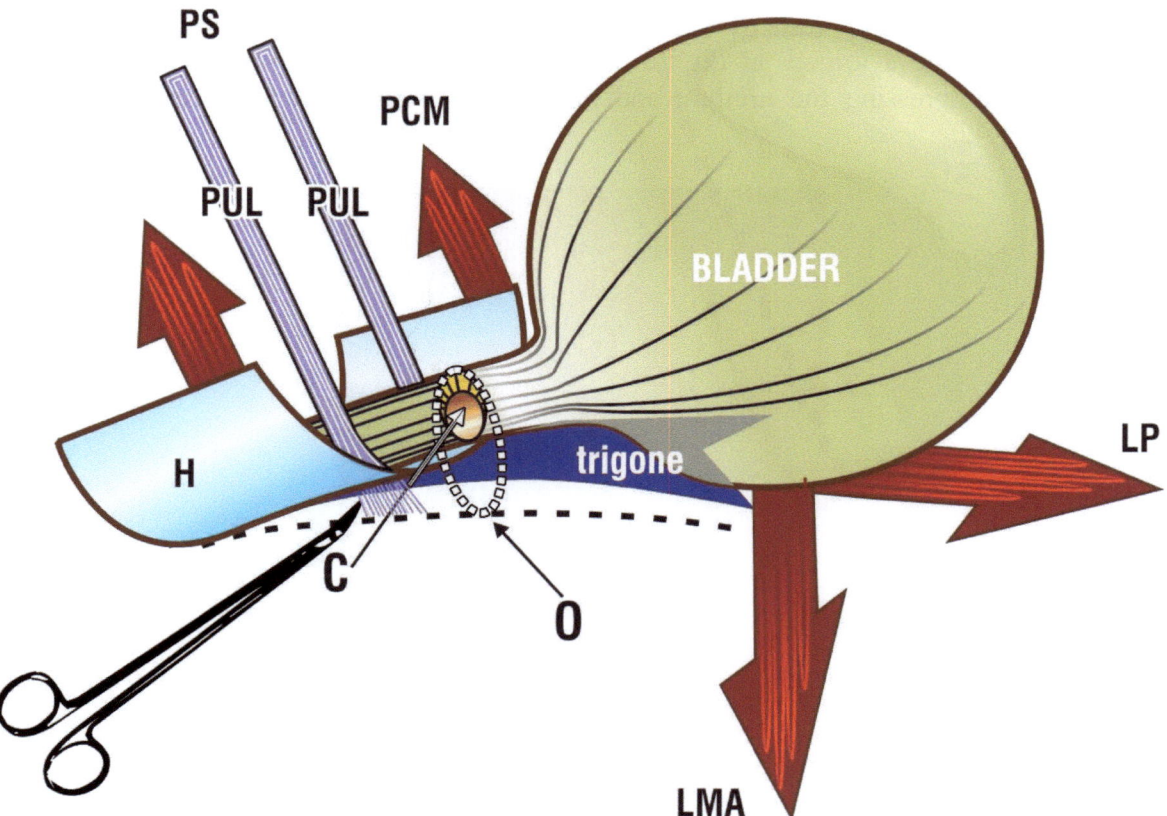

Fig. 5.42. Simulated surgery for SUI demonstration
(according to **Petros P., 2010**)

3D scheme: H – urethrovaginal fascia, BLADDER – bladder. Applying an unilateral pressure to the medium 1/3 level of the urethra mimics the effect of a suburethral mesh. The urethra returns from the "O" position – incontinence to "C" position – continence.

5.1.2.2. Clinical diagnosis of anterior vaginal prolapse (cystocele)

Anterior vaginal prolapse overlaps the notion of *cystocele*. Anterior wall prolapse is evaluated on the valve test (**Adekanmi O.A.,** *et al.,* **2003**).

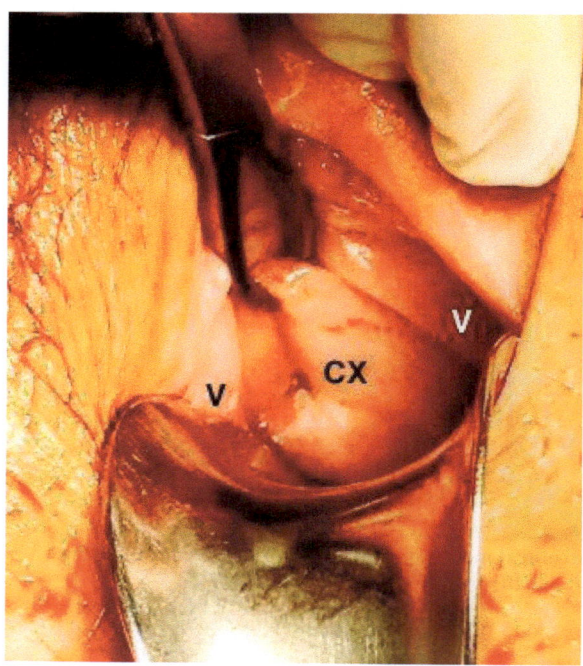

Fig. 5.43. Cardinal ligaments disinsertion
(according to **Petros P.E.P., 2010**)
3rd degree cystocele. Vaginal plications can be observed.
CX – cervix; V – vagina

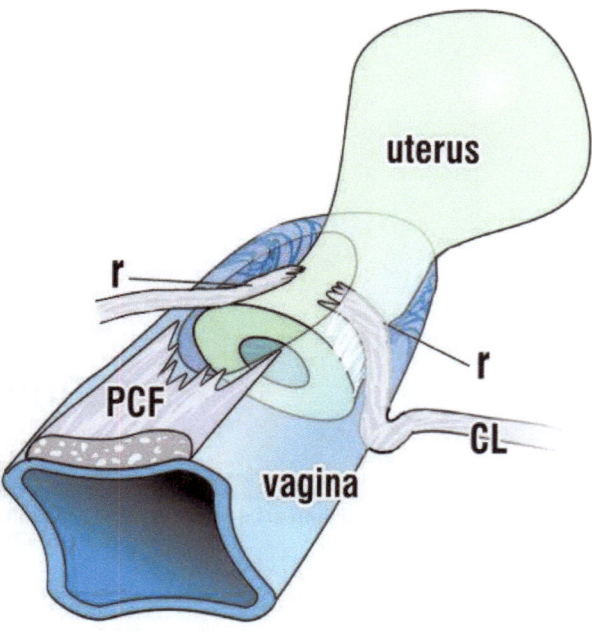

Fig. 5.44. Paracervix defect with cardinal ligaments and pubocervical fascia disinsertion
(according to **Petros P.E.P., 2010**)
PCF – pubocervical fascia; r – paracervix; CL – cardinal ligaments

The three types of cystocele should be clinically differentiated. The central defect cystocele has the disappearance of vaginal plications as a pathognomonic element, Fig 5.45. The central defect cystocele retains plications, although the anatomical defect is important, Fig. 5.46. In the case of high cystocele, through the disinsertion of pubovesical fascia from the paracervix, the anatomical defect presents as a prolapse in the immediate lower cervix, Fig. 5.43. and 5.44. (**Goeschen K.**, **2007**). The defect disappears if the lateral sides (the disinserted cardinal ligaments) are brought to the median line with two Chaput tissue forceps, Fig. 5.43. (**Falconer C.**, *et al.*, **1996**). However, most often, there is a mixed form of cystocele, in which several ligament defects coexist (**Petros P., 2010**).

5.1.2.3. Clinical diagnosis of uterine prolapse

Recognition of such a defect, especially if it is important, is easy, but difficulties arise in its quantification, with important scientific communication deficiencies. Classically, the uterine prolapse was classified into three degrees:
- first degree, cervix is lowered, but does not reach the vaginal introit;
- second degree, cervix is at the vaginal introit;
- third degree, cervix exceeds the vaginal introit (**Sîrbu P., 1981**).

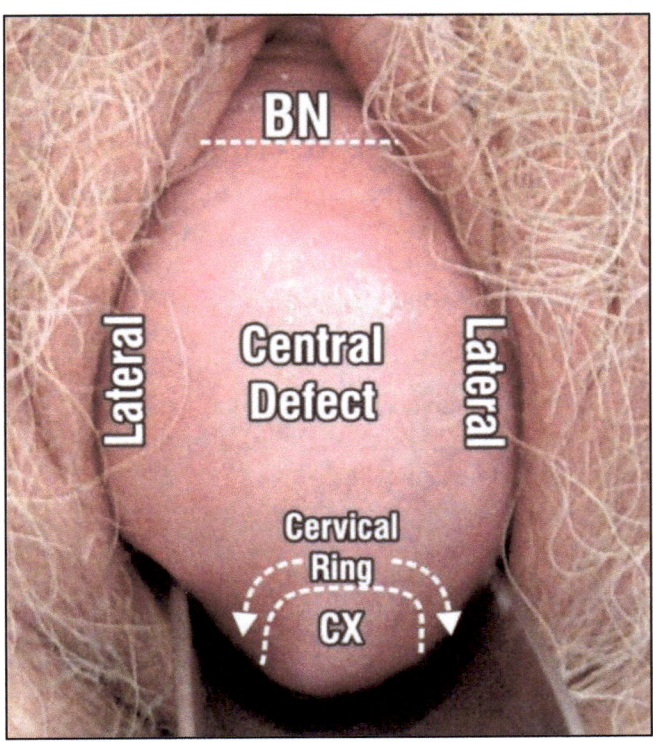

Fig. 5.45. Semiology of cystocele
(according to **Petros P.E.P., 2010**)
Cervical ring – paracervix, CX – cervix, BN – bladder neck

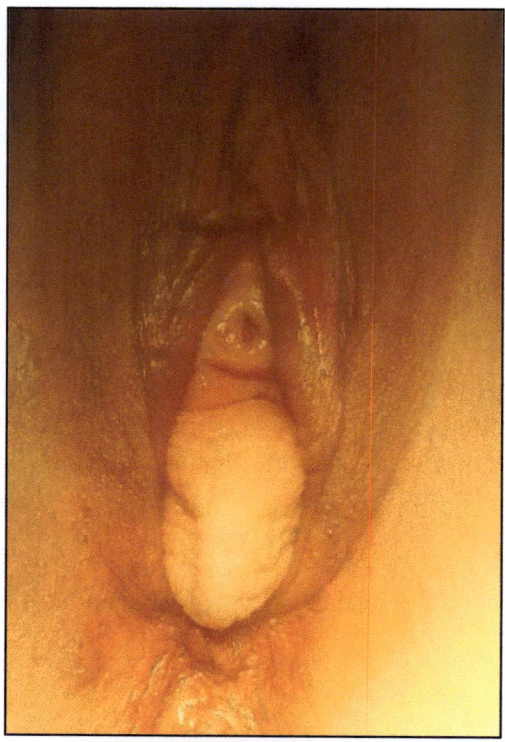

Fig. 5.46. Cystocele by lateral defect
(according to **Enache T., 2014**)

Currently, both classification systems are accepted: the Baden-Walker system and the POP-Q classification.

Baden-Walker System – the examination of the patient is done with a greater accuracy on the operating table to cancel the muscle tone (**Baden W.F. & Walker T.A., 1992**).

The system introduces the *"half of the vagina"* notion, Fig. 5.47. Thus, there are 4 degrees of prolapse:

First degree – cervix does not exceed the half of the vagina.
Second degree – cervix is located between the half of the vagina and the vaginal introit.
Third degree – cervix exceeds vaginal introit.
Fourth degree – total prolapse with complete vaginal eversion.

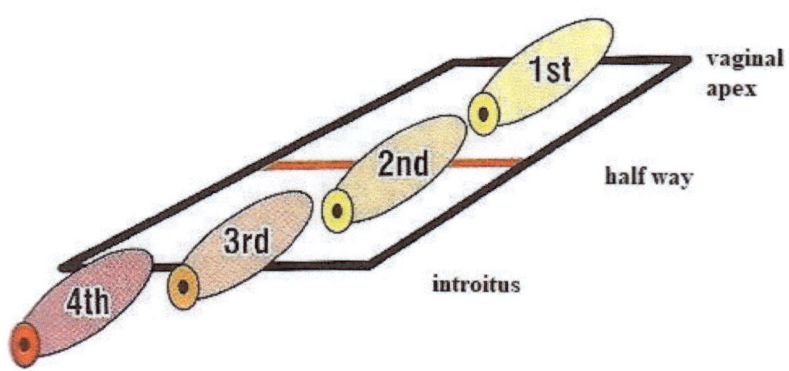

Fig. 5.47. Baden Walker system (according to **Petros P., 2010**)

The advantages of this classification system are simplicity and easy reproducibility. On the other hand, the description is not sufficiently explicit and refers only to uterine prolapse, ignoring the other associated defects.

POP-Q system (pelvic organ prolapse - quantification) – this classification was designed for a greater objectivity in the quantification of pelvic floor disorders (**Persu C., et al., 2011**). It is possible to obtain quantifiable data that facilitate scientific communication by using this system. Nine specific measurements are used, which are entered in an evaluation grid. Distances above the vaginal introit are noted with "-", and those that are distal to it, with "+". Nine specific points are measured, Fig. 5.46., and their values are written in an evaluation grid, Fig 5.47. The evaluation of these markers allows a five-stage classification.

a) Stage 0 – there is no prolapse: cervix can descend with maximum 2 cm of the total vaginal length.
b) Stage 1 – the most protruding part of the prolapse descends to maximum 1 cm above the hymen.
c) Stage 2 – prolapse is under 1 cm to the hymen (above or below).
d) Stage 3 – prolapse is at more than 1 cm below the hymen, but not more than the length of the vagina minus 2 cm.
e) Stage 4 – total prolapse with the complete vagina eversion, Fig. 5.48.

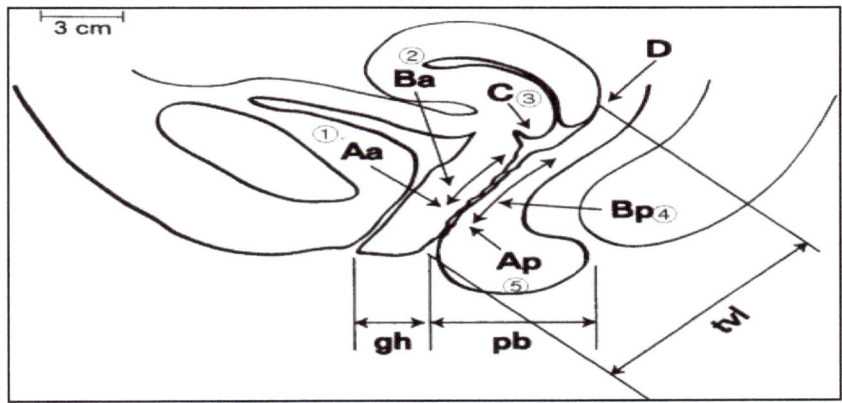

Fig. 5.46. POP–Q system and landmarks used

Anterior wall $_{Aa}$	Anterior wall $_{Ba}$	Cervix $_C$
Genital hiatus $_{gh}$	Perineal body $_{pb}$	total vaginal length $_{tvl}$
posterior wall $_{ap}$	Posterior wall $_{Bp}$	posterior vaginal fornix $_D$

Fig. 5.47. Grid for the introduction of values in Pop-Q system

Another great advantage of the POP-Q system is an integrative assessment of all pelvic floor disorders, not just the uterine prolapse.

5.1.2.4. Clinical diagnosis of vaginal vault prolapse

Vaginal vault prolapse is evaluated similarly to the uterine one. The difference consists in the disappearance of the cervix as a marker and the use of postoperatory scar in this respect, Fig. 5.49. POP-Q system can be successfully used, analogously to uterine prolapse.

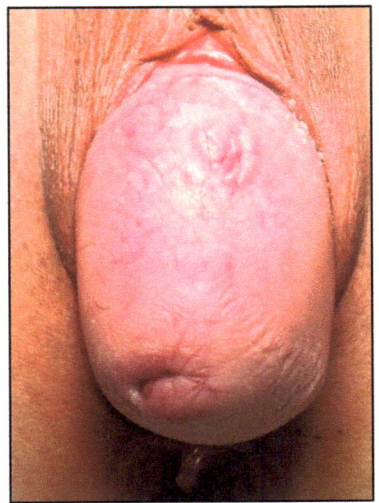

Fig. 5.48. POP-Q uterine prolapse stage 4
(according to **Enache T., 2014**)

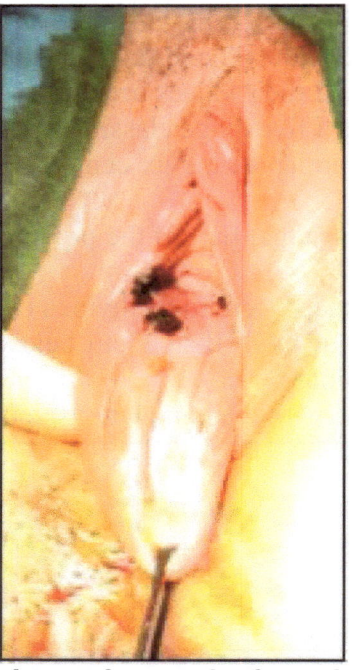

Fig. 5.49. Vaginal vault prolapse at three months after total vaginal hysterectomy
(according to **Enache T., 2014**)
Unabsorbed sutures can be observed

5.1.2.5. Clinical diagnosis of posterior vaginal wall prolapse (rectocele)

Posterior vaginal wall prolapse is subdivided into two categories: *elitrocele (high posterior vaginal prolapse)* and *rectocele*.

Elitrocele means the lowering of posterior vaginal fornix, above the rectum. Most often, the contents of the hernial sac are the ileal loops, hence the name of enterocele, which was used many times. Although the two notions are superposable, we prefer to use the term elitrocele to designate this pelvic floor disorder, as it correlates with the anatomic defect rather than the content, Fig 5.51. *Rectocele* is the posterior vaginal defect in the lower half, characterized by the anterior descent of this part.

At this level, posterior vaginal wall has a close relationship with the rectum, and, together with its movement, rectal wall also moves anteriorly, Fig 5.52. A complementary maneuver is the rectal examination that cranially delineates the anatomical defect (**Goeschen K.,** *et al.,* **2010**).

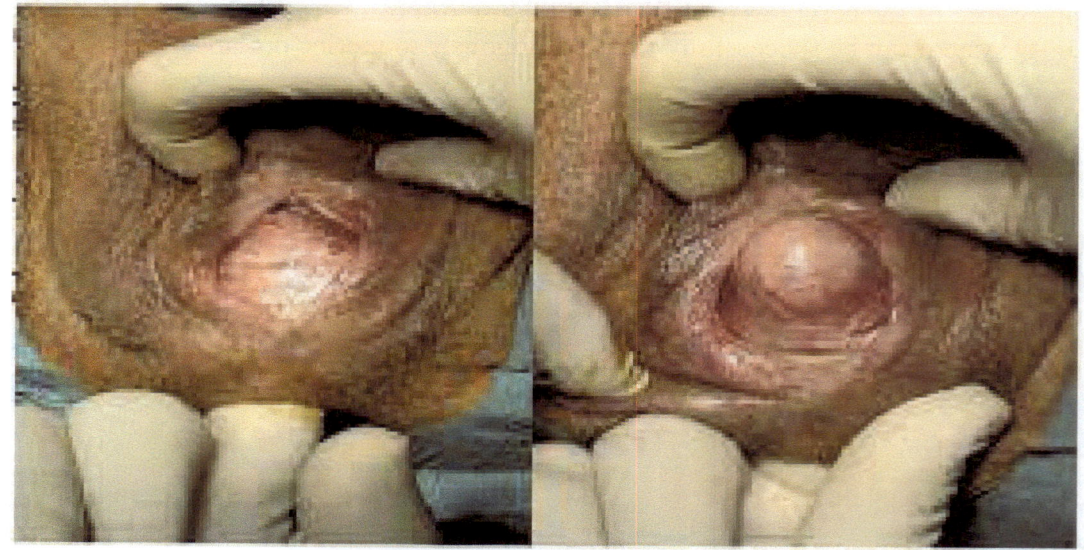

Fig. 5.50. Diagnosis of perineal body defect
(according to **Petros P., 2010**)

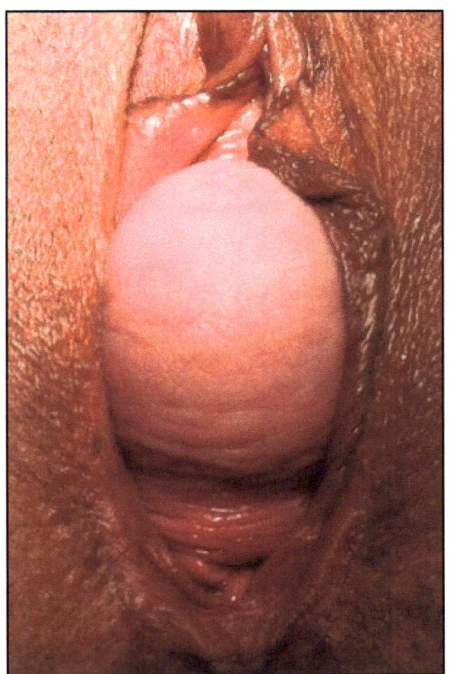 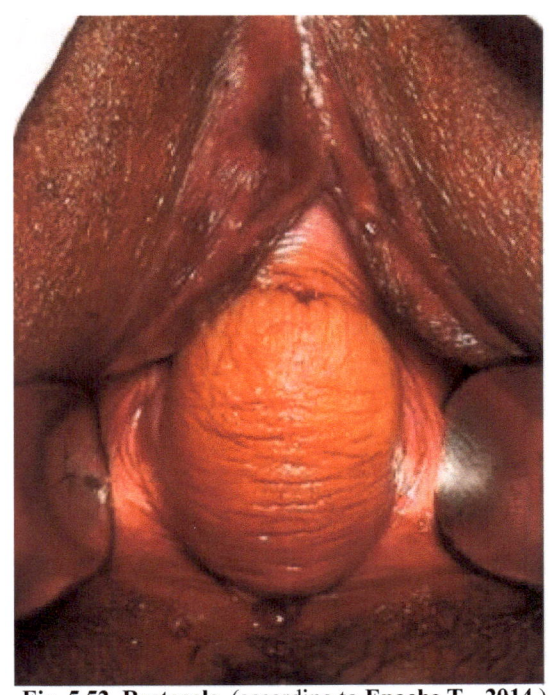

Fig. 5.51. High posterior vaginal prolapse – elitrocele (according to **Enache T., 2014**)

Fig. 5.52. Rectocele (according to **Enache T., 2014.**)

Diagnosis of the two forms is established during the examination with valves. Smaller defects require additional objectification maneuvers. The upper valve supports the anterior vaginal wall and the cervix, while the posterior valve retracts progressively. If the defect is not obvious, an isometric effort (strain) is recommended to the patient, in which case a hernial sac may be prominent. The POP-Q system can be successfully used for the evaluation of posterior vaginal prolapse (**Muir T.W.** & **Stepp K.J., 2003**).

The perineal body defect is achieved only through rectal tract. It is thus palpated, possibly with two hands, the index from one hand rectally placed and the thumb from the other hand placed at the level of vaginal introit, 2 lateral bodies, and the thinned central part. The protrusion of the rectum can be observed while the index finger is anteriorly moved Fig. 5.50.

5.2. *"Posterior fornix"* syndrome

This syndrome is represented by the emergence of a triad made up of urinary urge, chronic pelvic pains, and nocturia (more than 2 nocturnal micturitions), to which pollakiuria (micturition frequency > 8 times per day) can be associated, frequent cystitis can occur, bladder and rectum emptying disorders can appear, or, on the contrary, faecal incontinence can emerge.

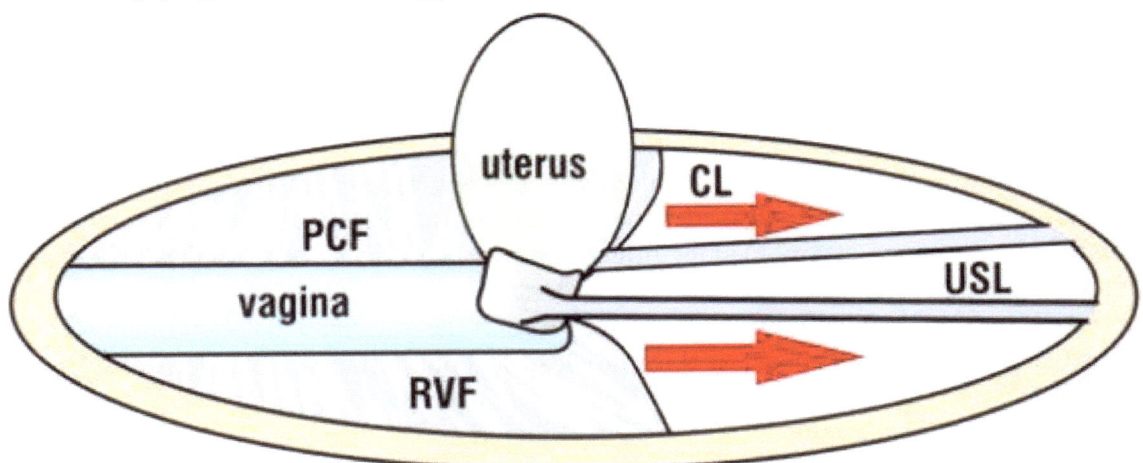

Fig. 5.53. Superior vaginal side support by fascias (according to **Petros P., 2011***a*).
PCF = pubocervical fascia, RVF = rectovaginal fascia, USL = uterosacral ligaments

Petros explains these disorders by the shortening of the vaginal proximal third due to tissue laxity and prolapse, Fig. 5.53.

5.2.1. Urinary urge

The vagina holds the bladder as a membrane stretched like a trampoline. The bladder is subjected to a vaginal feedback mechanism in that the tension of vagina stretching directly affects the baroreceptors in the bladder floor. Until the bladder is filled with a volume close to 300 ml, the counter tension of the vaginal stretching annihilates the stimulation of the pressoreceptors and, thereby, the appearance of the micturition reflex.

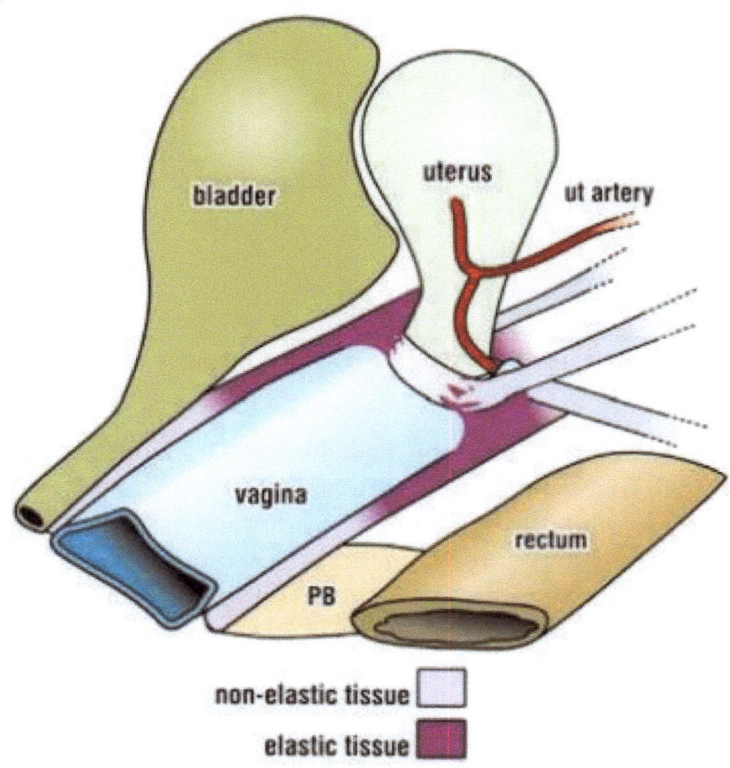

Fig. 5.54. Vagina support by fibromuscular tissue. At the cranial level of vagina, tissues laxer and richer in elastin can be found, which can be weak points and can favor prolapse and the occurrence of micturition instability
(according to **Petros P., 2011***a*)

Over this filling, the inhibition of baroreceptors can no longer be ensured by vaginal counter tension and the sensation of urinary urge appears.

Urinary urge is a symptom typical for posterior fornix syndrome and can be explained by the fact that the vaginal axis changes, at the same time shortening its length.

Logically, in situations in which the vagina is no longer properly anchored or lax in its central area which supports the bladder, the bladder floor prolapses even with a minimal urinary filling (less than 150 ml). The bladder floor support shortens and the bladder rotates towards the sacral cavity, a phenomenon that intensifies especially at night and during the supine position, Fig. 5.54. Therefore, the bladder floor, which contains the baroreceptors signaling the filling of the bladder, can no longer be totally sustained by the vagina. Baroreceptors of unsupported areas are stimulated early, even at low bladder filling and produce urinary urge, which is nothing but a prematurely activated micturition reflex. It can no longer be inhibited because the perineal muscles for repositioning the bladder floor can no longer stretch the vagina. This phenomenon cannot be reproduced urodinamically because it does not lead to contractions of bladder detrusor muscle, the so-called "urge" waves, and, through these, it cannot be recorded during cystotonometry.

While stress urinary incontinence is considered today curable, no clear remedies have been found for urinary urge. Drug therapy has many negative side effects, as for example, the anticholinergic treatment of urinary urge causes organic disorders that lead to the discontinuation of treatment by the patient. Another example is the botulinum toxin (*Botox*) intravesical injection, which annihilates the sensation of urinary urge, but causes bladder-emptying disorders that in some cases lead to the need for intermittent bladder catheterization.

5.2.2. Bladder voiding disorders

Micturition is a complex phenomenon, dependant both on the activity of perineal muscles and on the mobilization of the vagina, which must be elastically anchored in a certain anatomical position. The main phenomenon is represented by the pulling of the vagina posteriorly and lower, through which the bladder neck opens in a funnel shape (a phenomenon clearly demonstrated by lateral contrast cystography).

Logically, the posterior vaginal fornix loses its adequate anchoring to the levator plate through the laxity or lesion of the uterosacral ligaments (prolapse or elitrocele).

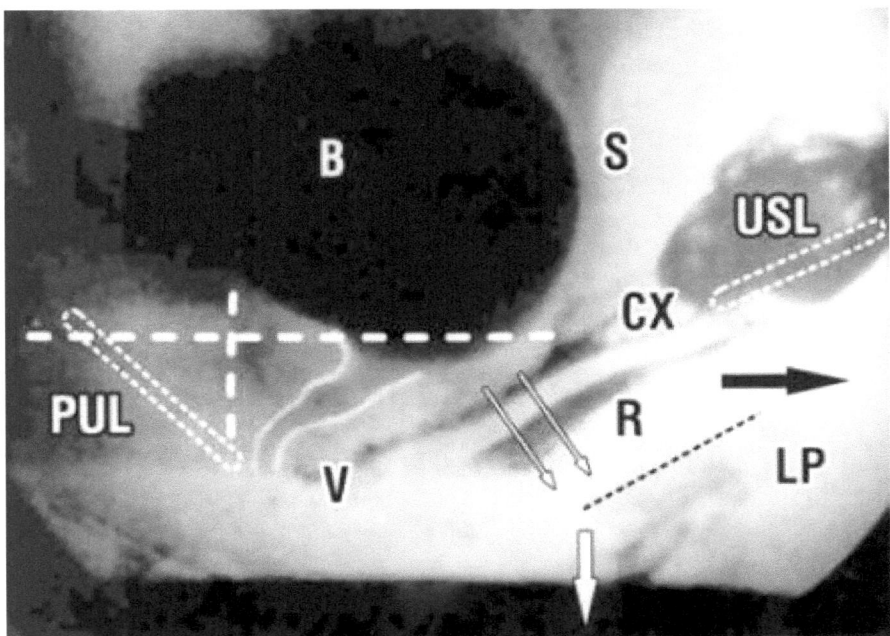

Fig. 5.55. Lateral contrast cystography highlighting the forces that influence the opening of the urethra during micturition
(according to **Petros P., 2011**a)
B = bladder, CX = cervix, LP = levator plate, PUL = pubourethral ligaments, R = rectum, S = sacrum, V = vagina

Not being anchored to the pelvic floor, the posterior vaginal wall cannot be pulled posteriorly and caudally (the muscular force cannot be transmitted correctly anymore), and thus the mobilization necessary for emptying the bladder during micturition, does not take place anymore. Therefore, the active mechanism of opening the bladder neck is prevented, and through this, micturition is made more difficult.

Due to the decoupling of the posterior vagina from the levator plate, the force vector to be transmitted to the bladder in order to provide the necessary motility for micturition is interrupted. As a result, micturition is *"interrupted and incomplete"*, thus producing urinary residue. It is normally between 30 and 40 ml and can reach up to 100-200 ml in pathological conditions.

The result is an incomplete, *"staged"* micturition, with the remaining of a substantial urinary residue. Patients describe a slow and discontinued urinary spurt, which implicitly leads to the chronic urinary residue formation and favors recurrent cystitis.

Poor transmission of perineal muscle force can only be positively affected by re-anchoring the vagina posteriorly to the levator plate, Fig. 5.55. Physical exercise, electrotherapy, and drug treatment will not yield satisfactory results in bladder emptying disorders.

5.2.3. Nocturia

Nocturia is a typical symptom in this syndrome. Patients report a tormenting nocturnal urinary frequency of more than 3 times, sometimes reaching 5 to 7 times.

5.2.4. Pelvic chronic pain

The last typical symptom of posterior vaginal fornix syndrome is deep pelvic pain with transmission to the lower coccygeus part. This is explained by the overloading of uterosacral ligaments and thereby of pain receptors contained in these ligaments. By extension of uterosacral ligaments over a certain limit, nerve endings that are inserted between their collagen fibers are under a continuous tension. This sensation is transmitted along the ligaments up to their insertion points (the bone area between the sacrum and the coccyx), causing deep pains in this area, pains which are often falsely interpreted by orthopedics and are resistant to any form of non-surgical therapy.

5.3. Clinical diagnosis algorithm according to "Integral Theory System"

The objective physical examination does not clearly define the connective elements injured. Peter Petros has developed an algorithmic system of diagnosing the pelvic floor disorders that combine the objective examination with symptomatology. The goal of this approach is to evaluate the affected structures as accurately as possible, which is a key element in subsequent surgical reconstruction. Generally, it is an excessive laxity of connective tissue, with the exception of a *"special case"*: *"the critical elasticity area"*, located at the bladder neck, which, due to some surgical corrections, causes an extensive fibrosis process and consequently a stiffening process (**Goeschen K., et al., 2010**). This diagnosis system uses three compartments in addressing pelvic floor disorders to clarify the complexity of the symptomatology. Each of these compartments contains some key ligament and fascial structures whose laxity is responsible for the anatomical defect and can be individually corrected, Fig. 5.56.

Anterior compartment
1. External urethral ligaments (EUL).
2. Uterovaginal fascia
3. Pubourethral ligaments (PUL)

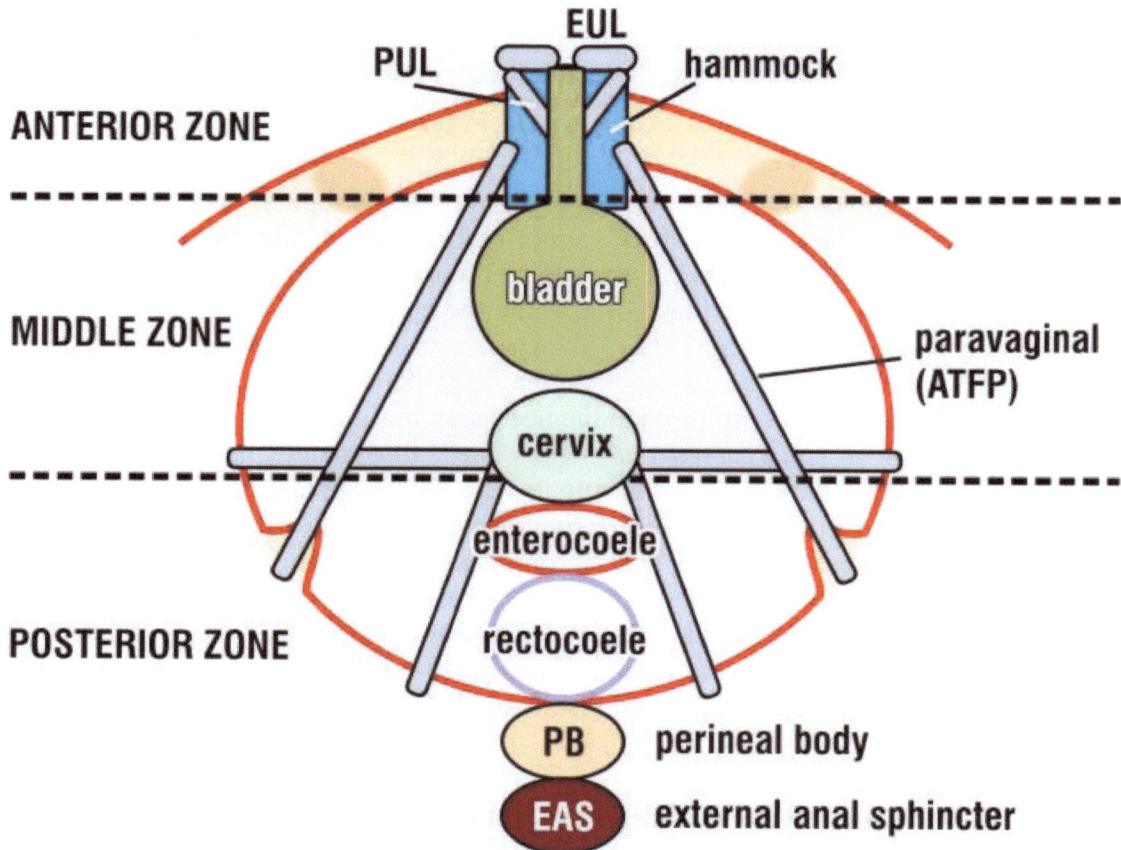

Fig. 5.56. "Key" structures in the occurrence of pelvic floor disorders
(according to **Petros P., 2010**)

Middle compartment
4. Arcus tendineus fasciae pelvis (ATFP)
5. Pubocervical fascia (PCF)
6. Paracervix/ cardinal ligaments – defects associated with the cranial disinsertion of pubocervical fascia.

At the limit of the two compartments, there is the zone of critical elasticity (ZCE), whose fibrosis and stiffening leads to a specific symptomatology.

Posterior compartment
7. Uterosacral ligaments (USL) and ligamentum cardinale (LC).
8. Rectovaginal fascia (RVF).
9. Perineal body – (PB). The clinical exploration is done algorithmically in two steps.

Step 1
Anamnesis and symptom evaluation

Symptoms are difficult to assess. Using a validated questionnaire introduces an objective assessment instrument. According to the Integral Theory, most of the symptoms can be found in the affecting of any compartment. Moreover, there is no correlation between the intensity of a particular symptom and the anatomical defect. Thus, the movement to the next step can be done after analyzing some symptoms and assessing them on an arbitrary qualitative scale, according to their intensity (**Petros P., 2010**).

Step 2
Objective examination

It is intended to identify areas potentially affected. The subjective elements are corroborated with the result of the objective physical examination and the deteriorated structures are established with a satisfactory probability, Fig. 5.57.

A. *Anterior compartment examination*

The anterior compartment extends from the external urethral meatus to the bladder neck. The urethral meatus is dehiscent with the appearance of urethral mucosa, usually denoting a EUL defect. The PUL assessment is done in two steps (**Petros P.P. & von Konsky B.R., 1999**) – initially the urine loss is detected while coughing, the patient being in a gynecological position, then anchoring unilaterally with a forceps at the level of the middle third of the urethra, the coughing effort is repeated. The disappearance of incontinence signifies the damage of this ligament. Urethrovaginal fascia damage is often obvious at the inspection – the urethrocele. By pinching it with a Chaput forceps, the loss of urine while coughing (if it exists) can be diminished, this maneuver being an objective assessment of the fascia damage (**Petros P. & Ulmsten U., 1990; Petros P., 2010**).

Symptoms commonly associated with anterior compartment disorders are stress urinary incontinence and faecal incontinence. Moreover, urinary urge and pollakiuria often appear. Bladder emptying disorders and nocturia may also be present, though to a lesser extent.

B. *Middle compartment examination*. It extends from the bladder neck to the anterior side of the cervix. The central pathological element is the cystocele. In the semiology presented, it is noted that anterior vaginal wall disorders overlap the ones of middle compartment.

Symptomatology is dominated by bladder emptying disorders. In an important percentage, urinary urge and pollakiuria can also be found, similar to the anterior compartment defects. Nocturia and faecal incontinence are less frequently associated. Although rare, pelvic pains can also be present (**Petros P., 2010**).

A special case is that of *"tethered vagina"*. It is met in patients operated for a perineal pathology (usually a suburethral mesh for SUI correction) and is characterized by important fibrosis around the bladder neck and near the vesical trigone. This process induces a stiff funneling of the bladder-emptying tract. The main symptom described is the involuntary loss of urine while changing position from clinostatic to orthostatic position. Posterior pulling of the bladder base associated with the coughing effort can be accompanied by urinary loss, although otherwise SUI does not coexist (**Goeschen K., et al., 2010**).

Posterior compartment examination. It is delimited by the cervix or the postoperatory scar in the cases of hysterectomised patients and the posterior perineal body and is the most difficult compartment to be evaluated and approached surgically. The associated defects are uterine or vaginal vault prolapse and posterior vaginal prolapse.

The posterior compartment disorders are the most troublesome from a symptomatic point of view and sometimes difficult to interpret. The lesions at this level can be associated with all types of symptoms that occur in pelvic floor disorders. Pelvic pains are met very frequently, sometimes representing the reason for the presentation to the physician. An important association is pollakiuria, urinary urge, and nocturia, Petros and Ulmsten reuniting them in a *"posterior vaginal fornix syndrome"* (**Petros P. & Ulmsten U., 1993**). Difficulties of bladder emptying appear in a high percentage.

Although they should represent the main correlation with the posterior compartment, faecal incontinence and obstructive constipation appear more frequently in relation to the anterior compartment damage and are not the most commonly met in this type of disorders. SUI can rarely be associated (**Petros P., 2010**).

5.4. Paraclinical investigations in pelvic floor disorders

A complete diagnosis leads to an appropriate therapeutic attitude. The clinical diagnosis is the most important step in the treatment of pelvic floor disorders, since an observed anatomical defect is correctly associated with a symptomatology. We can conclude that paraclinical explorations have only one secondary role, especially the one of excluding some self-contained pathologies.

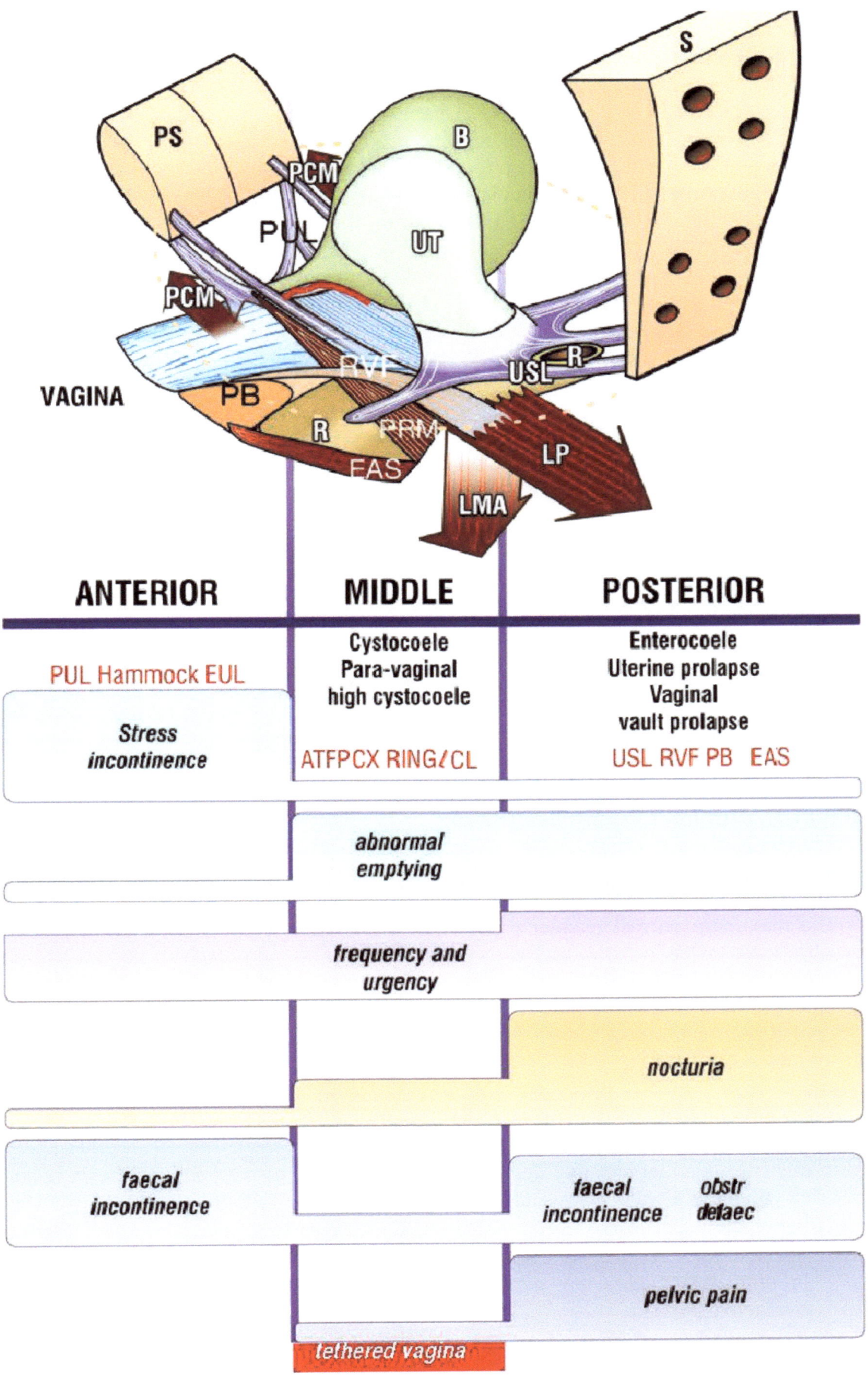

Fig. 5.57. **Pictorial diagnosis algorithm according to Integral Theory**
(according to **Petros P., 2010**)

5.4.1. Urodynamic investigations

The standardization of the techniques and terminology of urodynamic studies has been carried out since 1973 by the International Continence Society (ICS) (**Abrams P.**, *et al.*, **2002**; **Schafer W.**, *et al.*, **2002**).

There are three levels of complexity of urodynamic studies: uroflowmetry, essential urodynamic evidence (filling cystometry, pressure-flow studies) and complex urodynamic evidence (urethral profile, videourodynamics, ambulatory studies, neurophysiological tests).

In this chapter, for each type of investigation, the terms recommended by ICS will be presented together with the technical parameters to be specified when presenting the results, the technique of conducting the investigation as well as the most frequent artifacts that can be encountered during urodynamic investigations (**Calomfirescu N.** & **Manu-Marin A.V.**, **2004**; **Calomfirescu N.**, *et al.*, **2010**).

Before the urodynamic evidence, it is recommended that the patient does a urine culture and completes a micturition time chart. This urination calendar helps both to objectify urinary disorders, to interpret urodynamic data as well as validate them as representing a laboratory reproduction of symptoms in real life.

The micturition time chart offers incontestable data for the correct assessment of the patient's symptoms. For a period of 2-3 days, the patient is instructed to record at each micturition the following: time, urine volume, and any episodes of incontinence or urge micturition, in conditions of a normal water intake. It is recommended that the patient also notes the amount of fluid consumed. This calendar guides the subsequent anamnesis and avoids the erroneous perception of the patient's symptoms. It also provides clear data on the frequency of micturitions, diurnal and nocturnal, as well as about the average functional capacity of the bladder.

The data to be extracted from the micturition time chart are: the diurnal frequency of the micturitions (the number of micturitions starting from the first one in the morning until the last before bedtime), nocturia (the number of micturitions during the sleeping period, each one being preceded and followed by periods of sleep), frequency and volume for 24 hours.

5.4.1.1. Diurnal urinary frequency

The mechanisms that increase the frequency of micturitions are the following (**Blaivas J.**, *et al.*, **2009**; **Schafer W.**, *et al.*, **2002**):

a) Bladder with normal functional capacity

The maximum normal bladder capacity in the adult is between 300 and 600 ml, with gender variations, lower in males and higher in females. In this group, with normal volumes at each micturition, the increase in frequency of micturitions is determined by an increased water intake. This may be secondary to factors such as:

- polydipsia, can rarely have a psychogenic origin, more frequently due to some eating habits: tea, beer, etc.;
- diabetes;
- alteration of ADH production as in the case of diabetes insipidus.

b) Bladder with reduced functional capacity

In this case, bladder capacity determined under general or regional anesthesia is normal, but the urine volume is always below 300 ml. This may have the following causes:

− hyperactive detrusor;
− bladder residue due to subvesical obstruction or hypotonic detrusor and non-inflammatory causes that increase bladder sensitivity such as anxiety or idiopathic overactive bladder;
− inflammatory causes such as: acute cystitis or bladder lithiasis, or tumors such as carcinoma in situ;
− fear of urinary retention in elderly patients urinating with effort;
− fear of incontinence in patients with stress urinary incontinence and/ or hyperactive

detrusor, who urinate frequently to have a low vesical volume and to diminish the risk of incontinence.

c) Bladder with low anatomical capacity

In this case, the bladder capacity determined under regional or general anesthesia is low. The patient eliminates small quantities of urine every time. Capacity reduction may be due to the following:
- post-inflammatory fibrosis as in the case of urinary tuberculosis;
- non-infectious cystitis as in the case of interstitial cystitis;
- post-irradiation pelvic fibrosis;
- surgery (partial cystectomy, extensive bladder electro-resection). Measurement of urine volume over a period of 24 hours can highlight polyuria.

Polyuria is defined as an adult production of more than 2800 ml/ 24 hours.

The urine volume at night is defined as the total urine volume from the moment of falling asleep to the moment of awakening and includes the first micturition in the morning when waking up.

Night polyuria exists when a patient over 65 years old urinates at night more than 33% (for a young adult over 20%) of the total 24-hour urine volume.

The maximum bladder capacity is the maximum volume eliminated at a micturition. This term replaces the one of functional bladder volume that is more vague and confusing.

5.4.1.2. Urinary flow rate

It is a non-invasive method of studying the urinary flow dynamics. The technique of performing the urinary flow curve under standard conditions requires the sample to be taken when the patient has a normal sensation of urinating and is alone in the room and relaxed (**Schafer W.**, *et al., 2002*).

The curves obtained can be classified in continuous and intermittent. In their interpretation, it must be taken into account that the dynamics of the urinary flow is given by the result between the contraction of the detrusor and/ or the abdominal and urethral resistance (**Abrams P., 2006**).

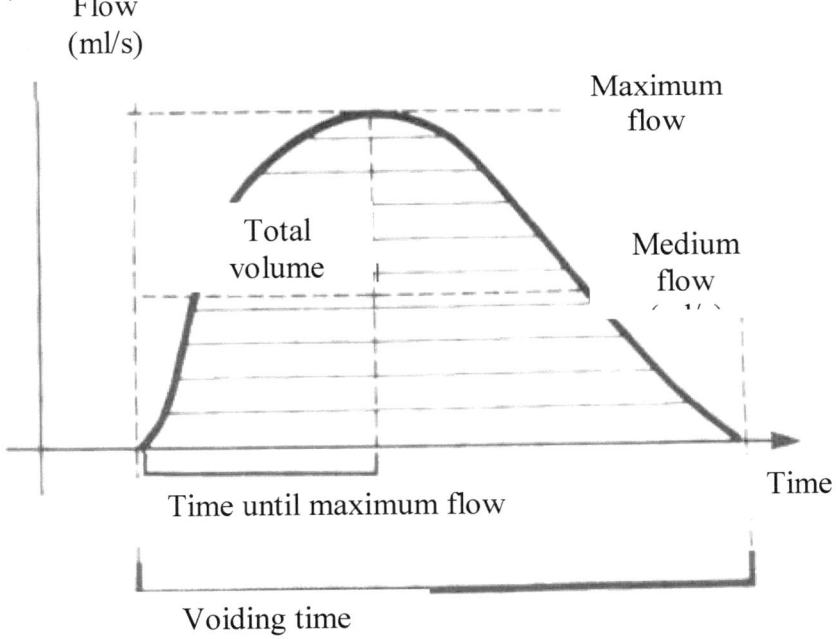

Fig. 5.58. Urinary flow curve with the terminology used

The aspect of the curve obtained is then evaluated by taking into account gender, age and urine volume (**Araki I.**, *et al., 2009*; **Calomfirescu N.**, *et al., 2010*). Numerous authors have developed nomograms used to appreciate the curve's appearance and to establish the diagnosis (**Schafer W.**, *et al., 2002*).

There are two types of urine elimination: continuous and discontinuous way (**Abrams P., 2006**; **Schafer W.**, *et al.*, **2002**).

a) Continuous elimination

The terms describing it are the flow and the curve aspect that can be continuous Fig. 5.58., or intermittent Fig. 5.59. (**Abrams P., 2006**).

Flow (Q), is the volume of liquid expelled in the unit of time, expressed in ml/s and is given by the following relationship (5.1)

$$Q(t) = \begin{cases} \frac{1}{\sqrt{2\sigma_1^2 \pi}} e^{-\frac{t^2}{2\sigma_1^2}} & pentru\ t < t_{max} \\ \frac{1}{\sqrt{2\sigma_2^2 \pi}} e^{-\frac{(t+2)^2}{2\sigma_2^2}} & pentru\ t \geq t_{max} \end{cases} \quad (5.1)$$

where:

- t_{max} - time until maximum flow is achieved;
- σ_1 for $\sigma < 0.7$;
- σ_2 for $\sigma > 0.7$.

Maximum flow (Q_{max}) is the maximum value of flow during the urine elimination and is given by the following function (5.2.)

$$Q_{max} = \frac{1}{\sqrt{2\sigma_2^2 \pi}} e^{-\frac{(t_{max}+2)^2}{2\sigma_2^2}} \quad (5.2)$$

The duration of evacuation (D_E) represents the time needed to eliminate urine.

The total urine volume (V_u) is the total eliminated urine volume, being the area under the curve (AUC) of urinary flow, calculated by the following relation (5.3)

$$V_u = \int_0^{D_E} Q(t) dt \quad (5.3)$$

The medium low (Q_{med}) is given by the report between AUC and the evacuation time (5.4)

$$Q_{med} = \frac{V_u}{D_E} \quad (5.4)$$

The normal aspect of the urinary flow curve is characterized by:
– the form of a bell lightly asymmetrical;
– Q_{max} reached in 5 s from the start or in 30% of the D_E evacuation period.

Regardless of the urine volume, the initial and final phase in the same individual differs by slightly increasing the standard deviation of the urine elimination function Fig. 5.58. (**Abrams P., 2006**; **Schafer W.**, *et al.*, **2002**).

The unstable detrusor, which is a disorder of the bladder storing function, is characterized by an increase in the parameters of the urinary flow curve due to the premature contraction of the detrusor that opens the bladder neck earlier. This action results in the Q_{max} being reached in a shorter time. The diagnosis is determined by filling cystometry (**Abrams P., 2006**; **Blaivas J.**, *et al.*, **2009**; **Schafer W.**, *et al.*, **2002**).

Subvesical obstruction is characterized by low values of Q_{med} and Q_{max}, with $Q_{med} > Q_{max}/2$) (**Abrams P., 2006**; **Blaivas J.**, *et al.*, **2009**; **Schafer W.**, *et al.*, **2002**).

Qmax is rapidly reached and is followed by a long slow slope that can end by terminal dribbling.

In this case, two aspects can be distinguished: compression given by prostate hypertrophy, described above and constrictive, urethral stricture, when the appearance is plateau with a small difference between Q_{med} and Q_{max} (**Abrams P., 2006**; **Blaivas J.**, *et al.*, **2009**; **Schafer W.**, *et al.*, **2002**).

Hypotonic detrusor, which is a disorder of the bladder storage function, is characterized by obtaining a low value of Q_{max}, which is reached late, sometimes in the second part of the curve. Diagnosis is determined by the flow/ pressure diagram (**Abrams P., 2006**).

b) Discontinuous elimination
Interrupted flow

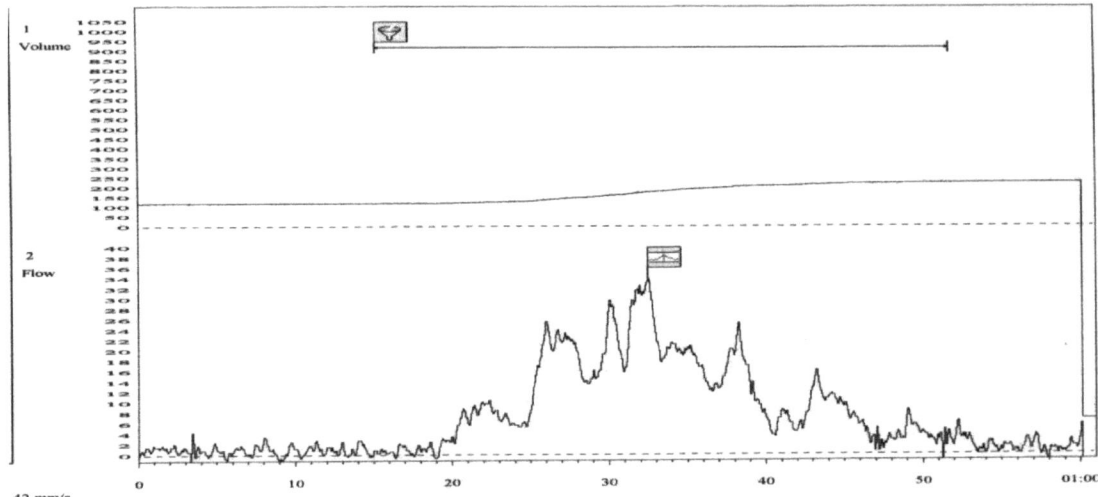

Fig. 5.59. Interrupted curve of urinary flow

The discontinued urinary flow curve is shown in Fig. 5.59. For its interpretation, the same parameters and the same terminology are used, as in the case of continuous elimination, but only that the duration of micturition is not equal to the one of evacuation, the latter not taking into account the interruptions (**Schafer W.,** *et al.,* **2002**).

Irregular path
It is due to abdominal contraction, it occurs in patients who, out of necessity or habitude, use their abdominal and diaphragmatic muscles to increase the urinary flow. The curve is generally almost continuous with slow variations and low amplitude.

To determine the etiology of this dysfunction, flow-rate studies are required.

The irregular path secondary to urethral hyperactivity
It is due to the involuntary contraction of the distal sphincter that may occur in neurological patients, being known as bladder sphincter dyssynergia, but also in patients without neurological history, when it is called "*micturition dysfunction*". The path is similar to that obtained by abdominal contraction, but variations are more extensive and faster.

Irregular path due to hypotony or fluctuating contraction of the detrusor
It is observed in patients with neurogenic or myogenic damage of the detrusor. The contraction of the detrusor does not produce a constant and sustained pressure but a fluctuating one. Frequently an interrupted curve is obtained.

Artifacts of urinary flow rate
Urinary flow rate artifacts can be determined by the variations in performance technique or the interpretation of results. In the performance technique, data may be altered due to the tendency of some patients to balance the urinary spurt during micturition, thus creating a false Qmax. Also, a false Qmax, this time reduced in value, may occur in cases of full bladder, when the force of contraction of the relaxed detrusor is temporarily low. Data interpretation can often be the altered when considering only Qmax, which can often be the result of an abdominal contraction, as well as when comparing flow rate curves in the same patient without taking into account the urine volume (**Abrams P., 2006**).

5.4.1.3. Study of urethral function
There are several ways to study the function of the urethra (**Abrams P., 2006**).
i) Pressure urethral profile:
- static;
- dynamic or of stress;
- micturition.

ii) Urethral leak point pressure (ULPP, VLPP) measurement
iii) Fluid bridge test
iv) Electrical conductivity measurements of urine

i) Static urethral pressure profile

It measures intraluminal pressure across the entire length of the urethra with the bladder at rest.

The parameters measured are the following:
- maximum urethral pressure – is the maximum pressure value, measured on the profile.
- maximum urethral closure pressure – is the difference between the maximum urethral pressure and the bladder pressure.
- the functional length of the profile – is the portion of the urethra across which the urethral pressure exceeds the bladder pressure.
- stress transmission rate – is the increase in urethral pressure under *"stress"* conditions, expressed as a percentage of the value with which bladder pressure increased at the same time.

When presenting the results, the following parameters should be mentioned:
- catheter infusion rate;
- catheter withdrawal speed;
- patient position;
- the medium with which the catheter was infused (liquid or gas);
- bladder volume;
- type of catheter used, size, position of catheter openings and orientation;
- type, cough or valsalva used must be mentioned for the stress profile.

The technique of performing the static urethral pressure profile

The most commonly used technique is that described by Brown and Wickham, which consists in measuring the pressure required to infuse a catheter with a constant rate (**Abrams P., 2006**).

It starts by bringing the system to zero, this being accomplished at atmospheric pressure, at the upper edge of the pubic symphysis. Then, the catheter is inserted into the bladder. The catheter can be between 4 Ch and 10 Ch and must have two lateral holes, at 5 cm from the top. The catheter should be infused at a constant rate, which requires connection to an automatic pump syringe. The infusion rate should be between 2 and 10 ml/min. Retraction of the catheter should be done with a constant speed rate, of less than 0.7 cm/sec using a mechanically activated engine system.

Testing is done with the patient in dorsal decubitus position. In some cases, it can be continued with a sample with the patient in vertical position that must show an increase of pressure, recorded by about 23%. The lack of pressure increase in position change may be a diagnostic test for stress incontinence.

Normal static urethral pressure profile

The normal values of the maximum urethral pressure obtained in a large group of patients and reported by Abrams in 1977 (**Abrams P., 2006**) are presented in Table 5.1.

Table 5.1. Value of maximum urethral pressure in functional patients
(according to **Abrams P., 2006**)

Age (years)	Man		Woman	
	Medium value	Limits	Medium value	Limits
< 25	75	37 – 126	90	55 – 103
25–44	79	35 – 113	82	31 – 115
44–64	75	40 – 123	74	40 – 100
> 64	71	35 – 105	65	35 – 75

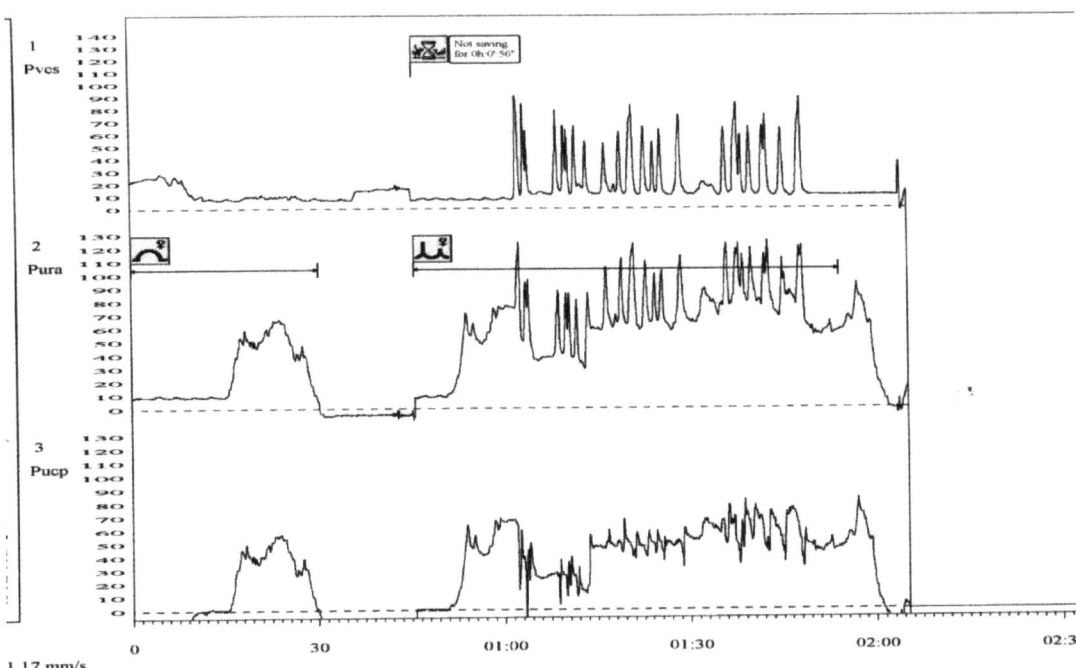

Fig. 5.60. **Normal aspect of static urethral pressure profile in woman**
In the second part, the test was reapplied, the sample being collected while coughing.
The difference of pressure was maintained positive.

Variations are observed according to gender and age.

Women, especially after menopause, present a decrease of maximum urethral pressure with age and a decrease in the length of the functional urethral profile (**Abrams P., 2006**). In woman, the aspect of the curve must be symmetrical at a correct determination, Fig. 5.60.

5.4.1.4. Classification of static urethral profile disorders

The static urethral profile disorders were classified by Abrams şi Calomfirescu as it follows (**Abrams P., 2006; Calomfirescu N. & Manu-Marin A.V., 2004**).

i) Presphincterial abnormalities

Most commonly appear in men with prostate or bladder defects when a prostatic plateau elevation or elongation occurs. In women, presphincterial abnormalities such as the elongation occur in patients in whom bladder neck suspension was practiced.

ii) Sphincter abnormalities

They are recorded in the area of maximum urethral pressure, half of the urethra in woman, the prostate-beak in man. Low pressure occurs following a trauma, atrophy, or a denervation. An abnormally high pressure occurs in case of sphincter hyperactivity or hypertrophy.

iii) Post sphincter abnormalities

Urethral strictures and meatus stenosis are not reliably highlighted by this method. Other pathologies are rarely encountered.

Stress urethral pressure profile

This concept, introduced by Asmussen and Ulmsten (1976), consists of simultaneous measurement of bladder and urethral pressure by means of a double lumen catheter, the catheter having openings both in the urethra and in the bladder. Both sensors, bladder and urethral, are first set to zero externally, at atmospheric pressure at the upper edge of the pubic symphysis. The catheter inserted into the bladder is then retracted through the urethra, very slowly (1-2 mm/sec), the patient coughing at regular intervals, Fig. 5.60.

This method measures the efficiency of the pressure transmission from the abdominal cavity in the proximal urethra, actually measuring the value of the urethral pressure (ure. p – ves. p) in dynamics. When the closing pressure becomes negative, the loss of urine occurs, so the method is ideal for diagnosing stress incontinence when performed in a patient with a full bladder (**Calomfirescu N. & Manu-Marin A.V., 2004**).

Urethral discharge point measurement

This technique was described by McGuire and globally defines the state of urethral function by measuring the bladder pressure to which urine loss occurs through the urethra. It uses the Valsalva maneuver to increase the bladder pressure, being also known as the Valsalva leak point pressure (VLPP) (**Calomfirescu N. & Manu-Marin A.V., 2004**).

Fluid bridge test

It was created to test the bladder neck. The principle consists in positioning the opening of a catheter immediately distal to the bladder neck. When the patient coughs, if the bladder neck opens, a fluid bridge is created between the bladder contents and the catheter opening, resulting in loss of urine.

It is not a reliable test, because it does not take into consideration the bladder neck movement resulting in false results, its value being also disputed by the video demonstration of urodynamics, the fact that postmenopausal patients have, in 50% of the cases, continence of damaged bladder neck (**Abrams P., 2006**).

Urethral electrical conductivity test

It is a variant of the fluid bridge tissue. The catheter is provided with two electrodes which, when connected to the fluid bridge, as described above, register an increase in conductivity (**Abrams P., 2006**).

Artifacts, limits, and indications of urethral pressure profile

Since the urethral pressure profile is an investigation performed at rest, it is hard to tell how much of the information obtained reflects one of the physiological situations, namely the filling of the bladder or the micturition phase. Changes that occur in bladder pressure during the investigation are another factor that determines artifacts. This way, the contractions of an unstable detrusor or the pressure of a detrusor with a low compliance will determine alterations in the urethral pressure profile. Therefore, concomitant measurement of bladder pressure is of great importance. Although it does not improve the diagnostic value of the test, it reduces the number of misinterpretations.

Due to the low specificity of stress urethral pressure profile, its importance is diminishing. Studies could not prove its diagnostic value neither in obstruction, nor in incontinence cases, or in vesical sphincter dyssynergia (**Abrams P., 2006**; **Calomfirescu N. & Manu-Marin A.V., 2004**).

The static urethral pressure profile maintains some indications:
- there is a strong association between sphincter alteration and maximum urethral closure pressure (MUCP) in post-prostatectomy incontinence;
- in patients with stress incontinence – a MUCP preoperatory value of less than 20 cm H_2O predicts a poor postoperatory outcome;
- in patients in whom a reanastomosis of the neo-urethral reservoir is searched, MUCP gives a valuable indication of the continence of the future reservoir; a value of MUCP greater than 50 cm H_2O forecasts a good result (**Abrams P., 2006**).

5.4.1.5. Cystometry

Cystometry studies the function of detrusor and the urethra in both phases, of storage and evacuation. The storage phase is studied through filling cystometry and the evacuation through micturition cystometry (**Calomfirescu N. & Manu-Marin A.V., 2004**; 9). Frequently, the two investigations take place one after the other.

Bladder pressure is measured concomitantly with the abdominal one (measured in the rectum), and, detrusor pressure is obtained by electronic subtraction.

Pressure measurement is done with a transducer that uses the principle of a liquid in a closed recipient (constant volume), that, on pressure variations, mobilizes a metallic membrane, which generates electricity that can be measured (**Calomfirescu N. & Manu-Marin A.V., 2004**).

Filling cystectomy

Filling cystectomy evaluates the storage stage based on the determination of four parameters (**Abrams P., 2006**; **Calomfirescu N. & Manu-Marin A.V., 2004**):

i) intracervical pressure (p_{icv})
ii) intra-abdominal pressure (p_{abd})
iii) detrusor pressure (p_{det})
iv) urine loss, the follow-up being made at the same time Fig. 5.61. Other optional determinations can be performed concomitantly:
  - bladder volume;
  - measurement of urethral pressure;
  - measurement of bladder pressure (p_{bla}),
  - EMG;
  - video- cystography.

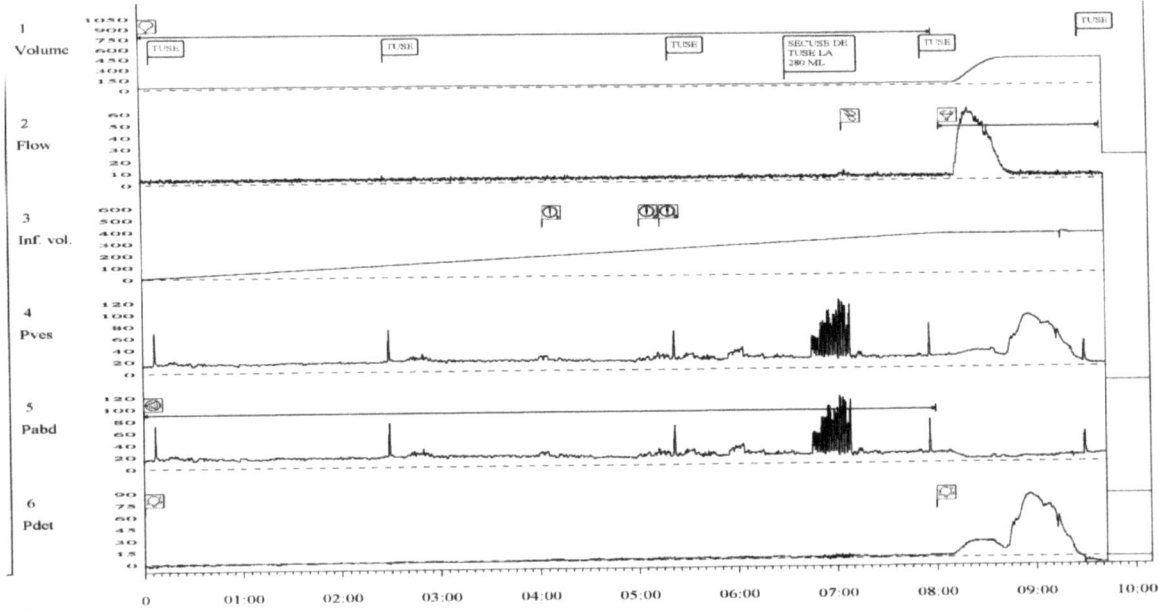

Fig. 5.61. Filling cystometry with recording control

Technique of measuring bladder pressure (p_{bla})
- Initially, all transducers are brought to zero at atmospheric pressure, at the upper edge of pubic symphysis.
- Urethral catheterization is done under local anesthesia busing 2 catheters, one epidural for the measurement of pressure and the second of 8 Ch for filling or one single catheter with 2 ducts. The catheter is inserted in the rectum. All the catheters are fixed on the skin with adhesive tape.
- The correct positioning of the catheters is controlled by asking the patient to cough.
- ❖ *Filling the bladder*

It can be done with water, serum, or contrast substance at room temperature (22^0C).

The filling speed can be slow (10 ml/min), medium (10-100 ml/min), or fast (100 ml/min). Because an increased filling speed decreases the bladder compliance, the standard speed accepted is of 50 ml/min.

The use of carbone dioxide for filling is not indicated because it is non-physiological, the gas is compressible, it dissolves in urine forming carbonic acid that is irritating, the bladder does not increase in weight by filling, an element that has a significance in the physiology of micturition, and does not make possible the continuation of the study with a flow-micturition pressure determination.

The position in which the patient urinates, vertical for men and sitting for women, describes most of the symptoms.

❖ *Residual urine*

Should not be evacuated before filling to observe the behavior of the bladder in real conditions. It is determined at the end of the flow-pressure micturition end of study (**Abrams P., 2006**; **Calomfirescu N. & Manu-Marin A.V., 2004**).

Technique of measuring abdominal pressure

Abdominal pressure (p_{abd}) is actually the perivesical pressure. Its determination can be transrectal or less frequently transperitoneal. After the enema, the catheter is inserted into the rectum about 10-15 cm and is connected to the manometer.

The wave caused by coughing is simultaneous in p_{bla} and p_{abd}, without causing variations in p_{det} (**Abrams P., 2006**; **Calomfirescu N. & Manu-Marin A.V., 2004**).

Technique of measuring detrusor pressure

The detrusor pressure (p_{det}) is determined by electronic subtraction of the abdominal pressure from the bladder pressure (5.5.)

$$p_{det} = p_{bla} - p_{abd} \qquad (5.5)$$

Correct determination depends on the quality of p_{bla} și p_{abd} pressures measurement. The accuracy of the determinations is based on the positioning of the catheters, the evacuation of any gas bubbles from the tubes and can be checked periodically by asking the patient to cough and observing the simultaneity of the coughing waves in p_{bla} și p_{abd}, Fig. 5.61. Coughing should not cause changes in p_{det}, but a small biphasic deflection is accepted as normal, being determined by the velocity difference of the transmission through the liquid in the tubes. In the same way, it will always be done during the test, by checking the quality of the recording and asking the patient to cough at every minute during the filling process. The simultaneity of waves caused by the coughing will guarantee a reliable recording. Under no circumstances will the system be reset to zero while the catheters are in the bladder or in the rectum. If they have not been properly emptied by the gas bubbles, they will be removed, washed (inside) until the gas is evacuated, reset to zero outside and repositioned (**Abrams P., 2006**; **Calomfirescu N. & Manu-Marin A.V., 2004**).

Cystometry must allow the sampling of data about:
- bladder sensitivity;
- detrusor activity;
- bladder compliance;
- urethral function;
- bladder capacity.

Bladder sensitivity
- ❖ *First desire to void – FDV –* occurs at about 50% of the cystometric capacity.
- ❖ *Normal desire to void - NDV –* the feeling to which the patient would empty the bladder in the first favorable place; occurs at 75% of the capacity.
- ❖ *Strong desire to void – SDV –* the persistent feeling of wanting to urinate, but without being afraid of urine loss; occurs at 90% of the capacity.
- ❖ *Urgency –* the persistent feeling of urge to urinate, accompanied by the fear of urine loss.
- ❖ *Pain –* the painful sensation during bladder filling occurs only in pathological cases.

Altered sensitivity of the bladder can be classified in the following:
- ♦ increased (hypersensitive), when the first sensation of urination occurs rapidly (100 ml) and persists until the normal sensation of urinating appears, limiting the capacity of the bladder to 250 ml;
- ♦ reduced, when the first sensation of urination appears late and persists until the normal sensation appears, the patient not experiencing neither an intense urge to

urinate nor urgency;
- absent, which occurs in case of a neurological pathology such as meningomyelocele or spinal cord trauma (**Abrams P., 2006**).

Detrusor activity

During bladder filling, it can be normal or increased.

Normal activity indicates a stable detrusor that does not have hyperactivity manifestations in the tests used. Detrusor muscle relaxes allowing the filling without intravesical pressure variations.

Increased activity indicates a hyperactive detrusor. During the filling stage, the detrusor has uninhibited contractions that cannot be suppressed. It is called an unstable detrusor in patients without neurological affection and detrusor hyperreflexia in those with a neurological history. These contractions may be spontaneous or may occur under certain circumstances such as position change, hand washing, telephone ringing, which should be performed as much as possible at the moment of cystometry (**Abrams P., 2006**; **Schafer W.,** *et al.,* **2002**; **Calomfirescu N.** & **Manu-Marin A.V., 2004**).

Bladder Compliance

Describes the relationship between bladder volume and bladder pressure (V/P) and is measured in ml/cmH$_2$O. Normally, a 400 ml bladder should not have a variation in pressure from empty to full, of more than 10 ml/cmH$_2$O, which means compliance greater than 40 ml/cmH$_2$O.

A low compliance can be determined by a too high filling rate. Checking this possibility is done by stopping the procedure for two minutes and resuming filling at a much lower rate.

The large compliance and high capacity detrusor cannot be classified as a hypotonic detrusor in filling cystometry, this being a diagnosis established by the flow-pressure test (**Abrams P., 2006**; **Calomfirescu N.** & **Manu-Marin A.V., 2004**).

Urethral function during filling

During the bladder filling phase, the urethral closure mechanism can be normal or incompetent (**Abrams P.,** *et al.,* **2002**; **Abrams P., 2006**; **Schafer W.,** *et al.,* **2002**; **Calomfirescu N.** & **Manu-Marin A.V., 2004**).

The normal urethral closure mechanism is established when the closing pressure is positive, even at times of abdominal pressure increase.

The incompetent urethral closure mechanism is defined as loss of urine in the absence of contraction of the detrusor. In this situation, two entities can be distinguished:
- stress urinary incontinence defined as loss of urine by increasing the bladder pressure to values higher than the urethral closure pressure in the absence of a detrusor contraction;
- urethral instability is a variation greater than 15 cmH$_2$O in the maximum pressure urethral closure, which can be a rare cause of incontinence.

The existence of uninhibited contractions of the detrusor does not allow the diagnosis of urethral closure mechanism's incompetence, because urethral relaxation in a bladder contraction is a normal phenomenon.

Bladder capacity

ICS uses the following terms to assess bladder capacity (**Abrams P.,** *et al.,* **2002**).
- Maximum cystometric capacity is the volume at which the patient feels she cannot postpone the micturition; it is a parameter difficult to appreciate if the patient has a reduced or absent bladder sensitivity, the investigator resorting, in this case, to data from the micturition time chart.
- The functional capacity of the bladder is the urine volume and is appreciated by using the micturition time chart that the patient completes before any urodynamic test.
- The maximum bladder capacity is determined while the patient is anesthetized. It may be different from functional capacity, especially in cases of unstable detrusor.

Micturition cystometry

Micturition cystometry deals with the relationship between urinary flow and intravesical pressure and is essential for a correct functional classification of micturition disorders (**Abrams**

P., 2006; **Calomfirescu N. & Manu-Marin A.V., 2004**).

During a flow-pressure test, intravesical pressure and urinary flow rate are measured dynamically, using the following notions (**Abrams P.,** *et al.,* **2002**; **Schafer W.,** *et al.,* **2002**):

♦ *premicturition pressure* is the pressure measured immediately before the isovolumetric contraction triggering;

♦ *opening time* is the time elapsed since the initial increase of the detrusor pressure until the spurt occurred;

♦ *opening pressure* is the pressure at the moment of the spurt, recorded as a debut spurt;

♦ *maximum micturition pressure* is the maximum pressure recorded during micturition;

♦ *maximum flow pressure* is the pressure recorded at the maximum flow rate;

♦ *maximum flow contraction pressure* is the difference between the maximum flow pressure and the premicturition pressure;

♦ *post-contraction period* describes the possible increases in pressure after the end of micturition.

Once the bladder filling is completed, whether due to the patient's sensation, or to the volume resulting from the frequency-volume calendar, it is advisable for the patient to start the micturition, Fig. 5.62., respecting her privacy and the position in which she usually urinates.

Interpretation of micturition cystometry is done by following the activity of the detrusor and the urethral function.

The detrusor activity can be classified according to the following (**Abrams P., 2006**; **Calomfirescu N. & Manu-Marin A.V., 2004**).

Normal activity, when though contraction, the detrusor empties the bladder with a normal flow.

Hypoactive activity, when the detrusor contraction is insufficient to empty the bladder or it empties it with a low flow. The value of diagnosis through this method decreases in case a subvesical obstruction exists. The detrusor's inability to empty the bladder and achieve a normal flow rate does not necessarily alter contractility. In this case, the following test can be done: during micturition, when the investigator thinks Q_{max} has been reached, he asks the patient to stop the micturition; the detrusor is not immediately inhibited and an isovolumetric contraction is obtained, which will result in increased bladder pressure. At this moment, detrusor pressure, noted with $p_{det}.iso.,$ offers data regarding its contraction force.

There is an acontractile activity when there is no change in the detrusor pressure during micturition.

Urethral activity during micturition can be normal or obstructive. The normal activity is when the urethra is completely relaxed during micturition.

Obstructive activity is due to a mechanical obstruction, the sphincter being completely relaxed, but the micturition is done with high pressures without variation. When it is due to an overactive urethra, bladder sphincter dyssynergia, intravesical pressure has high fluctuations.

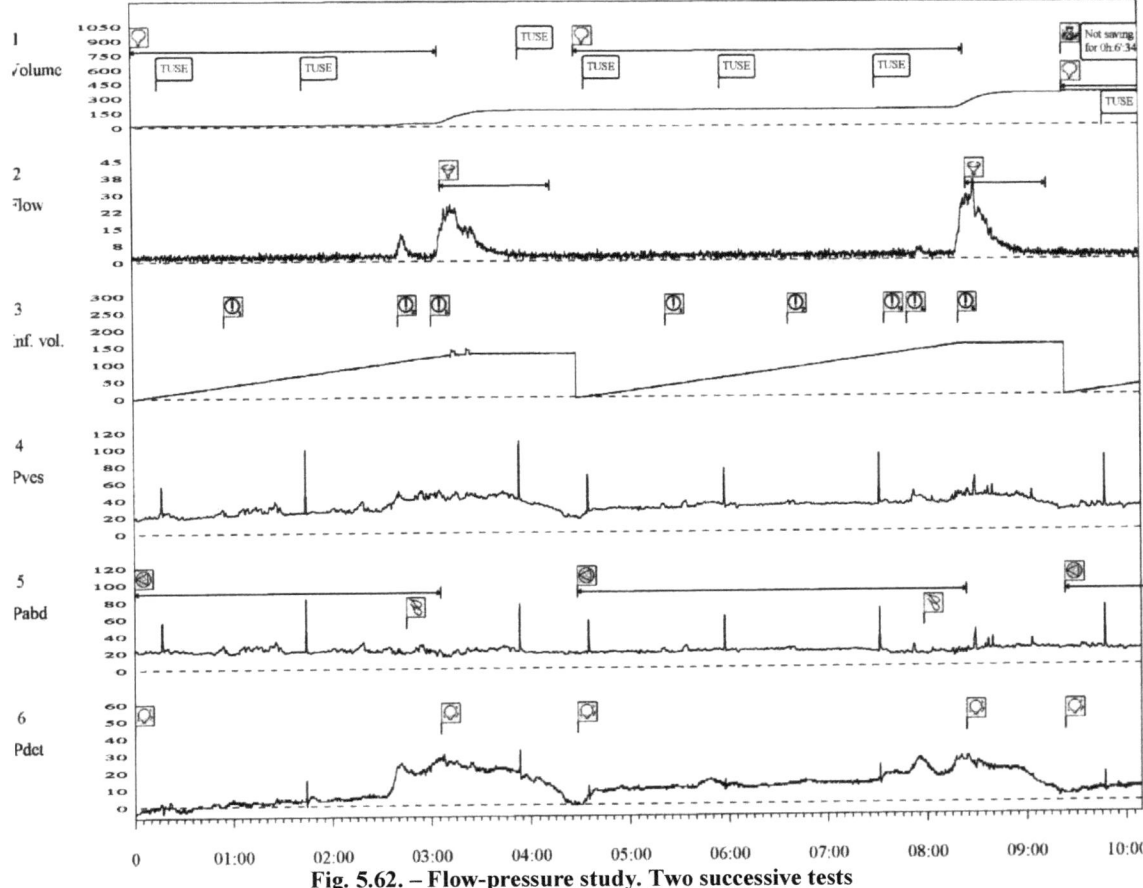

Fig. 5.62. – Flow-pressure study. Two successive tests

The presentation of the results of any type of cystometry must be accompanied by the specification of the following technical parameters (**Abrams P.,** *et al.,* **2002**; **Abrams P., 2006**):
- size of catheters, their types;
- the filling area and its temperature;
- speed of filling;
- position in which the filling was done;
- position in which micturition was done.

Artifacts of cystometry

They can be determined by psychological, physiological, or technical factors (**Abrams P., 2006**).

Psychological factors cannot be ignored no matter how much effort is made for the patient to be relaxed. The devices around the patient and, of course, the catheters will determine artifacts that, according to the sensitivity of each patient, will have a variable impact on the investigation. Therefore, it should not be forgotten that this investigation has the role of rebuilding the symptoms accused by the patient and we must always obtain the confirmation from the patient that the sample was representative for its symptoms at the end of the investigation.

Physiological factors that determine artifacts may be rectal contractions, which are difficult to prevent and can only be avoided in those with a full rectal ampulla through prior enema and abdominal contraction during micturition. To assess whether this is a patient's habit or a necessity, it should be noted that in case of obstruction, the abdominal contraction does not increase the flow.

The technical factors are related to the speed and volume of filling, the catheters that can slip during the investigation and the correctness of their preparation. A too high filling speed will cause uninhibited contractions, which will disappear when the pump is switched off for a moment and the filling is continued at a lower speed. An excessive filling of the bladder will result in a reduced flow, this being avoided by evaluating the patient's micturition time chart. The importance of the obstruction that catheters give can be appreciated by comparing the flow/pressure test with a free-flow that the patient performs before the investigation. The accuracy of catheter positioning and their gas bubble emptying is controlled by tracking the simultaneity of coughing-induced waves.

5.4.1.6. Videourodynamic tests

Videourodynamics uses urinary tract imaging equipments: an X-ray unit, an image amplifier, or an ultrasound (**Abrams P., 2006**).

Depending on the position and state of rest or micturition of the patient, the degree of filling of the bladder can provide the following information.

i) Full bladder in rest position – capacity, bladder contour, diverticula, passive vesicourethral reflux.

ii) Coughing – appreciates the bladder neck and its descending degree.

iii) Micturition:
- speed and degree of opening of the bladder neck;
- caliber and shape of the urethra;
- vesicourethral reflux.

iv) Micturition stop test:
- the speed and quality of the urethral closure mechanism;
- urinary retention in the prostate urethra;
- post micturition – residual urine.

Simultaneously with the determination of intraurethral pressure and EMG of the pelvic floor, the videourodynamic test provides a perfect demonstration of the mechanisms of continence and of micturition.

The indications of videourodynamics are the following (**Abrams P., 2006**; **Calomfirescu N. & Manu- Marin A.V., 2004**):
- suspicion of subvesical obstruction in a young patient;
- children with micturition dysfunctions;
- recurrent stress urinary incontinence in women, in preoperative assessment;
- vesicourethral dysfunction in neuropathy;
- post-prostatectomy incontinence prior to the implantation of the artificial sphincter;
- impaired renal function, with no intrinsic renal pathology, when urethral hyperactivity is suspected.

5.4.1.7. Outpatient urodynamic tests

Urodynamic ambulatory tests have been imagined and developed to achieve data collection under conditions identical to those in which the patient describes the symptoms by using the natural bladder filling (**Abrams P., 2006**; **Calomfirescu N. & Manu-Marin A.V., 2004**). A catheter is used with the transducer mounted on it (micro type transducer). It is inserted into the bladder, often having a second transducer on the same catheter to measure intraurethral pressure. The catheter is then connected to a microcomputer that the patient wears on her shoulder. The patient should note all the urinary events occurring during the recording, urge sensations, urine loss, and micturitions. These will then be correlated with the recorded data.

The technique is not fully studied, its value being appreciated by various authors. It is mainly used to investigate cases of urinary urge in which etiology could not be highlighted by the other tests (**Abrams P., 2006**). Blaivas argues that the bladder catheter itself may be the cause of unstable contractions, so this expensive method offers questionable results (**Blaivas J., *et al.*, 2009**).

Use of urodynamic data in clinical practice in patients with urinary symptoms

In case of pelvic organs prolapse, the study of the urodynamic pressure flow is considered important in assessing the cause of the micturition dysfunction of postoperatory retention. The preoperative study can evaluate the contractility of the detrusor and fit it into one of the five Schafer contractility classes. The post-micturition residue increases significantly (**Araki I., *et al.*,**

2009) after the prolapse correction operation, but returns to normal after the first month, if the contractility of the detrusor is altered. If the polyfunctional bladder residue does not decrease after a month, the question arises if the hypocontractile detrusor is the cause of this retention or subvesical obstruction because of an intraoperative barrier. The existence of a preoperative urodynamic test to evaluate the contractility of the detrusor helps the etiological diagnosis of postoperatory chronic retention (**Araki I.**, *et al.,* **2009**).

In the case of overactive bladder symptoms, it is admitted that in many cases they improve or disappear after the cure of prolapse. Clinical trials based on urodynamic tests have shown that symptoms of pollakiuria and urinary urge disappear in patients who do not have hyperactive contractions, a urodynamic hypertrophic detrusor and do not disappear in those who have contractions during bladder filling, in filling cystometry (**Araki I.**, *et al.,* **2009**).

For women with Stress Urinary Incontinence (SUI), NICE recommendations suggest that urodynamic tests are not necessary preoperatively in case SUI is "pure", meaning there are only symptoms of loss of urine during physical exercise.

In 2009, Digesu and co-authors (**Digesu G.A.**, *et al.,* **2009**) conducted a study on 3428 women aged between 24 and 81 and showed that only 8.9% were "*purely*" SUI and 52% of the women in this group of 3428 patients complained of urinary incontinence. The rest associated overactive bladder symptoms or altered emptying symptoms, to which urodynamic tests bring important data regarding the preoperative clarification of symptomatology and diagnosis.

Another study retrospectively re-evaluated the value of urodynamic tests performed before SUI curative operations (**Serati M.**, *et al.,* **2015**). The urodynamic results of a group of 2053 patients have been evaluated and the conclusion was that the surgical decision was altered or canceled in 19.2% of the patients with SUI, because of the urodynamic test.

The urodynamic tests are necessary for the etiological clarification of the patients' symptoms when other symptoms, especially the ones of bladder emptying, weak, discontinuous urinary spurt, post-micturition residue, are added to the ones of SUI. Investigating these symptoms is even more important in patients with prolapse.

Another category of patients requiring the urodynamic investigation of their urinary symptoms are those with a history of neurological disease, Parkinson's disease, multiple sclerosis, stroke, diabetes with neuropathy, spina bifida, myelomeningocele, trauma or vertebral tumors that have a neurological bladder (**Calomfirescu N.** & **Manu-Marin A.V. 2010**; **Calomfirescu N.**, *et al.,* **2010**).

5.4.1.8. Neurophysiological tests

Neurophysiological tests (EMG) are used in two situations in which they play a role in the medical diagnosis (**Abrams P., 2006**; **Calomfirescu N.** & **Manu-Marin A.V. 2010**).

1) Patients with micturition or retention difficulties in whom sphincter electromyography (EMG) reveals an abnormal sphincter electrical activity.

2) The detection of an abnormal activity of the pelvic floor during micturition by EMG determines the orientation towards a pelvic relaxation therapy in children with micturition dysfunctions.

5.4.2. Ultrasound

Although it is spectacular, the ultrasound evaluation does not bring many diagnostic elements. The path approached is transperineal. Thus, we have access to the exploration of the urethra and bladder neck, Fig. 5.63. and 5.64.

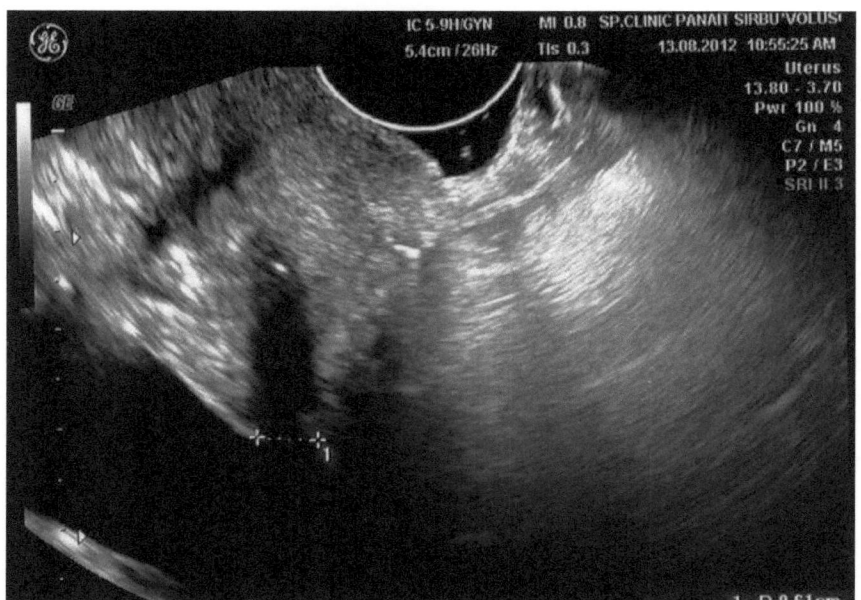

Fig. 5.63. Normal urethra at rest – ultrasound
(according to **Enache T., 2014.**)

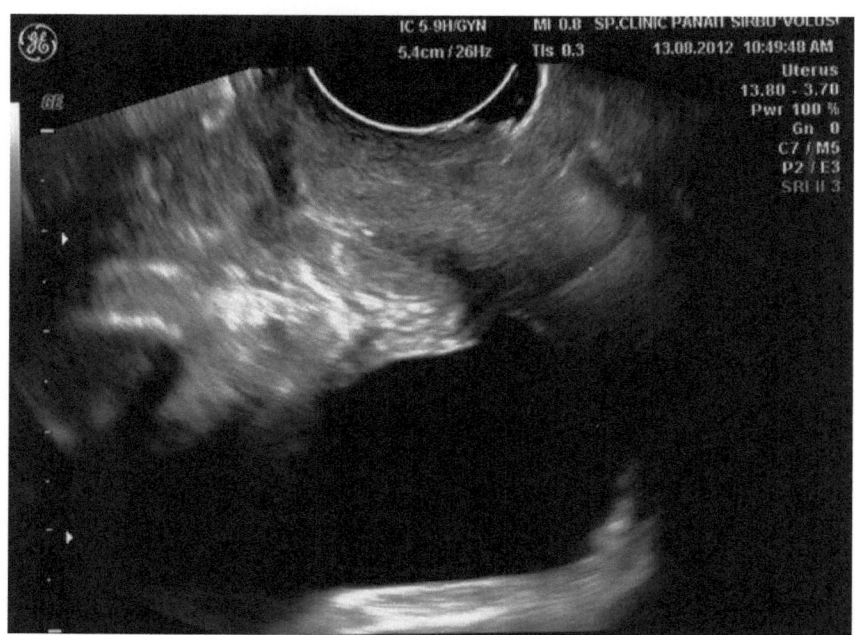

Fig. 5.64. Normal urethra at Valsalva maneuver – ultrasound
(according to **Enache T., 2014.**)

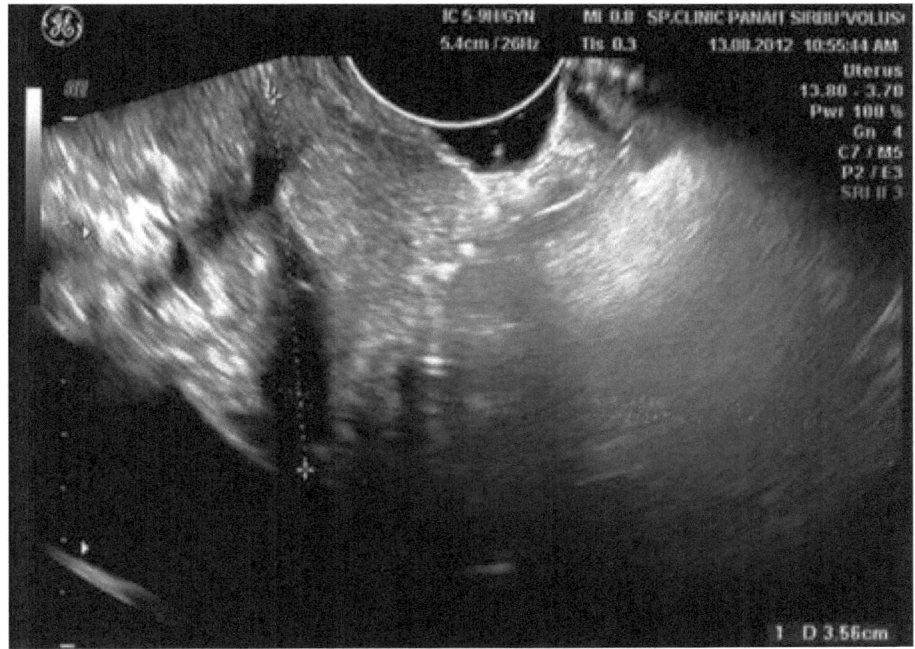

Fig. 5.65. Patient with SUI – funneling effect – ultrasound
(according to **Enache T., 2014**)

The internal urethral orifice and the urethral length can be measured. Bladder cavity funnel can also be evaluated by performing the Valsalva maneuver in patients with stress urinary incontinence Fig. 5.65. An overactive bladder in coughing effort is associated with SUI. In case of a competent urethra, the urethral closure can be observed in the medium third (**DeLancey J.O., et al., 2007**).

However, there is a certain benefit in the quantification of post micturition residue that can be measured accurately (**Petros P., 2010**).

5.4.3. Radiological examinations

Currently, many of the radiological examinations are no longer used in the diagnosis of pelvic floor disorders: simple kidney and bladder X-ray, intravenous urography, micturition urethrocystography. In 1986, Stanton and colleagues combined cystomanometry with the video-recorded parameters of micturition to exclude other bladder diseases (diverticula, etc.), but these explorations have a little contribution to the establishing of a diagnosis.

Exploration of the rectum with barium paste – defecography allows the assessment of faecal continence and objectification of faecal incontinence (**Morgan D.M., et al., 2007**). Even if the exploration brings some clarification, the interest is strictly scientific and is not used in the routine diagnosis of faecal incontinence, Fig. 5.66. and 5.67.

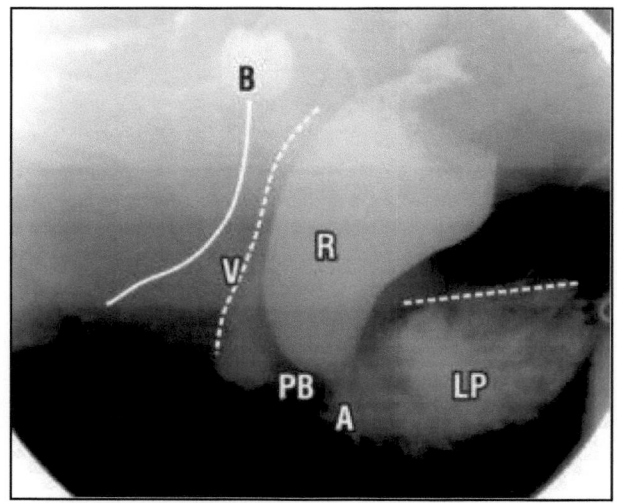

Fig. 5.66. Female patient with faecal incontinence at rest, in a sitting position
(according to **Petros P., 2010**)
B – bladder, V – vagina, R – rectum, PB – perineal body, LP – levator plate, A – anus

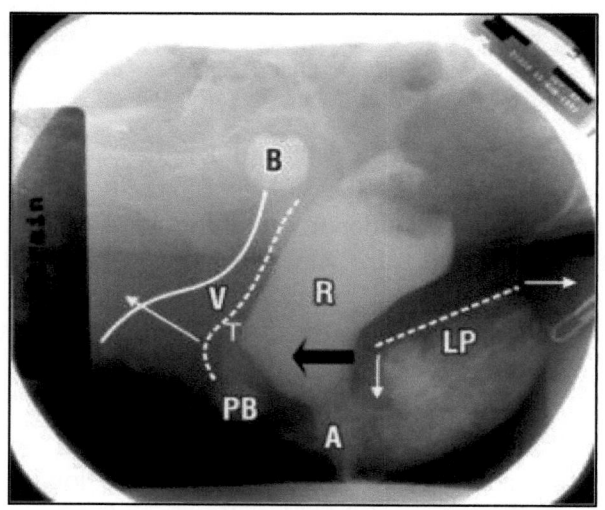

Fig. 5.67. The same female patient as in Fig. 5.66. in coughing effort. The barium substance can be observed entering the anus (A)
(according to **Petros P., 2010**)
B – bladder, V – vagina, R – rectum, PB – perineal body, LP – levator plate

5.4.4. Imaging examinations

Magnetic Resonance Imaging (MRI) images can offer important information regarding pelvic floor pathology and has many advantages: it is non-invasive and lacks unwanted side effects, explores many pelvic organs at the same time, dynamically highlights the changes of the pelvic floor muscles and the bladder and recto-sigmoid movements, helping, at the same time, in the direct measurement of the interacting pelvic structures and the relationship between them. However, it is also expensive and cannot be performed routinely. One of the major disadvantages of the MRI is that it is done in a clinostatic position, thereby reduces the gravitational effect exerted on the pelvic floor.

Especially in the case of uterovaginal prolapse, it can be underestimated and the measurements performed directly may be inaccurate. Elitrocele is an anatomical defect that is typically stressed by the orthostatic position, so it can be misinterpreted in the MRI. Rectocele is less influenced by gravity and more by the effort made during defecation.

This, in turn, is complicated to achieve objectively under voluntary conditions during the investigation and is dependent on how cooperative the patient is.

The contrast-based MRI examination consists of an investigation at rest and one during effort, requiring the contraction of the abdominal muscles and the relaxation of the pelvic floor. The cystography stage follows micturition and the defecography stage, defecation.

Finally, imagining information is collected during the maximum voluntary contraction of the abdominal muscles, especially to highlight elitrocele and rectocele. The last sequence of investigation highlights the degree of laxity of levator ani muscles and the lateral movement of puborectal muscles, which together with the detection of pelvic organs prolapse, finally demonstrates the rupture through the perineal urogenital hiatus.

The MRI examination remains an investigation that has not entered the routine circuit for the anatomical and dynamic diagnosis of perineal disorders because it is laborious and limited by the sensation of embarrassment which the female patient has during micturition and especially during defecation.

6. Conservative treatment of pelvic floor disorders

Conservative treatment of pelvic floor disorders practically overlaps the conservative treatment of stress urinary incontinence. Broadly, it also addresses other urinary disorders that can benefit more or less efficiently from conservative therapy. In the following, we will focus on the treatment of stress urinary incontinence alone, for which there are relevant studies on the improvement of symptomatology.

Urinary incontinence is a common problem throughout the world, but due to the feeling of shame, taboo, and ignorance of the possibility of treatment, only a small number of individuals suffering from incontinence seek professional help. Usually, patients seek help when the loss of urine leads to mental, physical, or social problems or discomfort to the patient or his/ her social environment.

Various forms of incontinence can be distinguished, such as stress urinary incontinence, mixed incontinence and incontinence due to detrusor hyperactivity (**Abrams P.,** *et al.,* **2002**).

The most prevalent form in women is stress urinary incontinence, accounting for 49% of all the cases. The next form after stress urinary incontinence is the hyperactivity of the detrusor, this being the second most prevalent cause (21%). In the above-mentioned symptoms, the combination between stress and urinary urge reflects mixed incontinence. Its prevalence is 29%.

Incontinence has many treatment options such as physical therapy, drug treatment, and surgical procedures.

Most patients can be treated satisfactorily. Guides have been published in several countries.

In the case of patients suffering from incontinence, physical therapy is often considered a priority treatment, due to its non-invasive nature, results regarding the relief of symptoms, possibility of combining physical therapy with other treatments, the low risk of side effects and tendency of low costs (**ICS., 2001**).

The important limitations are that success depends on the motivation and perseverance of the patient and the therapist and the time allocated to the therapy.

This article analyzes and discusses the diagnosis and therapeutic options of physical therapy for stress urinary incontinence, detrusor hyperactivity and mixed incontinence.

6.1. Medical evaluation

For the general practitioner (GP), who is in many countries around the world the first doctor whom the patient addresses for a consultation, it may be difficult to exactly identify the cause of urinary incontinence. Specialists, such as the urologist or gynecologist, can resort to specific diagnostic tests such as the urodynamic evaluation. Usually, GPs do not have access to such tests, so they rely on physical experience and examination.

When resorting to a therapist for the pelvic area, establishing a diagnosis as accurate as possible is important, and in this regard, it is important to discuss the impact of incontinence and the discontent that it causes to the female patient. The discussion on the estimation of the success or failure of physical therapy for the pelvic area is also very important.

Hyperactivity of the detrusor has a greater impact on quality of life than stress urinary incontinence, due to the unpredictability of the symptoms. Young people in particular consider the detrusor's hyperactivity to be very inappropriate.

After birth, stress urinary incontinence sometimes intertwines with a total denervation of the pelvic floor or with significant damage to the connective tissue and surrounding structures. In such situations, physical therapy has very little or no effect. Also, in patients with detrusor hyperactivity resulting from a neurological problem, the effect of physical therapy is minimal.

Other etiological factors such as age, hysterectomy, estrogen depletion during menopause, chronic diseases such as diabetes, sedentary disease, obesity, births, duration of labor and type of birth play a significant role in the onset and evolution of incontinence.

6.2. Physiotherapeutic evaluation

Based on the medical diagnosis of the reference physician, the therapist starts his physiotherapeutic diagnosis process. The aim is to establish, analyze and evaluate the nature and severity of the urinary incontinence and to determine if and to what extent the psychotherapeutic intervention can be effective (**Fantl J.A.,** *et al.,* **1996**).

The physical examination of the patient is important to check and support her profile in the medical history.

The objective of the physical examination is to understand:
- the functionality of the pelvic floor in relaxation and during activities that involve coordination, tone, endurance and strength;
- the conscious or unconscious possibility and degree of contraction of the pelvic floor muscles;
- the influence of other parts of the body on the function of the pelvic floor by inspecting during relaxation and while moving.

It is also important to consider other patient variables such as age, obesity, and normal birth, which have their impact on the intervention process.

6.3. Kinesiotherapeutic treatment

Generally, the least invasive procedure and the least problematic should be considered as a priority. After analysis and evaluation, the physiotherapist decides the treatment plan. The physiotherapist also estimates if a full recovery or just the compensation for certain more troublesome symptoms is possible. Moreover, he/ she determines the strategy, procedure, own methods of treatment to achieve the goal and whether he/ she has the abilities and competency to perform the task. The approach and treatment methods vary depending on the type of incontinence: stress urinary incontinence, detrusor hyperactivity, or mixed incontinence, but all these low risk interventions involve educating the patient in this respect as well as providing support for all the efforts and progress made (**Fantl J.A.,** *et al.,* **1996**).

Before starting the specific methods for pelvic floor therapy, it is important to know and appreciate the position and function of the pelvic floor and the way pelvic floor muscles contract and relax. In order to achieve (long-term) satisfactory results from this intervention, informing and supervising the therapist during the intervention is mandatory, especially with regard to the proper use of the pelvic floor muscles and behavior related to the micturition process.

6.4. Stress urinary incontinence

Physiotherapeutic methods for treating stress urinary incontinence are pelvic muscle training (PMT) with or without biofeedback, electrical stimulation, and/ or vaginal cones (**Abrams P., 2000**; **Berghmans L.C.M.,** *et al.,* **2000**).

A rational biological analysis for PMT in managing stress urinary incontinence is that a powerful and rapid contraction of the pelvic muscles will tighten the urethra, increasing the urethral pressure to prevent leakage during a sudden increase of intra abdominal pressure (**Wilson P.D.,** *et al.,* **2002**). DeLancey also suggested that an efficient contraction of the pelvic muscles could press the urethra towards public symphysis, creating a mechanical pressure increase. The contraction of the pelvic muscles also supports the pelvic organs. Synchronization can also be important. Bø suggested that a synchronized, rapid, and powerful contraction could prevent the urethral opening during an increase of intra abdominal pressure. Hence, PMT focuses in particular on improving the power and coordination of pelvic floor and periurethral muscles (**Wells T.J.,** *et al.,* **1991**).

The adequate PMT treatment should always include an assessment of the contraction and relaxation of the pelvic muscles, because the PMT effect depends on the correct contractions and relaxation.

Correct repeated contractions of the pelvic floor and the strengthening of the pelvic muscles in an intensive and long-term training program are essential for an efficient improvement through PMT. Until fatigue, the frequency and number of repetitive exercises recommended is the following: 8-12 maximum PM contractions, 1-3 sec to 6-8 sec maintenance/ relaxation, 3 maintenances of contractions for 30 sec, 3 times a day for at least 6 months.

It is very important to select the relevant beginning positions, appropriate to each individual patient, while the functional activities should be included in the training program as soon as possible.

Improving the power and total endurance of the pelvic floor does not guarantee proper functioning of the continence mechanism. The inclusion of a individually developed program of physical exercises is essential at home, as well as its integration into daily activities (**Wells T.J.,** *et al.,* **1991**; **Tapp A.J.S.,** *et al.,* **1989**).

Biofeedback consists of the technique through which information about contractions and relaxation of the pelvic muscles is set in a form intelligible to the patient in order to allow the self-regulation of these events (**Berghmans L.C.M.,** *et al.,* **1996**). This technique can be applied either by using electromyographic signals (EMG), manometry or by combining both. Biofeedback is based on exercises and a cognitive learning process. By using biofeedback, a patient suffering from incontinence can be trained to be selective in the use of pelvic floor muscles. By means of recording with an intravaginal or intrarectal electrode, the patient can see on a monitor if and to what extent the contraction or the relaxation of the pelvic muscles is possible and appropriate. Usually, from the beginning of the biofeedback therapy, the unitary motor activity (EMG) or the intravaginal/ anal pressure of the pelvic floor (manometry) is measured at rest during a maximum pelvic contraction (Pmax) and relaxation after Pmax.

For the treatment of stress urinary incontinence, biofeedback in combination with PMT seems as effective as PMT alone. However, in patients who suffer from urinary incontinence and do not understand how pelvic muscles work, who are unable to voluntarily contract or relax their pelvic muscles or have a low quality (intensity) contraction in the initial assessment, biofeedback is suggested as an important strategy to expedite this awareness (**Berghmans L.C.M.,** *et al.,* **1996**; **Bø K.,** *et al.,* **1990**).

Electrical stimulation is achieved through clinical equipment requiring electrical connection or portable battery powered equipment. Although relevant studies report relatively weak statistical results, there is a well-founded biological reason in the use of electrical stimulation. In stress urinary incontinence, the purpose of electrical stimulation is to improve the function of the pelvic floor muscles, while for patients suffering from urge incontinence, the objective is to inhibit the detrusor hyperactivity (**Berghmans L.C.M.,** *et al.,* **1998**).

In the case of stress urinary incontinence, electrical stimulation is channeled into restoring local reflex activity by stimulating the pudendal nerve fibers in order to create a contraction of the pelvic floor. Electrical stimulation causes a motor response in patients in whom a voluntary contraction is not possible because of the insufficiency of the pelvic floor, if the nerve is intact (**Eriksen B.C., 1989**).

In the case of women suffering from stress urinary incontinence, appropriate vaginal cones are sometimes used in combination with PMT. All cones are identical in size, but they grow in weight. The idea is that the stronger the pelvic muscles, the greater the cone's weight to stimulate the pelvic muscles to hold the cone inside the vagina.

In the case of Urge Incontinence, it is likely that the specific treatment for pelvic muscles facilitates and rebuilds Detrusor Inhibition Reflex (DIR) by selectively contracting pelvic muscles (**Yamanishi T.,** *et al.,* **2000**). Treatment for pelvic muscles contains PMT and specific or general relaxation exercises. Different from the stress urinary incontinence mechanism in patients with detrusor hyperactivity, selective contractions of pelvic muscles during therapy are concentrated on the inhibition of involuntary contractions of detrusor muscle (reflex inhibition).

In many patients with hyperactivity of the detrusor muscle, there is a permanent hypertonia of the pelvic floor, due to which the contractions can no longer be exercised. The training of the contraction but also of selective relaxation of the pelvic muscles is then an important step. Once accomplished, the selective contraction of pelvic muscles focuses on facilitating DIR. After testing a patient's ability to maintain contractions for at least 20 seconds by fingers palpation by a psychotherapist, patients are trained how to relax the muscles for a period of 10 seconds. Learning how exercises for pelvic muscles can be performed during daily activities complete the exercises program.

Recent studies show that electrical stimulation, in cases of urge incontinence, at either hospital or home, is effective in 70% of the cases. This can be the first-line treatment in patients with hyperactivity of the detrusor muscle (**Wang A.C., et al., 2004**).

Thus, physical therapy is proven effective in the treatment of urinary incontinence, and therefore physical therapy is the first-line treatment for patients with urinary incontinence, managing to reduce the costs and risks of therapy and to select patients who can only benefit from the surgery.

7. *Surgical treatment of pelvic floor disorders*

The treatment of pelvic floor disorders implies a careful prior assessment (**Thompson J.D., 1997**). Selection of cases with surgical indication is sometimes problematic, in terms of both postoperatory results and comorbidities. Young female patients with minimal anatomical defects and whose symptoms are not very noisy, who eventually want more children, can benefit from conservative treatment. Moreover, alternative treatment options must be sought for elderly patients who seek for treatment and in whom surgey is contraindicated.

Regardless of the outcome of the objective examination, the most important element is the patient's perception of her own suffering and consequently the extent to which her quality of life is affected. Surgical treatment should be applied when there is a sufficient degree of morbidity (**Thompson J.D., 1997**).

Complementary measures, such as the treatment of chronic associated diseases, weight loss, smoking cessation, and local estrogen treatment can be considered both conservative treatment and preoperative preparation (**Petros P., 2010**).

7.1. General principles of surgical treatment of pelvic floor disorders

According to "*Integral Theory*", reconstructive surgery involves the restoration of form as close as possible to the original anatomy, which should lead to the regaining of the function (**Petros P., 2010**). Unlike excisional surgery, this type of surgery implies increased difficulty. The final goal of restoring the anatomy must also take into account the structure and role of each structure involved. An increasing number of patients wish to preserve the sexual function in old age.

One of the key structures of the pelvic floor, which is most frequently used in surgery, is the vagina. This is an elastic tubular membrane whose resistance is given by the fibromuscular layer (**Petros P., 2010**). Surgical reconstruction should consider these characteristics. Classic surgical techniques are followed by a high percentage of cases of dyspareunia, because most of these methods involve the resection of a mucosal vaginal fragment (**Francis W.J. & Jeffcoate T.N., 1961**). The vagina has no regenerative capacity, and the stretching and tensioning of the urogenital tissue leads to a decrease in resistance of up to 30% (**Hiroshi Y. & Evans F.G., 1973**).

Pathogenic treatment of pelvic floor disorders should reconstitute altered structures without modifying the anatomy and function of other tissues and organs. This implies a proper surgical tactic and the appropriate technique. An important problem is the choice of the surgical approach. Determinant factors include the surgeon's abilities, habit, and the nature of pathology. Thus, vaginal, abdominal, or laparoscopic approach can be chosen (**Brubaker L., et al., 2008**).

Synthesizing, some principles to be followed during the surgical treatment can be stated (**Petros P., 2010**; **Sung V.W.**, *et al.,* **2008**).
1. Restoring perineal anatomy, following a pathogenic therapy as much as possible, by strengthening the support means, ligaments, fascia, or by creating new ones to functionally replace those injured.
2. Preservation of pelvic organs function: physiological micturition and defecation, adequate sexual activity.
3. Choosing the approach and the optimal surgical technique for both the patient and the surgeon.
4. Preserving the vaginal anatomy and elasticity. Vaginal mucosa excision should be avoided as much as possible in order to keep its structure and be tensioned by the muscular vectors that continuously act upon it.
5. Avoiding the tensioning of the structures to elude postoperatory complications that lead to a decrease in the quality of life through pain, dyspareunia, the occurrence of the "*non-expandable vagina*" syndrome.

Following a chronological evolution of the treatment of this pathology, we can divide the surgical techniques into two categories: classical surgeries and alloplastic material surgeries.

Classical surgeries

These interventions developed in the last century try to restore the anatomy by techniques to compensate for ligament or fascial laxity. It is difficult, in principle, to supply affected tissue using virtually the same material. Even if in a certain disorder, specific ligaments and fascias are affected, the general characteristics of collagen in all age-related resistance structures and other coexisting diseases imply a vulnerability of the whole connective tissue. Therefore, classical surgeries use structures similar to those affected for the correction of static disorders and induce their excessive tensioning by pulling. These elements predispose to an increased rate of relapse.

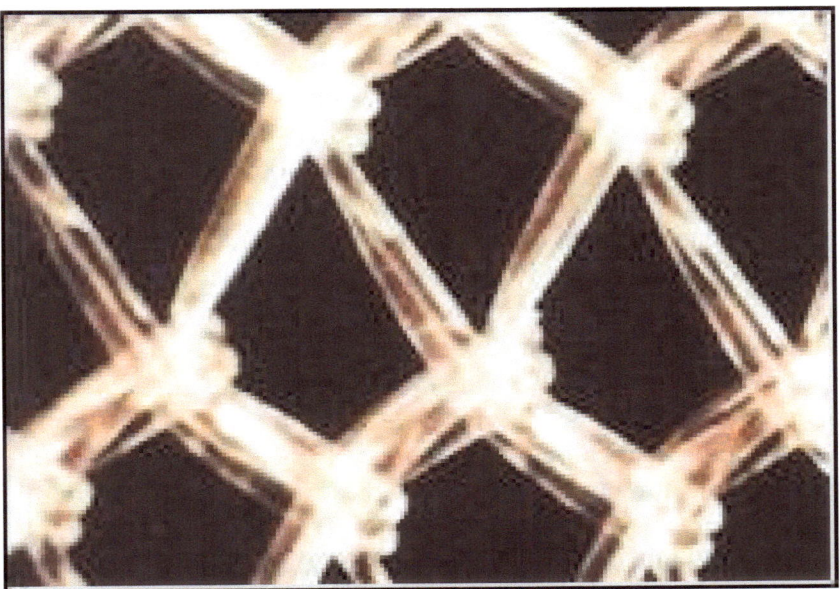

Fig. 7.1. Model of macroporous monofilament mesh of 100-150 microns thickness
(according to **Petros P., 2010**)

Also in this type of surgeries, techniques that used homographs, such as the fascia lata tensor can be included, these being the base of using heterographs (**Sîrbu P., 1981**). The reason for their presentation in this paper is the need for knowing all the therapeutic means, also taking into account the limitations imposed by the FDA in recent years, which has led some surgeons to cautiously adopt alloplastic material techniques. We believe that classical surgeries are still current in many experienced centers, with success rates comparable to newer techniques. Also, with very few exceptions, as in the treatment of stress urinary incontinence, there was no consensus on optimal surgery for each defect. However, we consider that regardless of the adopted technique, it is important to respect the five principles outlined above. One of the basic principles outlined by Petros P. is the preservation of the uterus during the treatment of pelvic floor disorders.

Alloplastic material surgeries

This type of surgery has developed especially since 1990, with the emergence of synthetic materials that can be tolerated by the organism and laparoscopy. The underlying principle of the new surgical approach is the *substitution* of ligaments and affected fascias with a solid structure to restore their role. The main synthetic material used is polypropylene, which is inert from the immunological point of view (**Ulmsten U., et al., 1996**). Polypropylene meshes have developed a lot in the last 20 years and various structures and sizes have resulted.

The best results were obtained with monofilament and macropores meshes of 100-150 microns (**Amid P.K., 1997**). Through this macroporous monofilament structure, the mesh reaches relative weights of less than 20 grams per square meter (*light mesh*).

The mechanism underlying the formation of some neoligaments is the reaction of foreign body. The invasion of macrophage meshes which begin to synthesize collagen and glycosaminoglycans, thus forming a conjunctive scar that provides resistance (**Petros P., 2010**). This neostructure is permanently subjected to remodeling, so that, over time it can lead to some complications: erosions, retractions, rejection reactions. Exceptionally, fistulae or extensive intravesical adhesions are mentioned, Fig. 7.1.

By synthesizing, polypropylene materials must meet the following criteria:
- should be macroporous, in order to facilitate their penetration by collagen tissues;
- should have a lower mesh weight (*light mesh*) and a lower impact surface;
- should have a soft consistency and not stiff, but cannot be broken by pulling;
- should not be too elastic or modify form too much when subjected to tension;
- should not be allergenic and carcinogenic;
- should be safely sterilized;
- should have no sharp edges to damage the surrounding tissues.

A subject of debate is how to insert these prostheses. Several surgical approaches have been invented, some of them becoming standard, others being heavily challenged. Finding optimal methods is a topic of great relevance (**Maher C., et al., 2010**).

Peter Petros set out some fundamental rules to follow in the surgical reconstruction of pelvic floor disorders, regardless of the approach chosen.

1. Preserving the anatomy and elasticity of the vagina. The vagina is an organ and should not be excised. The appropriate elasticity is required for its function. Even if the vagina appears widened at the end of the surgical correction, it generally decreases until the period of 6 weeks is reached. The basic substance of the vagina, collagen along with glycosaminoglycans is readapted to the new force vectors and readjusts its shape *if the surgical technique allows it*.

2. Do not remove the uterus. The uterus acts as the springing point of a Gothic arch. Almost each pelvic ligament is anchored to it. Moreover, the descending arm of the uterine artery is the main vascular source for proximal parts of the cardinal and uterosacral ligaments. They should also be preserved.

3. If a ligament is weakened, it must be shortened and reinforced. It should be shortened so that the muscular vectors can contract efficiently and reinforced with an alloplastic material to synthesize new collagen. Prolapse occurs because the tissues are damaged. Suturing damaged tissue means more damaged tissue. That is why the surgical techniques that use *"native tissue"* can only be efficient if they are strong enough. This explains the high relapse rates of these techniques.

We believe that in order to be able to accurately assess a surgical technique, it must be known and performed correctly, this way having a correct opinion on the results. For this reason, we preferred to present both the laparoscopic and the vaginal approach, although the two methods have their firm supporters and detractors, so the scientific perspective is strongly divided. Studies conducted so far have not approached a technique in favor of the other, and probably in the years to come will be intensely debated. Pending clear conclusions, we consider that any procedure that results in an improvement of the patient's suffering must be taken into consideration.

7.2. Surgery for anterior compartment

Correction of anterior compartment concerns the functional reconstruction of pubourethral and external urethral ligaments and suburethral fascia. Surgery at this level is the most common, both in classical and alloplastic techniques.

7.2.1. Classical surgical procedures

The history of classical surgical procedures for anterior compartment contains many techniques that have become obsolete with the development of alloplastic materials. Some of them are still used in some cases and in some centers in which there is experience. However, most of them were abandoned, but they have been the base for the development of surgical treatment, sensing the importance of urethral angulation, a hundred years ago, as evidenced by Petros' *Integral Theory* (**Petros PE Papa, 2010**). Even the technique of polyurethane suburethral mesh is derived, from the principles point of view, from techniques of suburethral prosthesis that angulated the urethra. Aldrige surgery uses an aponeurosis fragment of external suburethral oblique muscle, and the Goebbel-Stoeckel technique used a musculoaponeurotic system membrane from the pyramidal muscles and the aponeurosis of the external oblique muscle. Current techniques are mentioned below.

7.2.1.1. Kelly Procedure

It is a correction intervention of cystocele and urethrocele, most often concomitant, which is frequently used in female patients with stress urinary incontinence. Kelly plication of the urethra is designed to reduce its diameter, while the pubovesical fascia plication is intended to support the bladder and the urethra.

Surgical steps

1. The patient is placed in a gynecological position. The vulva, vagina, and perineum are prepared for the surgery, respecting the aseptic and antiseptic measures. Cervix is spotted with a forceps and a transversal incision is made (Crossen incision) at the vaginal mucosa insertion in the cervix. A lot of attention should be paid so that the incision is not too deep, up to the pubocervical fascia, Fig. 7.2. (**Sîrbu P., 1981**).

2. Vaginal mucosa is carefully dissected on the median line, anterior to the pubovesical fascia, up to approximately 1 cm from the urethral meatus. The edges of vaginal mucosa are tensioned by spotting with Chaput tissue grasping forceps. Kelly plication of the urethra is performed at 1 cm from the urethral meatus, classically with non-resorbable "U"-shaped suture along the lateral edges of the urethra, Fig.7.3. The last suture is used at about 2 cm from the vesicourethral angle.

3. Surgery can continue with the pubovesical fascia plication, in case of an associated cystocele, with 0 wires of a slowly resorbable material passed over in the same manner, but carefully, so that they are passed only over the fascia and not over the bladder wall, Fig. 7.4. As in the previous case, the passing over of the wires starts at 1 cm from the urethral meatus.

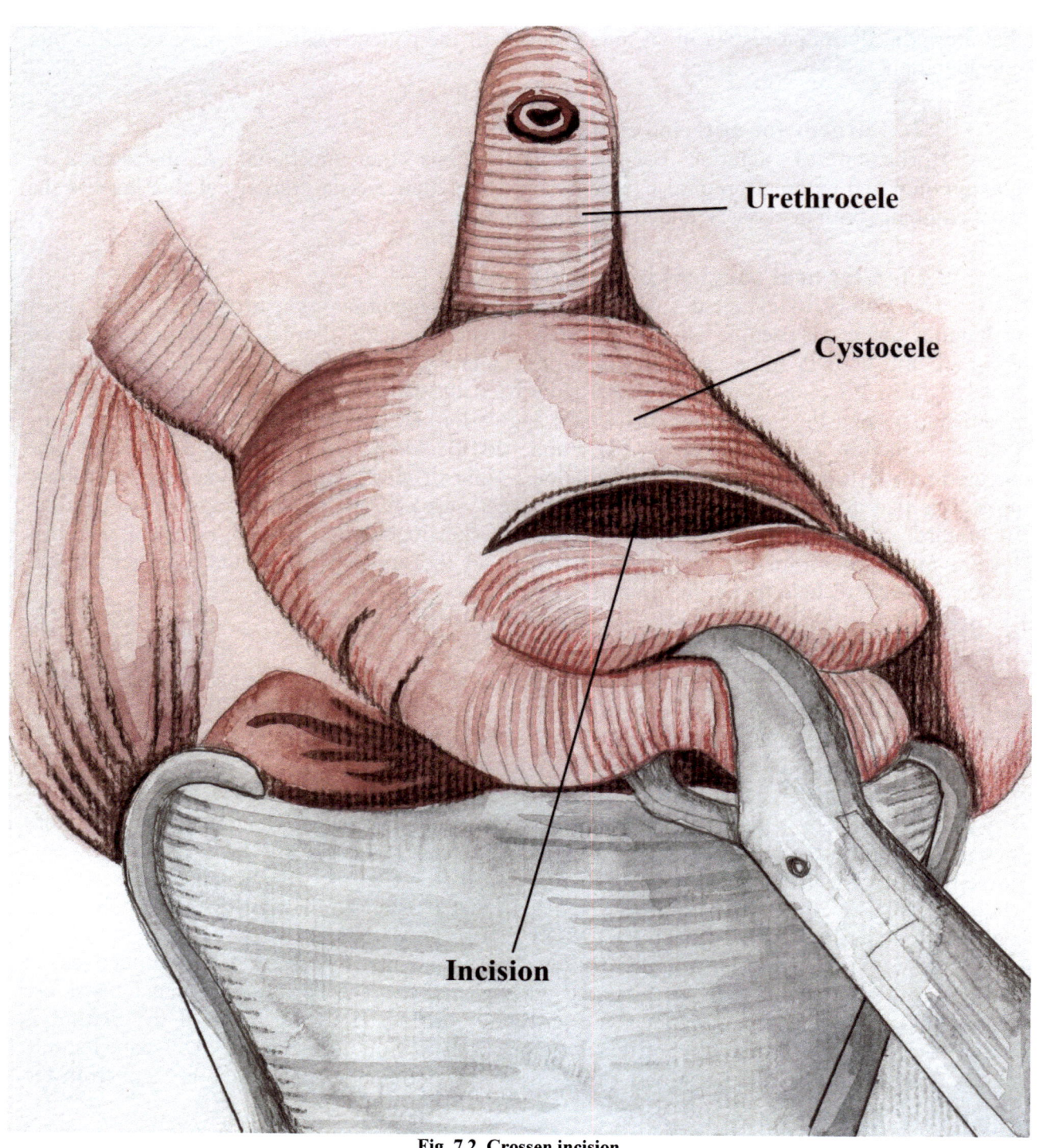

Fig. 7.2. Crossen incision
(*drawing by Vanessa Mureşan*)

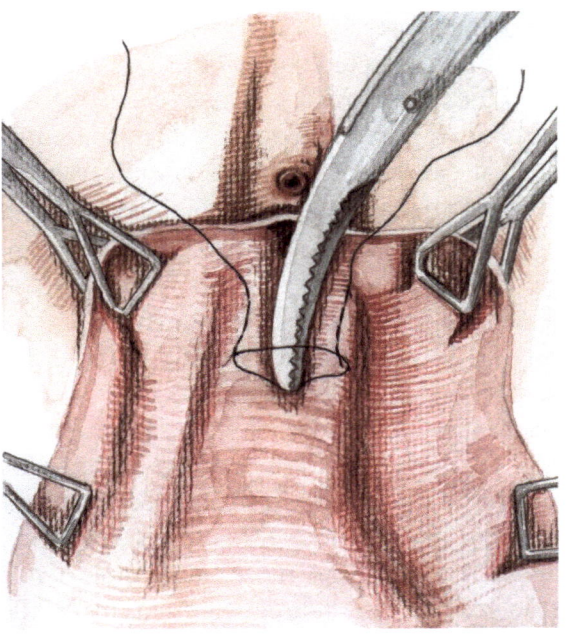

Fig. 7.3. Placing the wire in an "U" shape
(*drawing by Vanessa Mureşan*)

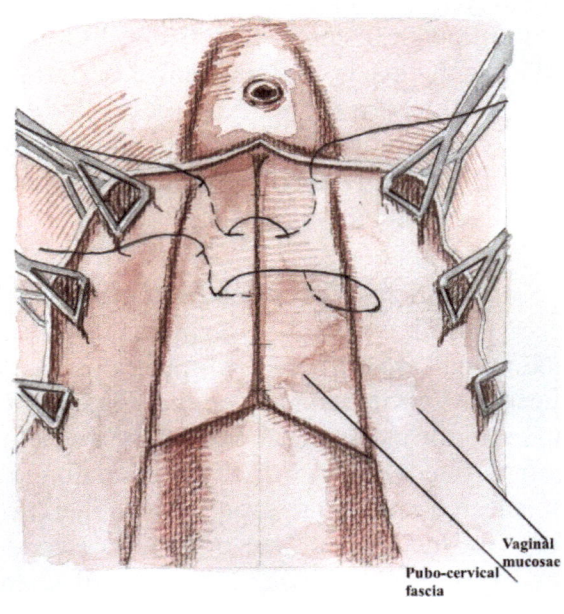

Fig. 7.4. Suture of pubocervical fascia
(*drawing by Vanessa Mureşan*)

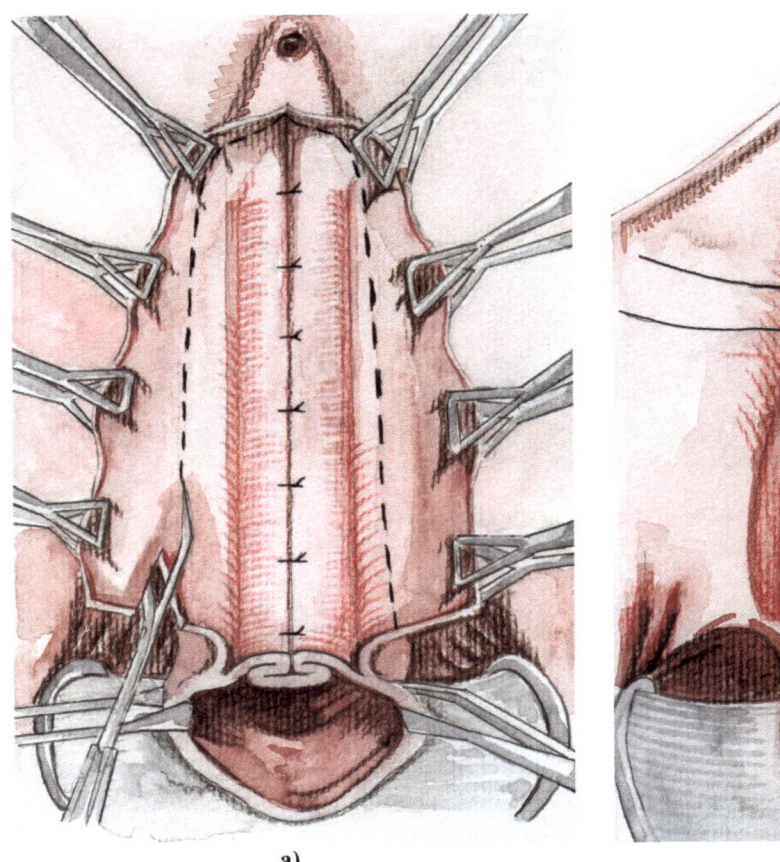
a)

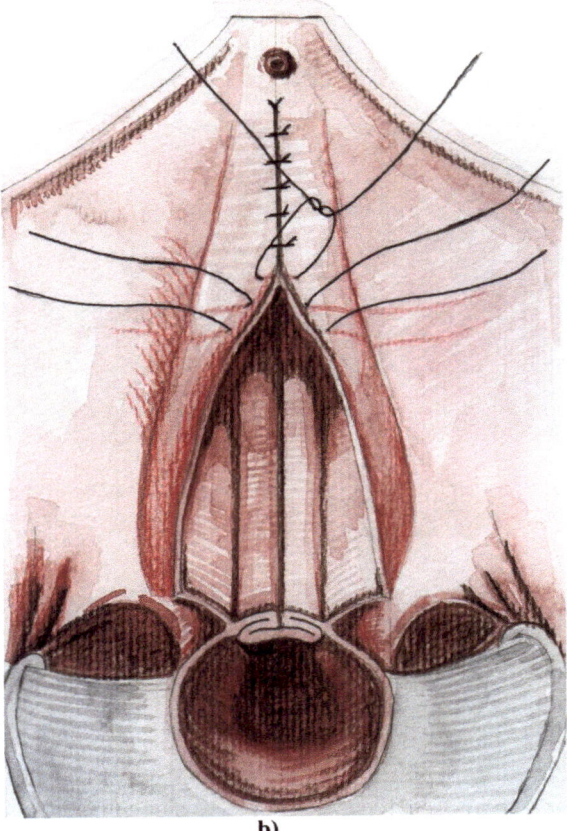
b)

Fig. 7.5. Reducing both the urethrocele and cystocele
(according to **Wheeless C.R.** Jr. *&* **Roenneburg M.L., 2017**)
a) excision of vaginal mucosa fragments, b) suture of remaining mucosa

4. Plication of the fascia is continued until the urethrocele and the cystocele are completely reduced. During the plication, the edges of vaginal mucosa are kept in tension.

Finally, the excess of vaginal mucosa is removed and the edges of vaginal mucosa can be sutured with 0 slowly resorbable suture, separate sutures or interrupted suture, **Fig. 7.5** *a* and *b*. Although this is the classical description of the technique, we consider that excision of the vaginal mucosa should be avoided, this associating with both a greater frequency of dyspareunia and varying degrees of decrease in sexual satisfaction that can lead to anorgasmia (**Petros PE Papa, 2010**). If a Foley catheter has not been installed at the beginning of the surgery, it is finally mounted.

7.2.1.2. Marshal-Marchetti-Kranz Procedure and Burch Procedure

Both types of interventions involve the elevation of the urethrocystic junction in the intra-abdominal area. There are operations that actually change the pressure applied on the urethra during a Valsalva maneuver and do not produce the intraurethral or intravesical pressure changes, and are not indicated in case of cystocele or urethrocele. Of the classical operations for anterior compartment defects, these have a pathogenic correction mechanism, which makes them current in selected situations, even in the context of the existence of alloplastic materials. For example, they are met in multiple operated cases at the suburethral level, where mounting a new mesh involves increased risks and reduced chances of surgical cure. An indirect angulation of the urethra-indirect urethropexy can be attempted with the help of these two techniques.

Surgical steps

1. A Pfannenstiel incision is made and Retzius space is penetrated. The bladder and vesicourethral angle are identified by palpation with the Foley catheter.

The left hand is inserted intravaginal and the periurethral space is identified, where a non-resorbable monofilament suture is passed over (for example Prolene 0) each side, paying attention to the often appreciable bleeding in the Santorini plexus, Fig. 7.6. *a* and *b*.

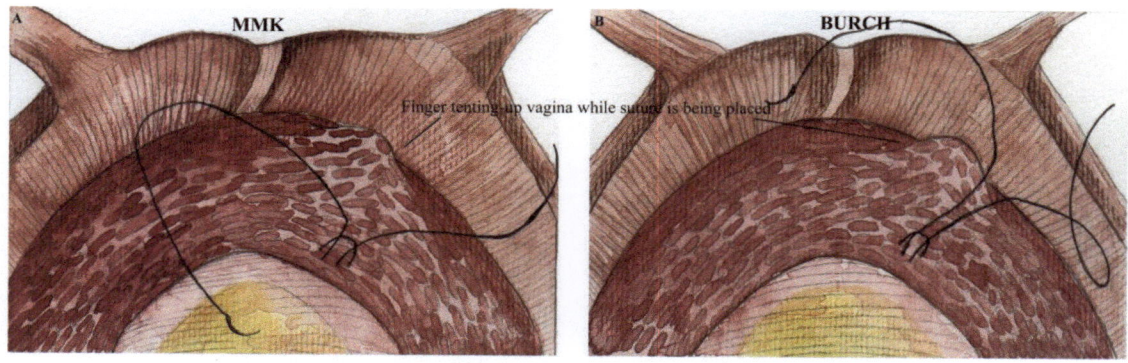

Fig. 7.6. Passing over of the periurethral wire
(*drawing by Vanessa Mureşan*)
A) MMK procedure; B) Burch procedure

2. The next moment, the other end of the wire is anchored. In Fig. 7.7.A (Marshal-Marchetti-Kranz – MMK procedure), the periurethral passed over wire is brought to the pubic symphysis periosteum, while in Fig. 7.7.B (Burch procedure), the wire is brought to Cooper ligament.

3. 1 or 2 wires are passed over each side without being connected. The wires are connected while the anterior vaginal wall is lifted on each side. In MMK procedure, the wires are connected to the symphysis periosteum, while in Burch procedure, the wires are connected by placing a finger between the Cooper ligament and the periurethral tissue, Fig. 7.8. and 7.9.

4. Once the wires have been tied, the retro-symphysis space is checked with the anatomical forceps tail. This remains wide enough if the wires applied on the vaginal wall are placed at least 1 cm outside the median line, otherwise the vaginal suspension may compress the urethra below the pubic symphysis edge and may produce urinary retention postoperatory.

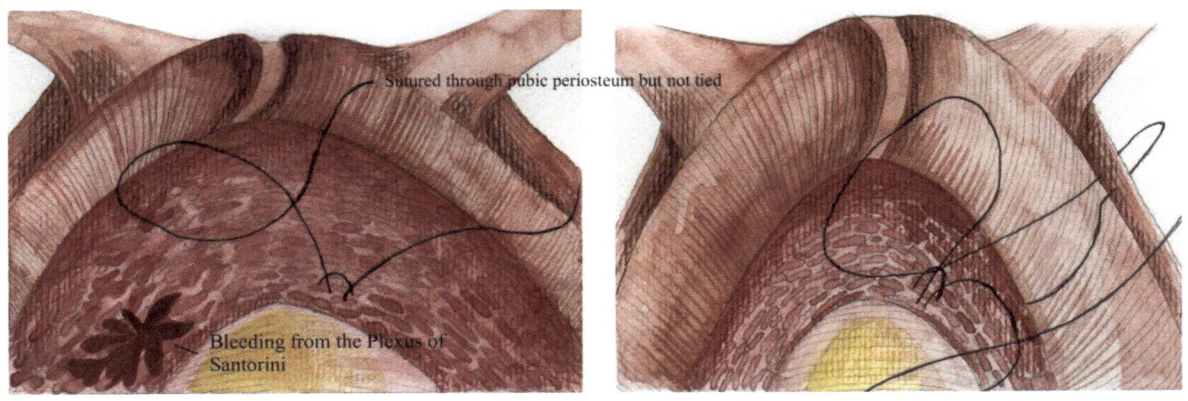

Fig. 7.7. Passing of suture (*drawing by Vanessa Mureşan*)
A – through periosteum of pubic symphysis. B – at the level of Cooper ligament

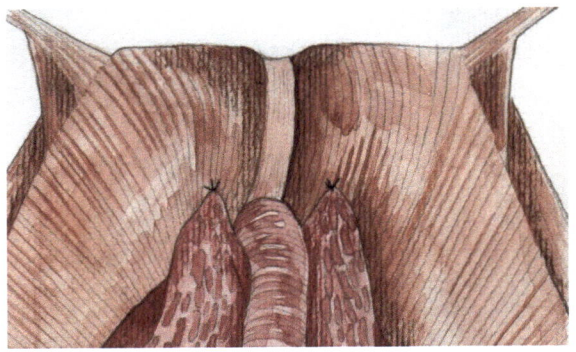

Fig. 7.8. Ligature of sutures using MMK procedure
(*drawing by Vanessa Mureşan*)

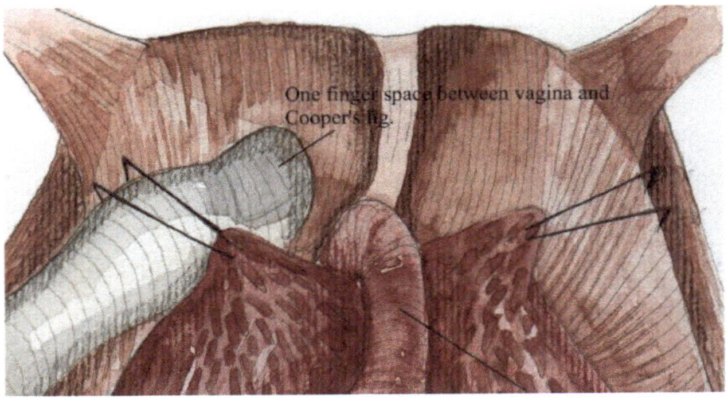

Fig. 7.9. Ligature of sutures using Burch procedure
(*drawing by Vanessa Mureşan*)

7.2.1.3 Direct urethrocystopexy

The procedure is better known as "*Pereyra procedure*" (**Pereyra A.J., 1959**). The procedure is rarely encountered at present; however, there are some centers in which it is still actual. Direct urethrocystopexy involves the anchoring of the urethrocystic junction with 2 non-resorbable sutures to the aponeurosis of the external oblique muscle. Anchoring is done through a digital retropubic tunnel.

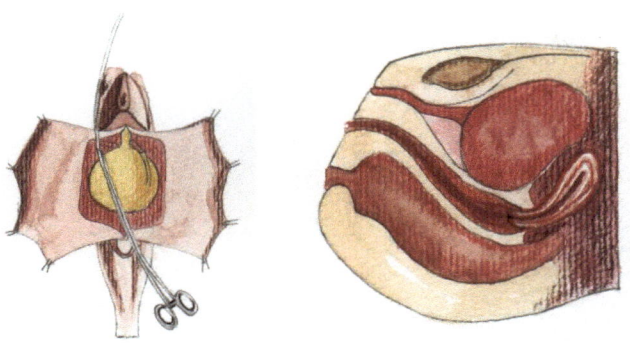

Fig. 7.10. Creating the tunnel in direct urethrocystopexy
(*drawing by Vanessa Mureşan*)

A satisfactory angulation of the urethra is achieved but has the disadvantage of the stiffening of the position of the urethra with a partially obstructive effect, Fig. 7.10.

Surgical steps

1. Although a Crossen incision is classically described, the intervention with a subcutaneous median incision may be initiated up to the urethrocystic junction.

2. Bilateral digital dissection with the realization of a tunnel on each part of the urethra, retro-symphysis, up to the level of the anterior abdominal wall.

3. A non-resorbable suture is passed over at the level of the cystourethral junction and its ends are passed through the previously realized tunnel up to the external oblique muscle aponeurosis. A disadvantage is the difficulty of establishing an optimal tension, with the risk of over-correction, the patient becoming a retentionist.

4. Suture of the vaginal and abdominal tract. Mounting a Foley catheter.

7.2.2. Surgical techniques using alloplastic material

The current trend is to completely replace the classic procedures. Polypropylene slings are used in the surgical correction of the compartment defects. They are 30 to 35 cm long and have a width that varies between 7 and 15 mm. With the aid of the suburethral-mounted sling, the urethral support ligament apparatus can be reconstructed vectorally. The principle of suburethral suspension was inspired by Goebell-Stoeckel procedure in 1917, which used a sling created from the external oblique muscle aponeurosis. Surgery with polypropylene sling softly anchors the medium third of the urethra, thus reconstituting the physiological mechanism of occlusion. There are currently 3 most often used techniques, all using a *vaginal approach* (**Murphy M., 2008**). In the onset of alloplastic techniques, we have often adopted the Goeschen working method that starts with two paramedian longitudinal incisions between which a tunnel is made instead of the classical median longitudinal incision.

7.2.2.1. Retropubic suburethral sling

The retropubic suburethral sling, TVT (Trans Vaginal Tape), is a procedure invented by Petros and Ulmsten in 1988, which involves the insertion of a retropubic suburethral sling with the distal ends, passed through some paramedian buttonholes at the level of external oblique muscle aponeurosis. The ends are then sectioned and left free, thus achieving the *"tension-free"* lax anchoring of the urethra, Fig. 7.11.

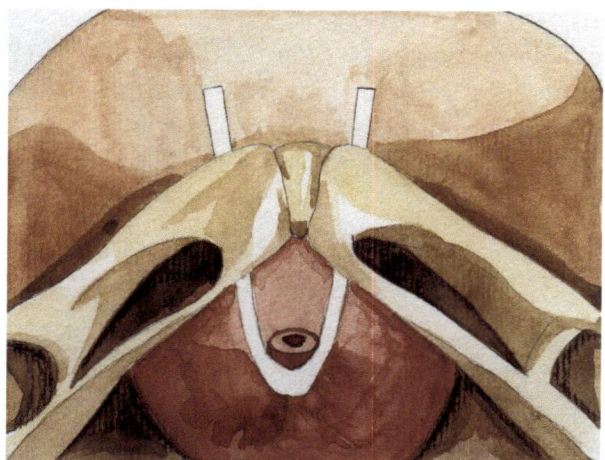

Fig. 7.11. TVT (*drawing by Vanessa Mureşan*)

Surgical steps

1. The procedure starts by making two paramedian longitudinal incisions in the middle third of the urethra and laterally to it, on both sides. The urethra is detected by palpating the catheter, and the optimal area is determined by identifying the balloon corresponding to the bladder neck and by calculating the distance to the external urethral meatus. According to Anglo-Saxon anatomical literature in the lateral part of the vagina where a channel - *sulcus vaginalis,* appears.

2. A transverse tunnel between the two incisions, located between the vaginal mucosa and the urethra, is performed with an Overholt forceps. By the repeated opening of the forceps, a caliber of the tunnel correspondent to the sizes of the mesh is achieved. Urethral lesions may

appear at this level. The medium part of the mesh is inserted in this tunnel, the ends remaining freely externalized at the level of the two incisions.

3. Creating a retropubic tunnel with a *"tunneling"* between the two incisions and the suprapubic abdominal skin. The instrument will cross the Retzius space, the aponeurotic layer, and the subcutaneous tissue. As an additional protective measure, some surgeons prefer the insertion of a stiff catheter through the urethra and into the bladder and its movement contralateral to the side where the *"tunneling"* passes. The ends of the mesh are inserted through these tunnels and they are exposed at the level of skin incisions. The vascular lesions represent the main risk of these surgical steps by snapping *"corona mortis"* or the femoral vein. Although rare, these accidents can have a vital impact.

At the end of these surgical steps, a cystoscopic control is recommended to exclude the bladder wall perforation.

4. Suture of vaginal cuts, best in double layer to avoid erosion. The closing of the first layer bursa with a short surge prevented at the level of vaginal mucosa are practiced. 2/0 resorbable multifilament suture is used.

5. The insertion of 300 ml physiological serum and the verification of bladder continence by tensioning the mesh are achieved. The maneuver is performed with a stiff catheter, possibly a Hegar 8 dilator, inserted into the urethra, to ensure that the mesh does not become obstructive. Surgery is completed by sectioning the free ends at the level of the skin and by its suturing, without including the ends of the mesh in the sutures.

The urinary catheter is usually kept for 48 hour postoperatory to avoid the occurrence of a vesical globus secondary to edema or to possible hematoma. However, there are various recommendations that urinary catheter can be removed starting from two hours after the surgery. Postoperatory evolution is generally favorable, and if properly executed it rarely has recurrences. The patient can be discharged at the latest 72 hours postoperatory.

7.2.2.2. Tissue fixation system for the treatment of stress urinary incontinence

Tissue Fixation System (TFS) is a surgical kit and a technical solution for surgical correction of pelvic floor disorders proposed by Peter Petros. The underlying principle of this tissue fixation system is the anatomical reconstruction of the main ligaments involved in perineal pathology. Neoligaments are formed by the introduction of alloplastic material slings, which by impregnation with collagen become resistant. The kit contains an applicator, and an unexpandable mesh of 7.5 mm width, which has an anchor with a one-way adjustment mechanism attached at its ends. The mesh is made of light macroporous monofilament polypropylene, Fig. 7.12.

The anchor is made of plastic material, its tip being inserted in the tissue, where it remains fixed. There is a system at the base of the anchor that allows the sliding of the mesh in one direction, thus allowing its tensioning and shortening with the reinforcement of the respective ligament. When the applicator is pulled out, the mesh remains fixed in the same position.

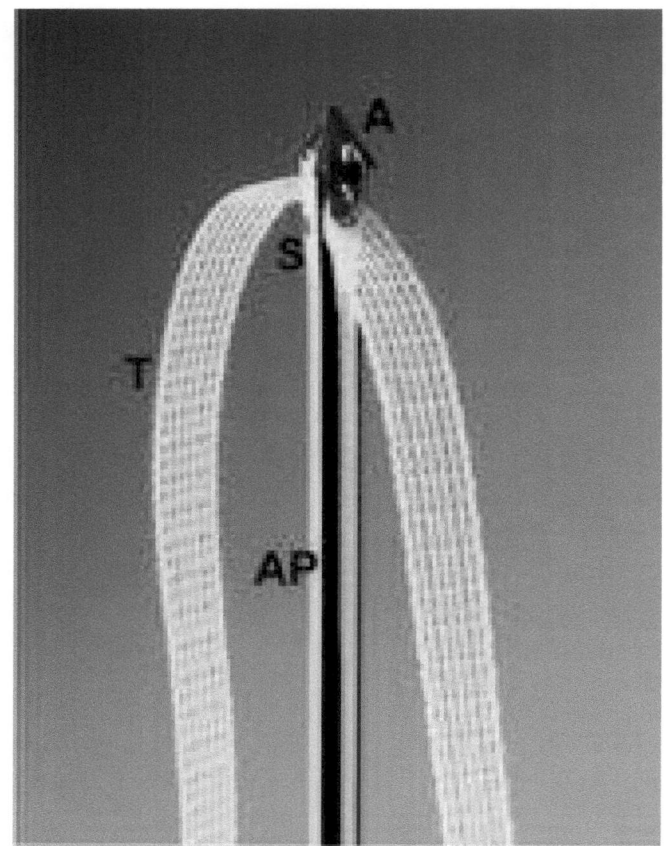

Fig. 7.12. TFS
(according to **Petros P. 2010**)
with the permission of TFS Surgical
AP – applicator; T – tape; A – anchor; S – system of tape tensioning

This system is intended for the reconstruction of 5 ligaments: pubourethral ligaments, arcus tendineus fasciae pelvis, cardinal ligaments, uterosacral ligaments and perineal body. TFS applies only to the level at which a ligament deficit is found. The anchor is inserted into the ligament or adjacent to it. Following the conjunctive reaction, a structure is created that will take over the affected ligament function Fig. 7.13.

By the anchoring type, TFS establishes a minimum contact with the vaginal wall, being applied transversely. The advantage is that it does not influence the movements of the vaginal membrane in the anterior-posterior direction, movements that are essential for the opening, closing and tensioning of the bladder and rectum, Fig. 7.14. and 7.15.

The restoration of the pubourethral and external urethral ligaments is important for the correction of the anterior compartment. Peter Petros described the following surgical steps.

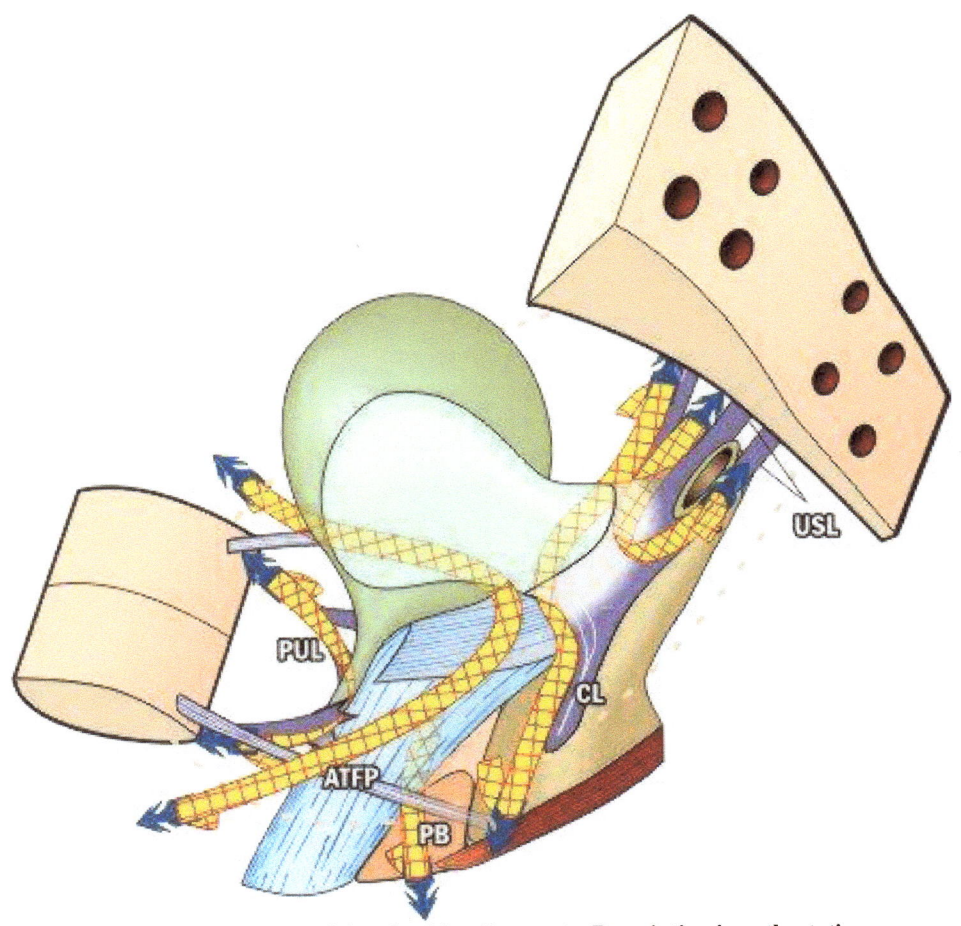

Fig. 7.13. TFS in repairing the 5 key ligaments. Description in orthostatism
(according to **Petros P.**, 2010)
PUL – pubourethral ligaments; ATFP – arcus tendineus fasciae pelvis, CL – cardinal ligaments; USL – uterosacral ligaments; PB – perineal body

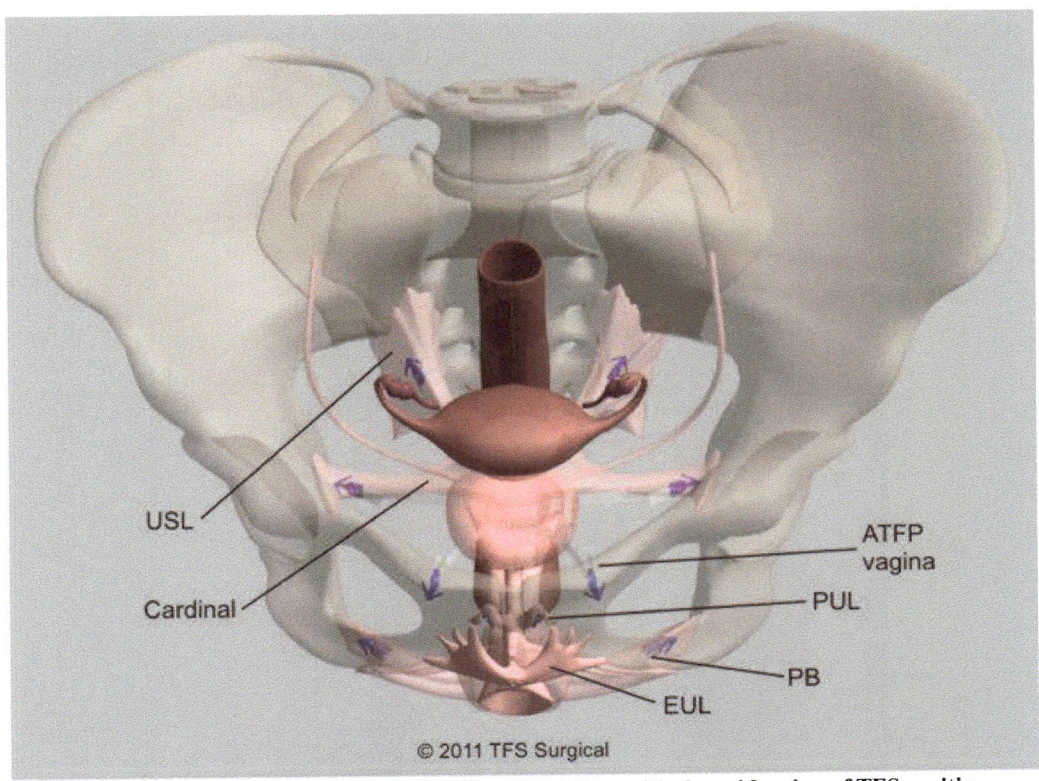

Fig. 7.14. 3D overview of the pelvis in orthostatism with the evidencing of TFS position
(with the permission of TFS Medical)
PUL – pubourethral ligaments; ATFP – arcus tendineus fasciae pelvis; Cardinal – cardinal ligaments; USL – uterosacral ligaments; PB – perineal body; EUL – external urethral ligaments

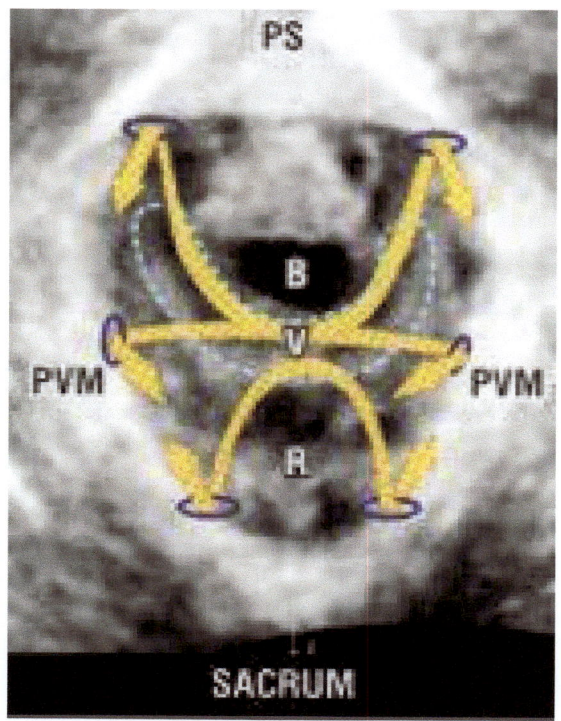

Fig. 7.15. View of the pelvis from cranial position with the cross-sectional orientation of the TFS
(according to **Petros P., 2010**)
PS – pubis, B – bladder, V – vagina, R – rectum, PVM – pubovisceral muscle (levator hiatus)

Surgical steps

1. A median, urethral-centered incision, approximately 2 cm long, starting from 5 mm of the urethral meatus is performed.

2. Dissection with dissection scissors is performed retropubically in the direction of the ipsilateral shoulder until a perineal membrane resistance is encountered. A perforation of the membrane of about 1.5-2 cm is done with the dissection scissors on the index guide.

3. The applicator is inserted on the index guide, or if the space is too narrow, on the scissors guide. Tissue is penetrated with the tip of the anchor and the way it was fixed is verified. Once the anchor is firmly attached, the applicator is removed and the same procedure is repeated contralateral, Fig. 7.16.

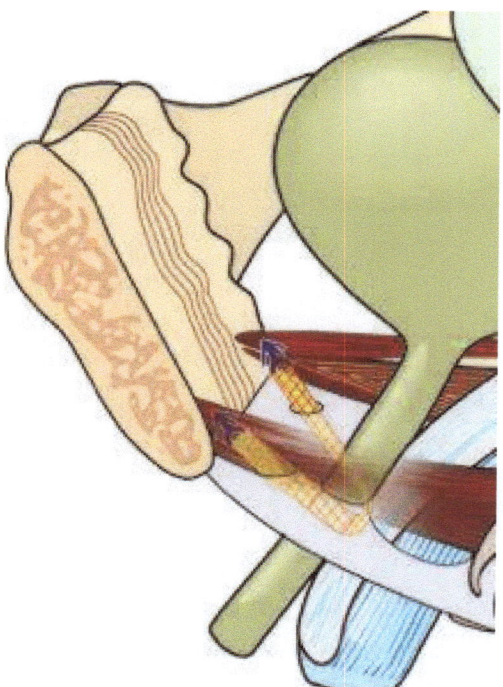

Fig. 7.16. Repairing pubourethral ligaments by TFS
(according to **Petros P. 2010**)

4. A Hegar 8 dilator is inserted into the urethra and then the mesh is tensioned so that it does not become obstructive. Tensioning is done until a resistance is detected.

5. The bladder is filled with fluid and a control cystoscopy is performed to ensure that there is no bladder perforation. If after cystoscope extraction, fluid leakage is still observed, it means that the mesh is too wide. Hegar dilator is reinserted and the mesh is recalibrated. It should never be tightened without cauterization of the urethra with a dilator. The moment the position of the mesh is considered final, the applicator is removed, and it remains fastened.

6. Suture of the vaginal cut with separate wires is performed.

In addition to this procedure, *reconstruction of external urethral ligaments*, meaning of distal occlusion mechanism, can also be performed. This procedure is complementary to the one described above and is performed during the same Surgical steps, through the same incision.

Surgical steps

1. A Foley catheter of 18fr is inserted.

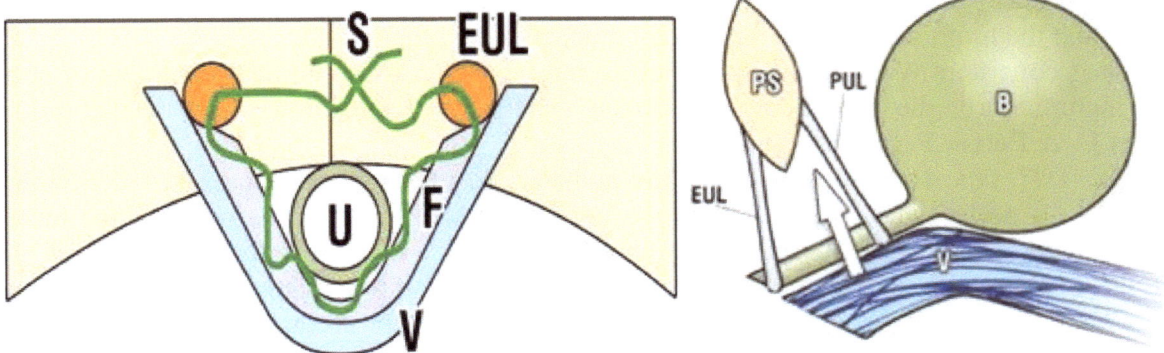

Fig. 7.17. Repairing the external urethral ligaments
(according to **Petros P., 2010**)
EUL – external urethral ligaments; U – urethra;
F – urethrovaginal fascia; V – vagina

Fig. 7.18. Correction mechanism of pubourethral and external urethral ligaments
(according to **Petros P., 2010**)
EUL – external urethral ligaments; PUL – pubourethral ligaments; PS – pubis; V – vagina; B – bladder

2. A continuous suture is performed, which passes through the two external urethral ligaments and the urethrovesical fascia, Fig. 7.17. The knot is gently tensioned.

3. Suture of vaginal mucosa.

The final goal of surgical reconstruction is the restoration of the normal position of the urethra, by pushing it backwards and achieving the effort urinary retention, Fig 7.18.

The patient can be discharged the same day.

Results after TFS.

Sekiguchi reported a 91% success rate using local anesthesia (**Sekiguchi Y.**, *et al.*, **2009**). In a randomized trial, Sivaslioglu reported a 89% success rate for TFS and 78% for TOT. There were no significant complications in the TFS group, except for an anchor movement case (**Sivaslioglu A.A.**, *et al.*, **2012**).

7.2.2.3. Transobturator suburethral tape

1. History and concept of suburethral tape

In 1998, during the first days of the development of TOT ("Transobturator Tape"), a suburethral fascia was created using a synthetic material mesh, suspended on one side and the other of the urogenital hiatus, anchored to the inner edge of the levator ani muscle, mimicking the natural suburethral fascia. Initially, the tape was only sutured to the inner obturator muscle fascia on either side of the urethra and only later was inserted through the obturator fossa in the form of a non-tensioned structure, similar to the retropubic tape.

In accordance with Petro' work (**Petros P., 2007**), the tape should be placed immediately below the middle third of the urethra, away from the bladder neck. The anatomical description of the obturator fossa demonstrates the absence of nervous, vascular, and visceral structures lower from the levator ani muscle insertion on the inner side of the internal obturator muscle. The device was inserted by OUT-IN method and Delmas' anatomical studies, followed by the ones of Spinosa, confirmed that this route is safer than the IN-OUT one. The most difficult part was to find a method by which the tape does not slip towards the bladder neck and remain at the medium third of the urethra. The technique described for the first time in 2001 (**Delorme E., 2001**), has not yet been perfected, and the follow-up of the patients revealed two erosions of the bladder by the tape and 3 patients who suffered from urethral obstruction due to the fact that the tape was leaning against the bladder neck: they complained of urinary urge, recurrent urinary infections and bladder emptying dysfunction. Further anatomical studies have led to the choice of the safest and most efficient ways to insert TOT. This safe procedure can be called horizontal TOT or retropubic TOT. In the following, we will describe this procedure: OUT-IN horizontal TOT. First results of horizontal TOT with a 1 to 3 year follow-up have confirmed the efficiency in treating incontinence and low morbidity (**Castaing T. & Abello D.E., 2012**).

The concept of transobturator tape combines the principles outlined above and the clinical experience:

- reproduces the position and orientation of the suburethral fascia covering the urogenital hiatus, behind the urethra, from one puborectal muscle to the other.

- it is consistent with the theory of Petros and Ulmsten on the surgical treatment of stress urinary incontinence, the tape being positioned exactly at the medium third of the urethra (**Ulmsten U. & Petros P., 1995**).

The TOT tape is held in place by the aponeurotic muscular structures of the obturator foramen. It is a perineal procedure. The procedure takes place in the space between the levator ani muscle fascia, cranial, perineal membrane, inferior, obturator foramen, lateral and paraurethral space with the medial urethra, Fig. 20 and 21. This anatomical space does not contain vascular, nervous, or visceral structures. The transobturator urethral tape is more lax than the retropubic one.

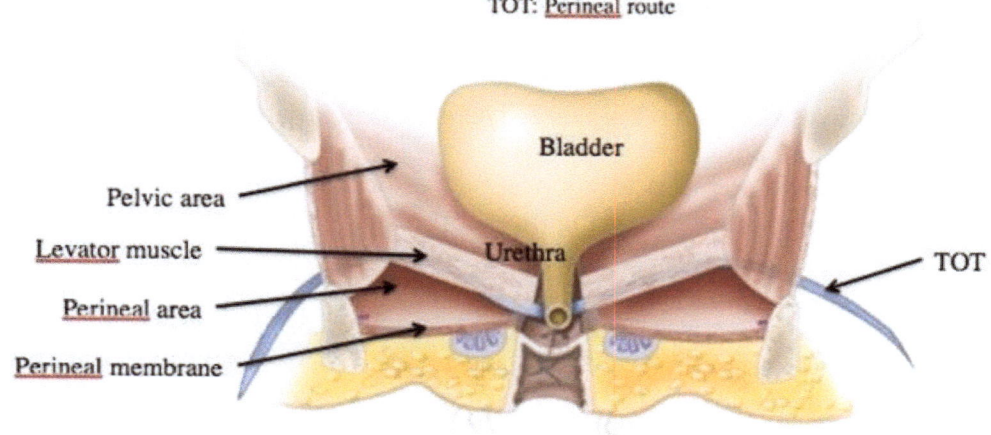

Fig. 7.20. Anatomical overview of the TOT tape placement in the perineal space (Delorme E.)

It has 2 advantages. Risk of visceral injury, bladder, digestive structures; vascular, Santorini vesical venous plexus, iliofemoral and neurological vessels, obturator and pudendal nerves, is reduced (**Latthe PM., 2008**). Furthermore, the transobturator urethral suspension is theoretically less susceptible to cause urethral obstruction than the retropubic suspension, but TOT still seems less effective in the treatment of urinary incontinence due to sphincter deficiency (**Rechberger T.**, *et al.,* **2009**; **Myung-Jae J.**, *et a.,* **2008**).

2. Anatomy

The first anatomical studies published or communicated about TOT are essentially based on Delmas' work (**Delmas V., 2003**; **Delmas V., 2002**). Anatomical structures of the obturator foramen, from superficially to deep, are represented by the large adductor muscle, external obturator, obturator membrane and the internal obturator muscle. On its median side, the obturator foramen is divided into two parts by the parietal insertion of levator ani muscle. The upper part, above the levator insertion line, is located in the pelvic subperitoneal space. At this level, at the superolateral angle, there is the obturator tunnel that is crossed by the obturator pedicle. The lower part of the obturator foramen borders the perineal space. The levator ani muscle cranially delimits the perineal space, which is also delimited inferiorly by the perineal membrane and laterally from backwards to downwards by the ischiopubic ramus and the internal obturator muscle, the median limit being the urethra and the periurethral space. This perineal space does not contain vascular, nervous, or visceral structures. The tape should be placed in this space. In the perineal area of the obturator foramen there are only two anatomical structures subjected to a certain risk during tape insertion.

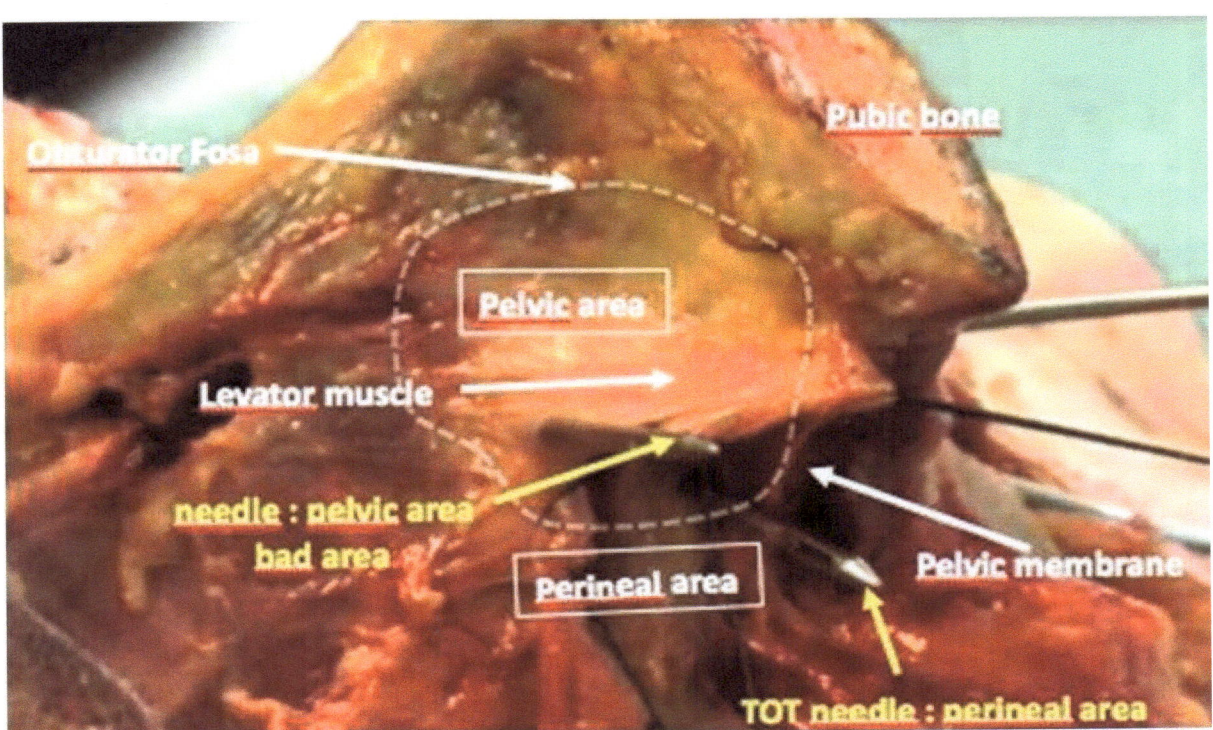

Fig. 7.21. Anatomical aspect in cadaver regarding the placement of TOT tape in the perineal space (Delorme E.)

The first structure is the urethra, which must be identified and protected during the passage of the tunneling instrument.

The second structure is the pudendal pedicle and especially its terminal branch, the dorsal nerve of the clitoris. This nerve follows the median angle of the ischiopubic ramus from downwards to backwards. During the OUT-IN passage of the instrument, the ischiopubic ramus protects the pudendal nerve. The root of the thigh can be found lateral from the obturator fossa, where the two terminal branches of the obturator nerve are located. The anterior branch is far away from the area in which TOT is inserted, but the posterior branch is much deeper than the previous one and closer to the TOT tape trajectory. Therefore, the tape must be mounted as close as possible to the ischiopubic ramus (**Spinosa J.P.,** *et al., * **2005**).

The goal of the horizontal or retropubic TOT is the safety, Fig. 7.22. In case of horizontal TOT, the tape is located at the medium third of the urethra, so that there is no risk of it sliding towards the bladder neck. The needle inserted through the OUT-IN method should be horizontal, behind the pubis, and not oblique. Many surgeons use an oblique approach for the insertion of TOT tape, Fig. 7.22. The oblique path transverses the lateral tunnel of the urethra, increasing the risk of vaginal erosion. The oblique path is directed toward the bladder neck and not the medium third of the urethra. This increases the risk of bladder damage or malposition of the tape so that it closes the bladder. This may induce micturition disorders or urge incontinence.

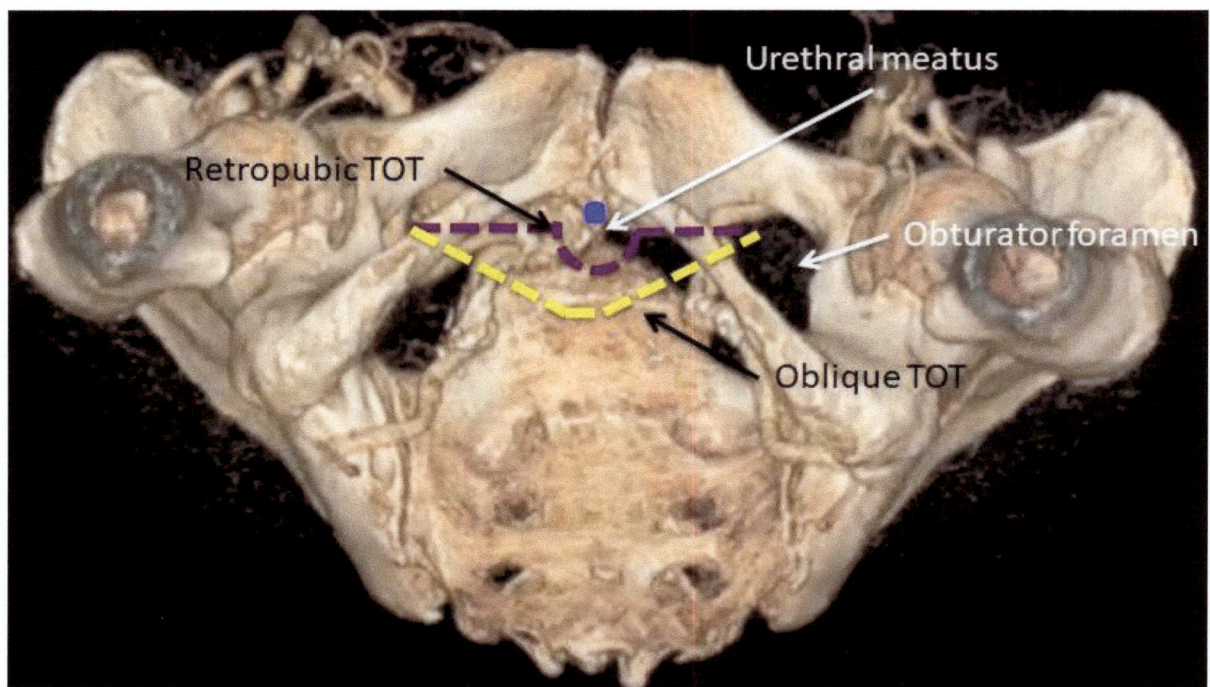

Fig. 7.22. Anatomy of pelvis in MRI: retropubic and oblique trajectory of TOT tapes (Delorme E.)

The tape is held in the correct position by two mechanisms, Fig. 7.23.:
- the trajectory is horizontal, crossing the obturator muscles and pointing towards the downwards side of the pubis;
- the needle punctures the perineal membrane lateral from the urethra and near the urethral meatus. At the same point, the retropubic tape punctures the perineal membrane.

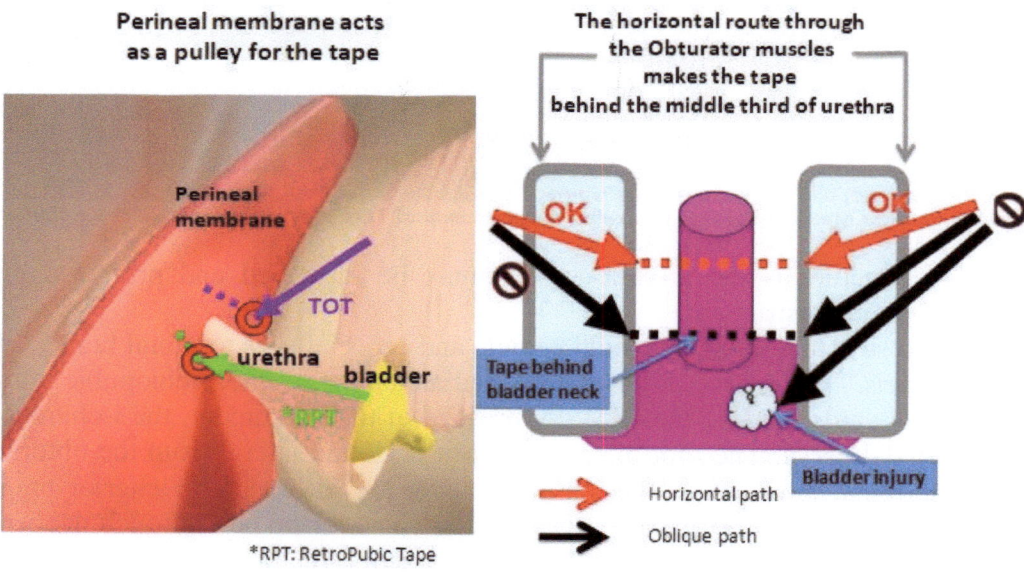

Fig. 7.23. Retropubic trajectory and report of the tape with the perineal membrane (Delorme E.)

This procedure reduces the risk of classical complications described by TOT classical procedure, Fig. 7.24.:
- pain at the root of the thigh and injury to the rear branch of the terminal part of the obturator nerve;
- vaginal erosion lateral from the urethra;
- bladder damage;
- tape malposition at the bladder neck level.

The RETRO-PUBIC TOT route DECREASE THE RISK OF COMPLICATIONS

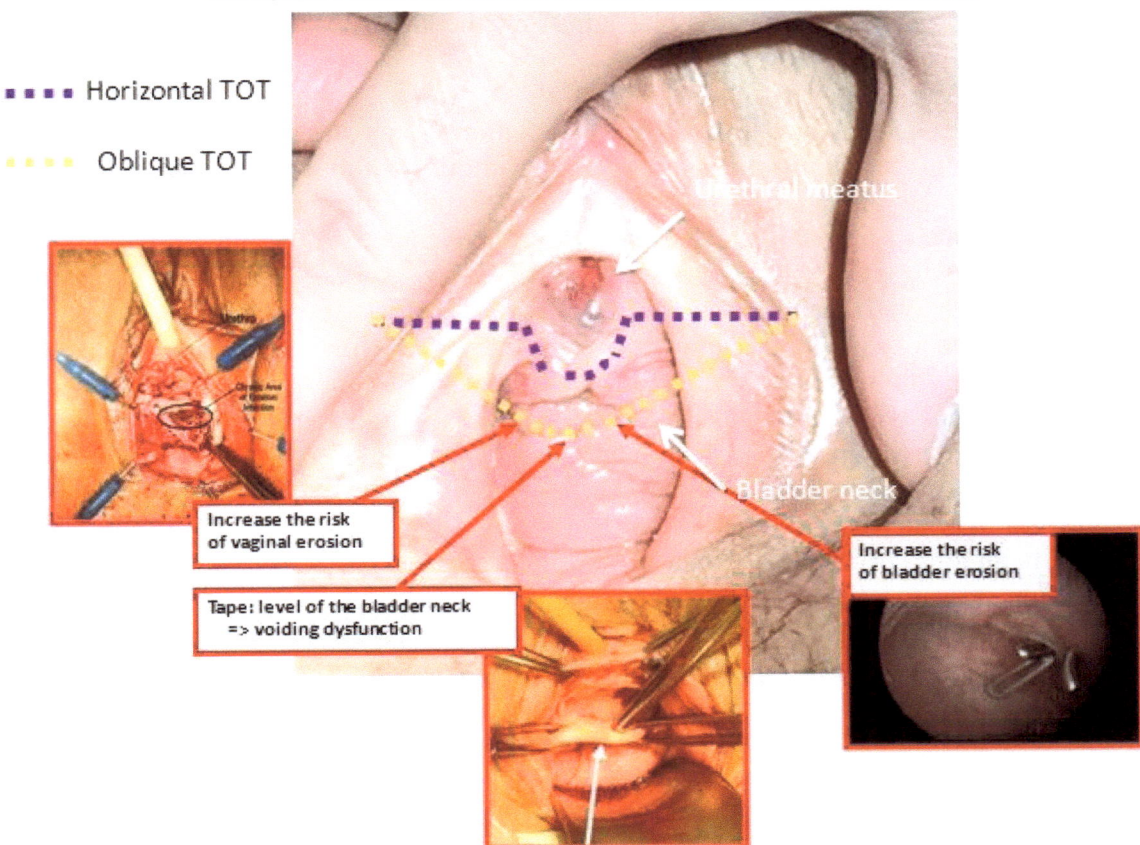

Fig. 7.24. Risk of complications related to oblique path (Delorme E.)

3. Surgical procedure, tunneling instrument with exterior-interior approach

a) Alloplastic material and surgical instruments

The tunneling instrument is a needle with a functional part designed in the form of a special dimension curve, provided with a fastening system that allows the pulling of a tape through the obturator foramen. There are many types of tunneling instruments with different systems for fixing the tape at the top. The tape is usually made of polypropylene embroidered monofilament. Tapes are either highly elastic, requiring a plastic sheath for insertion, or have low elasticity so that no plastic sheath is required.

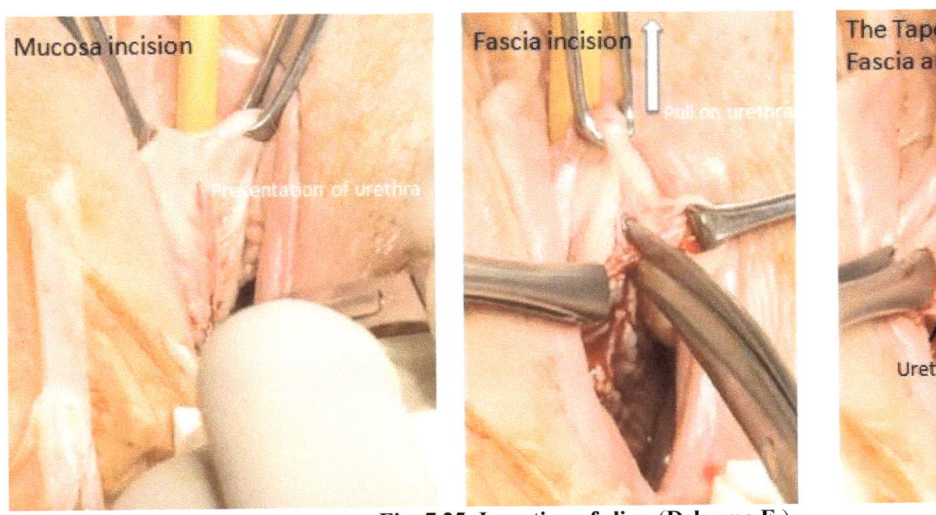

Fig. 7.25. Insertion of sling (Delorme E.)

a) incision of vaginal mucosa *b)* incision of fascia *c)* correct placement of sling

c) Anesthesia

All types of anesthesia are possible; adjusting the final position of the tape does not require the patient's participation.

c) Patient positioning

The patient is placed in a gynecological position. A position in which the thighs are moderately flexed on the trunk is also acceptable without additional risks, since through the OUT-IN technique, the blind passage of the needle of the instrument is very short and the markers do not change their position according to thigh movements.

d) Surgical steps

1) Catheterization of the urethra is started to reduce the risk of urethral injury.

2) Vaginal mucosa is spotted with two Allis tissue forceps, on both sides of the meatus, so that it expands widely under the urethra. The incision starts at 5 mm from the urinary meatus. It is a retro-urethral incision comprising the whole thickness of the vaginal wall, which must be wide enough to allow the insertion of the surgeon's finger Fig. 7.25.*a*. The lateral dissection starts from the urethra and must be between the fascia and the urethra, never between the fascia and the mucosa, as it increases the risk of vaginal erosion, Fig. 7.25.*b* and *c*. Dissection stops at the perineal membrane, because at this level, the needle of the instrument will act as a pulley, directing the tape towards the medium third of the urethra, Fig. 7.23.

3) A cutaneous incision is applied at the level of the horizontal line that passes through the clitoris and intersects with the external edge of the ischiopubic ramus. Usually, a straight needle is used, but it is also possible that a helicoidal transobturator needle is used. The instrument's trajectory is obtained by directing it towards the urinary meatus, Fig. 7.26. A finger is inserted as a sentinel at the level of the previously realized tunnel. However, the finger is located on the posterior side of the pubis, thus the perineal membrane being respected. The index placed on the vaginal incision has the role of protecting the urethra from the needle by pushing it towards backwards, upwards, and medially.

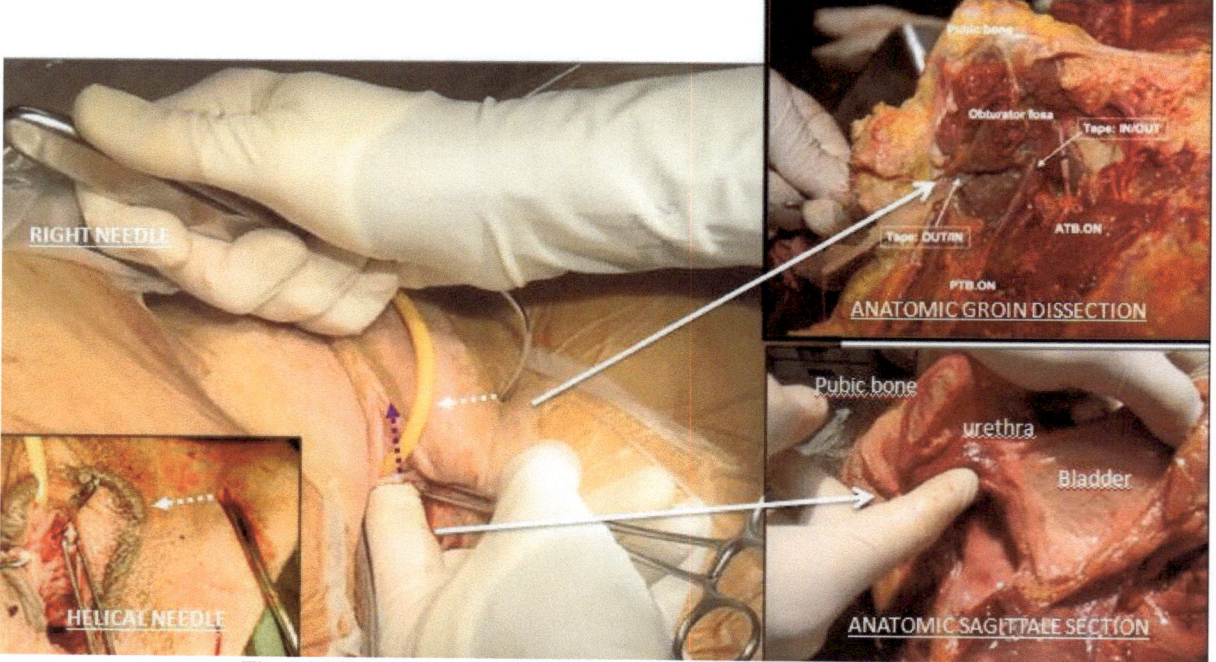

Fig. 7.26. Procedure of insertion of transobturator needle (Delorme E.)

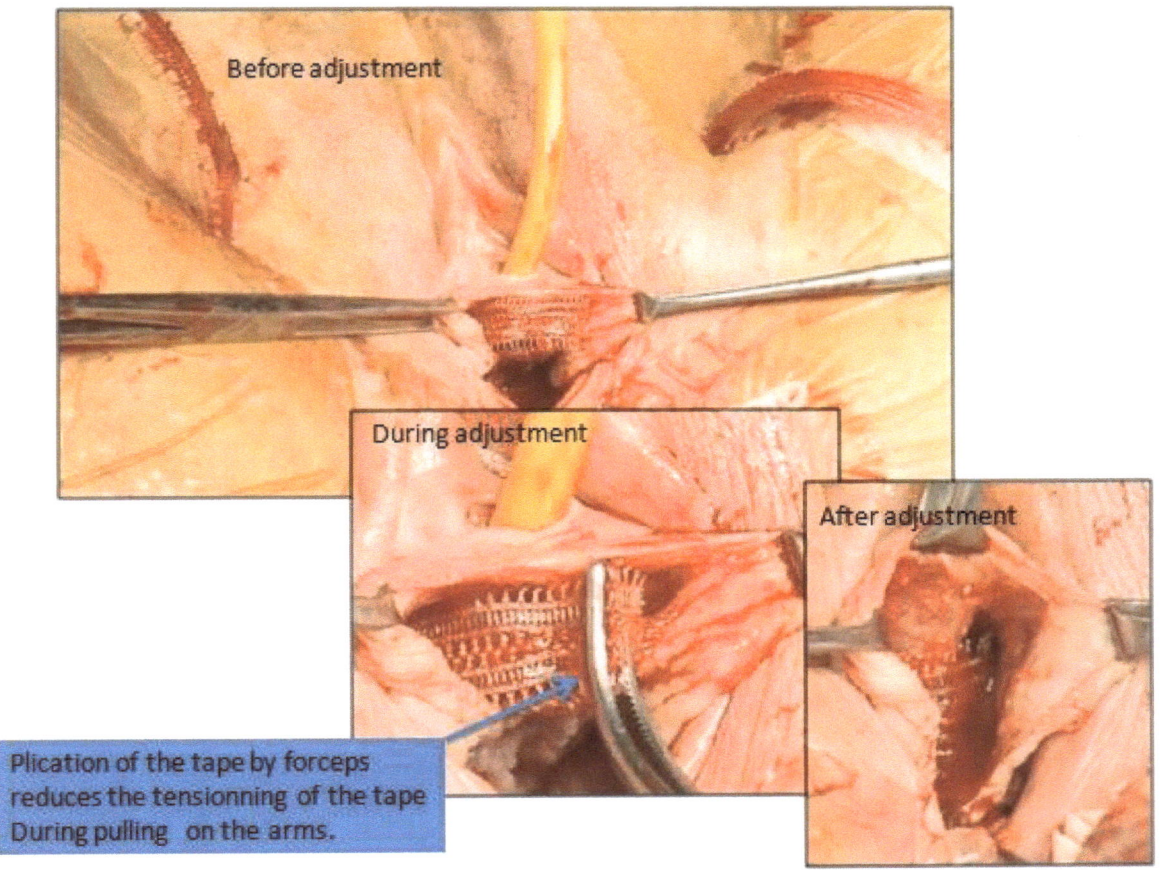

Fig. 7.27. **Calibration of TOT tape** (low-elasticity sling) (**Delorme E.**)

4) The horizontal tunneling path of the instrument is done in 3, Fig. 7.26.

The first step is the intimate contact of the tip of the instrument with the ischiopubic ramus and the following of the bone structure from the inner side.

Step 2 takes into account the moment the needle leaves the bone surface, needle direction suddenly changes in intimate contact with the tip of the finger that is on the inner side of the pubis and not laterally under the ischiopubic ramus. The blind trajectory of the needle is very short, only from the moment it leaves the bone surface and encounters the surgeon's finger. During this trajectory, the obturator muscles are punctured.

Step 3 takes into account that the needle is pushed through the perineal membrane towards the vaginal incision by the surgeon's finger. The needle of the instrument punctures the perineal membrane laterally from the urethra, in a sharp angle, between the ischiopubic ramus and the urethra, so that is reaches the median third of the urethra.

This maneuver is to trace the trajectory of the instrument to the perineal level to remain inferior to the levator ani muscle fascia and to reach the lateral side of the urethra, in the medium third.

Once the maneuver is performed, it is advisable to check the integrity of the vaginal mucosa, so that the tip of the instrument did not puncture it. The end of the tape is fixed by the tip of the instrument, and, by its retraction, the mesh reaches the intended position.

5) The adjustment and tensioning of the suburethral tape is difficult and depends on its elasticity. There is no easy and reproducible technique to propose. The only advice is to always use the same type of tape. In the case of a slightly elastic tape, a visible space should be left between it and the urethra, Fig. 7.27. A very elastic tape should be placed as close to the urethra as possible, but not to be tensioned.

The excess mesh at the level of the skin is cut off. Skin incisions are sutured with some resorbable sutures. The obturator incisions should not be sutured, but care should be taken to separate skin from the tape. If the incisions are small and vertical, they will tend to close naturally when the lower limbs are brought back horizontally at the end of the procedure. The suture material can induce a kind of discomfort. The vaginal mesh is not required.

e) Postoperatory care

The urinary catheter is removed at the end of the procedure or the next day after it. The post micturition residue is measured by ultrasound or by cystoscopy. If there is no significant post micturition residue, which usually happens, the patient can be discharged.

As a result, it can be stated that the technique of inserting a transobturator tape, OUT-IN procedure, although simple, must follow the surgical steps accurately.

For the safety of the intervention, the surgical technique should consider the following steps:

- the vaginal incision must be deep to ensure a dissection in the anatomical plane between the urethra and the retro urethral fascia;

- the trajectory of the tunneling instrument should be directed towards the medium third of the urethra: this being achieved by pointing the tip to the urethral meatus until it can be palpated with the tip of the index finger of the surgeon on the posterior side of the pubis; the tip is in horizontal position.

- the tunneling instrument should remain in contact with the ischiopubic ramus during the maneuver.

- the tip of the index finger should be inserted at the level of the vaginal incision to protect the urethra and then to accompany the tip of the instrument towards the vaginal incision.

Technique for oblique TOT suburethral tape

Hereinafter we present the oblique variant of mounting a TOT-type transobturator suburethral tape. One of the surgeon's concerns should be to prevent the movement of the tape backwards and cranial, by translation, thus avoiding the occurrence of the syndrome of tethered vagina. Even though the technique described above limits this movement, we present the artifice associated to the oblique translation technique to avoid this shortcoming. It involves two paramedian incisions and the creation of a tunnel between the two, so that there are no spaces for movement, Fig. 7.28. (**Frohme C.,** *et al.,* **2014**; **Petros P., 2010**). The technical artifice was invented by Klaus Goeschen, as a modification of the original technique of Emmanuel Delorme (**Delorme E.., 2001**).

Surgical steps

1. It starts by making two paramedian longitudinal incisions in the area of the medium third of the urethra and laterally to it, on both sides. The urethra is observed by palpating the urinary catheter, and the optimal area is determined by identifying the balloon corresponding to the bladder and by calculating the distance to the external urethral meatus.

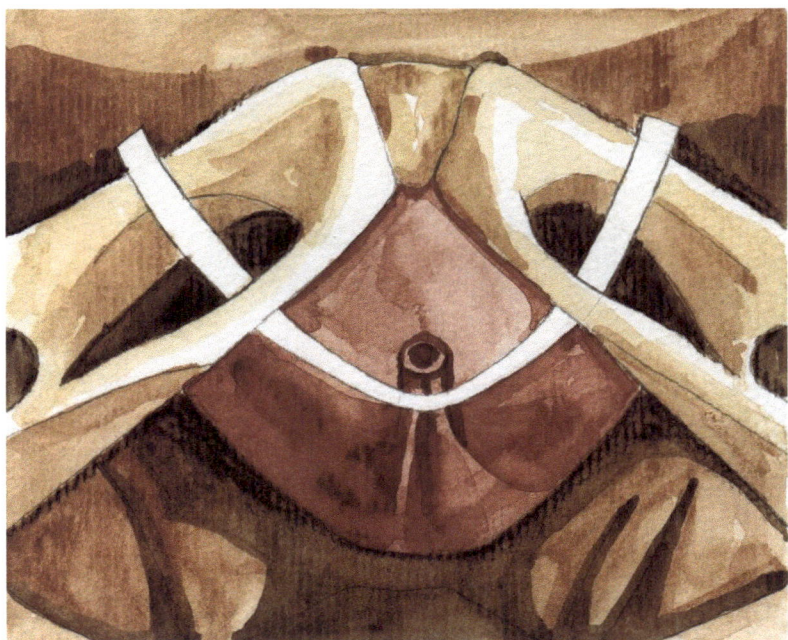

Fig. 7.28. TOT (*drawing by Vanessa Mureşan*)

According to Anglo-Saxon anatomy literature, incisions are made in the lateral side of the vagina, where a channel, *sulcus vaginalis*, appears.

2. Realization of a transverse tunnel between the two incisions, located between the vaginal mucosa and the urethra, by using an Overholt hemostatic forceps. By the repeated opening of the forceps, the size of the channel is determined, correspondent to the size of the tape. Urethral lesions may occur at this level. The medium part of the tape is inserted in this tunnel, the ends remaining freely exteriorized at the level of the two incisions, Fig. 7.29. (**Petros P., 2007**).

3. Bilateral lateral digital dissection is performed while highlighting the internal side of the ischiopubic ramus, its superior external edge, up to the internal obturator muscle fascia. On the internal side of the internal obturator muscle, towards the medial angle of the obturator foramen, a thickening of the homonymous fascia can be palpated, which is represented by „*arcus tendineus fasciae pelvis*", Fig. 7.30. (**Spinosa J.P., 2005**).

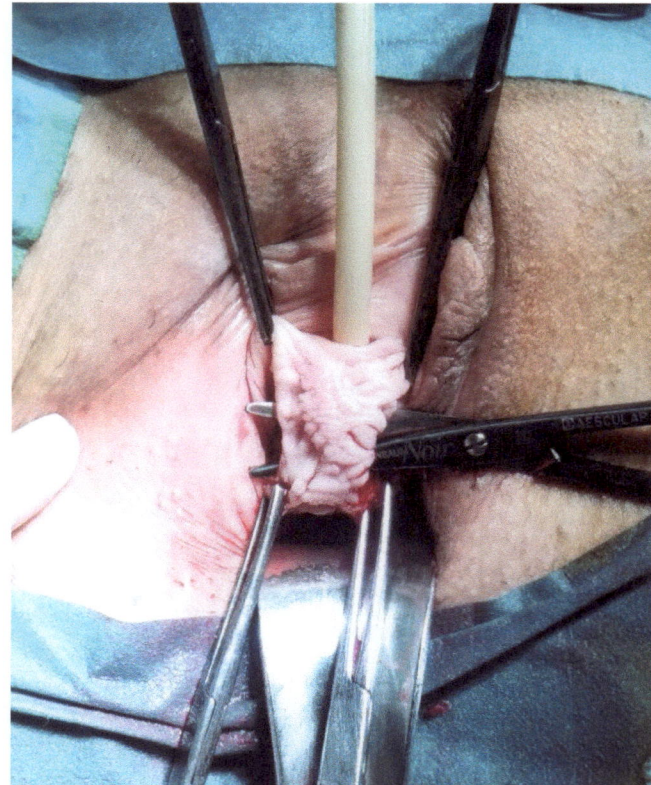 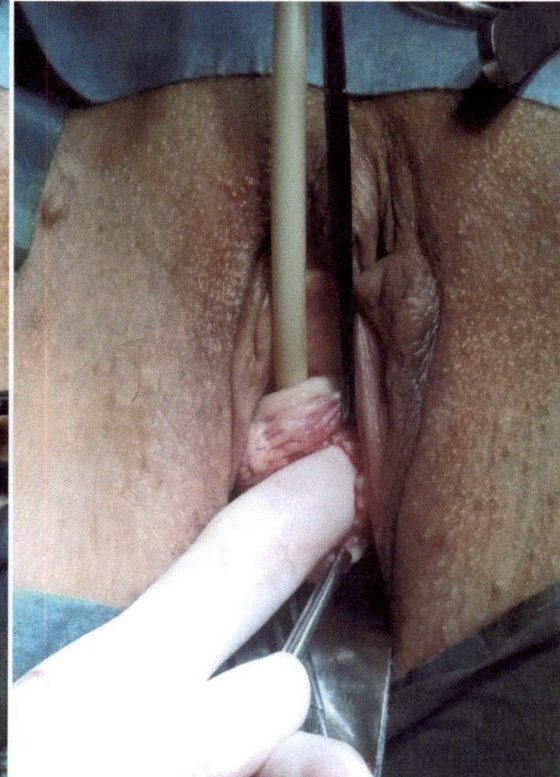

Fig. 7.29. Realizing the transverse tunnel between the 2 paramedian incisions (from the archive of **Enache A.**)

Fig. 7.30. Paramedian incision and lateral digital dissection towards the internal side of internal obturator muscle (from the archive of **Enache A.**)

4. An incision is made bilateral, at the level of the skin, at 2-3 cm lateral from the clitoris knee and at 1.5 cm lower from the origin tendon of the long adductor muscle. The instrument that the helix obturation membrane will be perforated with will be oriented with the tip towards the incision, the handle making a 45-degree angle with the vertical. The tip of the helix correspondent to each side, right and left, is inserted through each incision, Fig. 7.31., while the index finger of each hand, left for left side and right for the right side of the patient is in contact with the fascia of the internal obturator muscle. The tip of the helix will be inserted by applying pressure with the thumb of each hand, the contralateral hand being caught on the handle of the instrument and only having the role of maintaining the 45 degrees angle, Fig. 7.32. Thus, the distance between the tegument and the internal obturator muscle is crossed by passing through the following anatomical layers: subcutaneous fat, fascia and external obturator muscle, obturator membrane, fascia and internal obturator muscle. The tip of the instrument in permanent contact with the index will be exposed to the vaginal incision. Through its ears, the edges of the tape and the extraction of the helixes will lead to their transobturator insertion, Fig. 7.33. At the end of this time, a cystoscopic control is recommended to confirm the integrity of the bladder wall.

5. Suture of vaginal cuts, is best done in double layers, to avoid erosion. The closing of the first layer is performed using a bursa suture and the second layer with a contiuous suture for the vaginal mucosa.

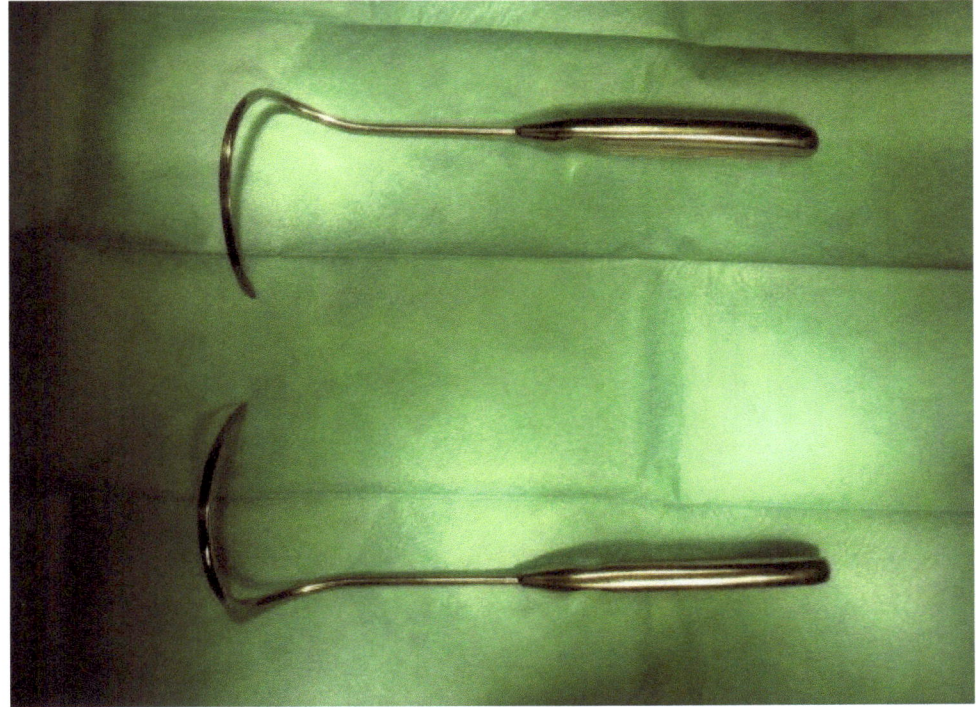

Fig. 7.31. Helixes

A 2/0 resorbable multifilament suture is used, Fig. 7.34.

6. Insertion of 300 ml of physiological serum and verification of bladder continence by tensioning the tape. The maneuver is performed with a stiff catheter inserted into the urethra to ensure that the tape does not become obstructive. The operation is completed by cutting the free ends at the level of the skin and its suturing, without catching the ends of the tape in the suture wires.

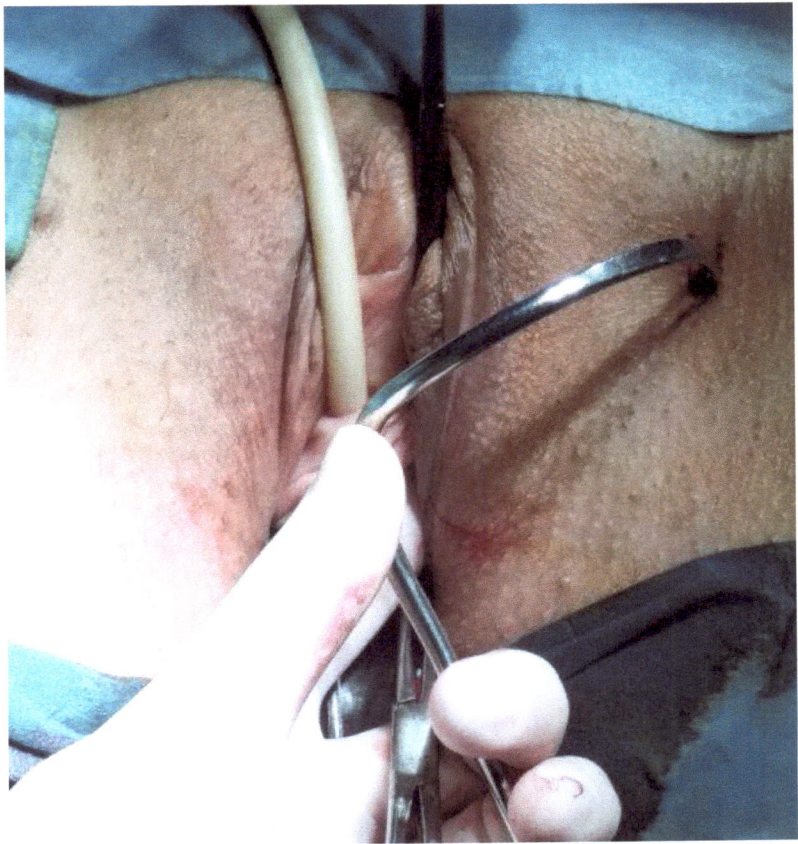

Fig. 7.32. Inserting the helix transobturator
(from the archive of **Enache A**)

151

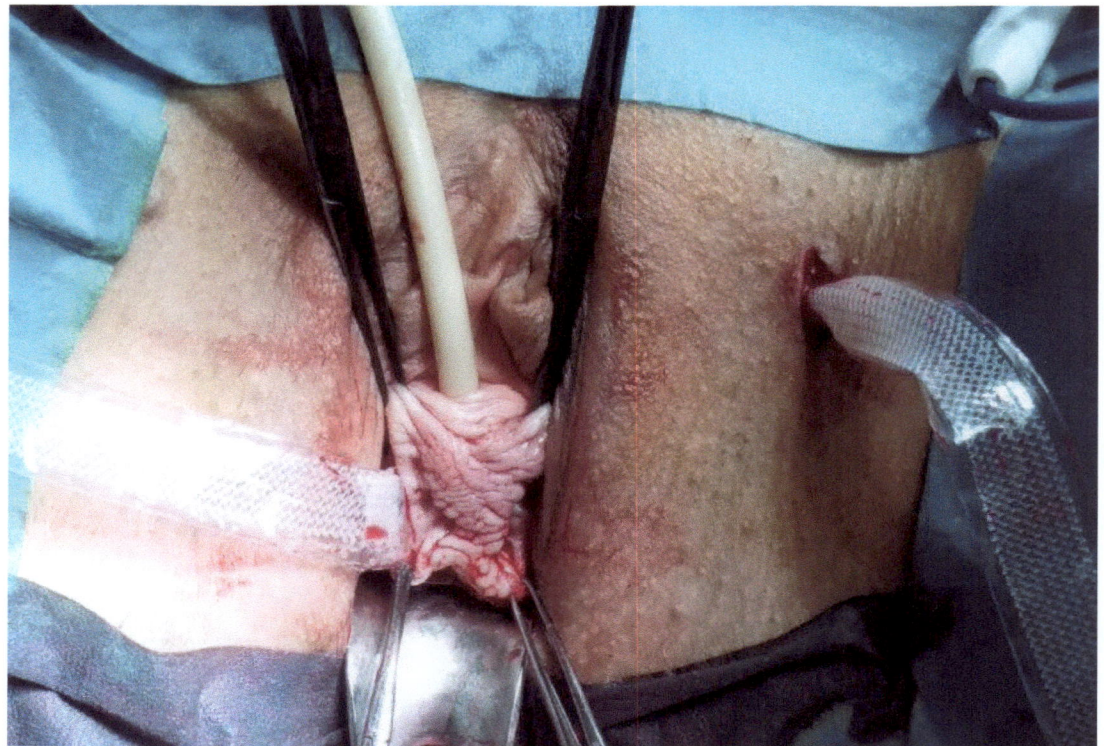

Fig. 7.33. Passing the tape transobturator and through the suburethral tunnel
(from the archive of **Enache A.**)

There are less complications of the technique, the incidence of vascular lesions being minimal due to the distance from the main vascular packs at this level, at least 2-3 cm from the femoral vein and the internal obturator vasculonervous cluster.

As in the case of TVT, the urinary catheter is maintained for 48 hours. In case of physiological micturitions, without a postmicturition residue, the discharge of the patient is at 72 hours.

7.2.2.4. Mini-sling

Mini-slings have seen a strong development in recent years, with an expanding industry, although still in experimental stage. Their main advantage is the single incision in the vaginal mucosa (without a skin incision). These are different from the classic slings used in TOT and TVT in that they are much shorter (about 8 cm compared to 40 cm long).

There are different anchoring systems at the ends, and some can even be adjusted intraoperatively, as is the case of Petros' TFS.

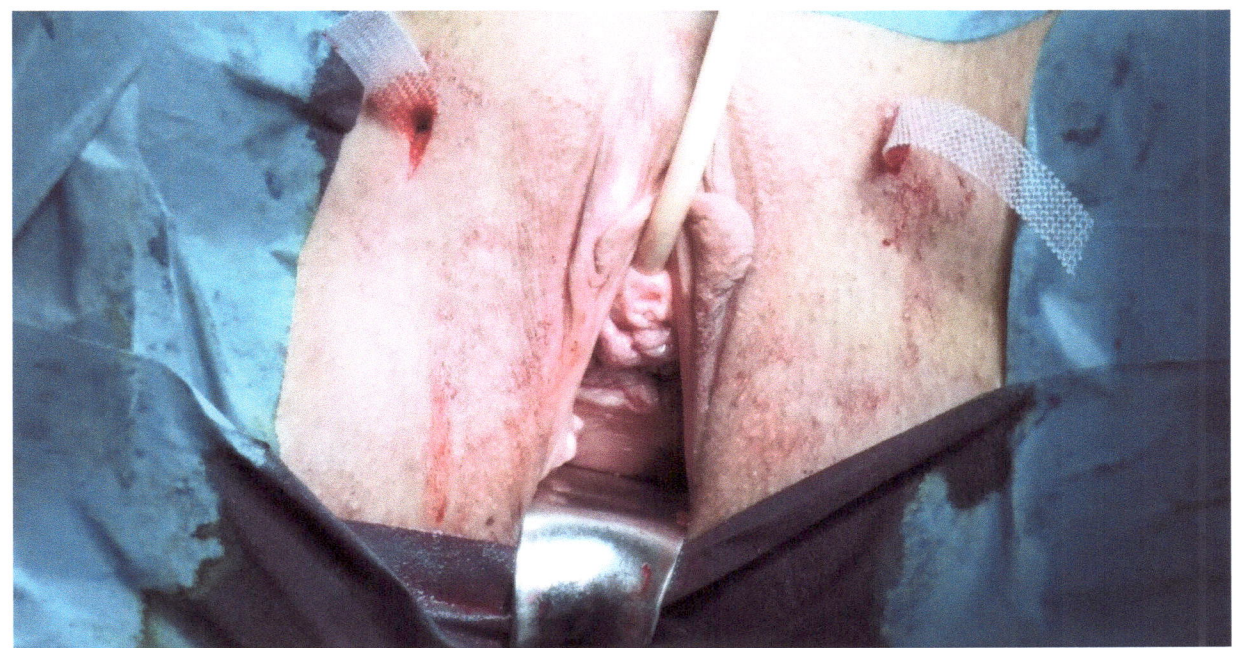

Fig. 7.34. Appearance of suburethral sling after closing the vaginal cuts
(from the archive of **Enache A.**)

Mini-slings can be anchored both retropubically, in the urogenital diaphragm, and transobturator, into the internal obturator muscle.

The retropubic mini-mesh is "U"-shaped and reconstitutes pubourethral ligaments, as in TVT. Transobturator mini-mesh has an almost horizontal direction and restores the suburethral fascia.

Mini-slings companies claim they are less traumatic, require limited dissection and thus lower risk of urethra and bladder injury. In addition, postoperatory micturition disorders would also be rarer. However, there are very few studies to support these assumptions. The rate of postoperatory success, meaning of continence, is in several studies between 74% and 95% at 6 and 12 months after surgery (**Pickens R.B.,** *et al.,* **2011**; **Lee K.S.,** *et al.,* **2010**; **Kennelly M.J.,** *et al.,* **2010**; **Serels S.,** *et al.,* **2010**; **Debodinance P., Delporte P.,** *et al.,* **2010**; **Moore R.D.,** *et al.,* **2009**; **Schellart R.P.,** *et al.,* **2014**). Another study of 173 patients followed up for 3 years shows a subjective healing rate of SUI (Stress Urinary Incontinence) of 84% (**Yildiz G.,** *et al.,* **2016**).

A meta-analysis of 15 randomized trials comparing mini-slings with classical slings highlights that both the objective and the subjective treatment of SUI are superior in the classical slings category. The symptoms of postoperatory hyperactive bladder are similar in the case of mini-slings and transobturator slings, but slightly increased in the case of retropubic slings. The percentage of erosions in the vaginal region of the mesh is similar for mini-slings and transobturator meshes, but lower for the retropubic ones (**Schimpf M.O.,** *et al.,* **2014**).

Considering all these aspects, mini-slings are not a routine therapeutic option in the SUI treatment.

7.3. Middle compartment surgery

From a pathogenic point of view, surgical techniques for the correction of middle compartment defects aim at substituting the following connective structures: pubocervical fascia, arcus tendineus fasciae pelvis, and pericervical ring through which the pubocervical fascia is inserted into the cervix. Clinical manifestations are anterior vaginal prolapse through central and lateral mechanisms.

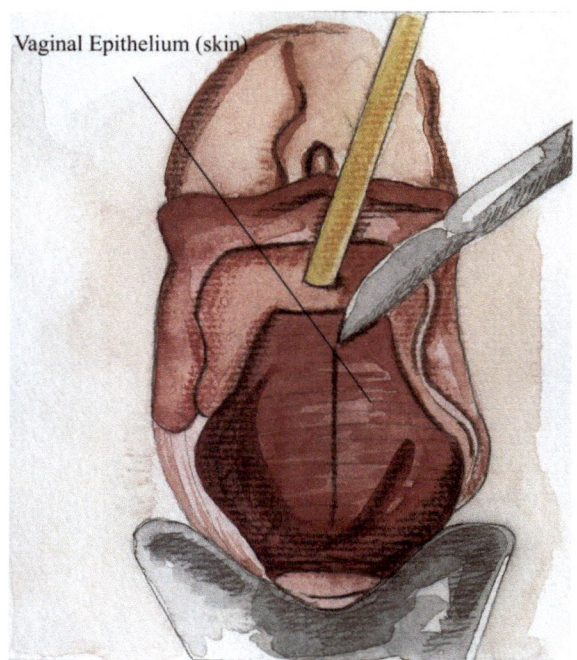

Fig. 7.35. Longitudinal incision
(*drawing by Vanessa Mureşan*)

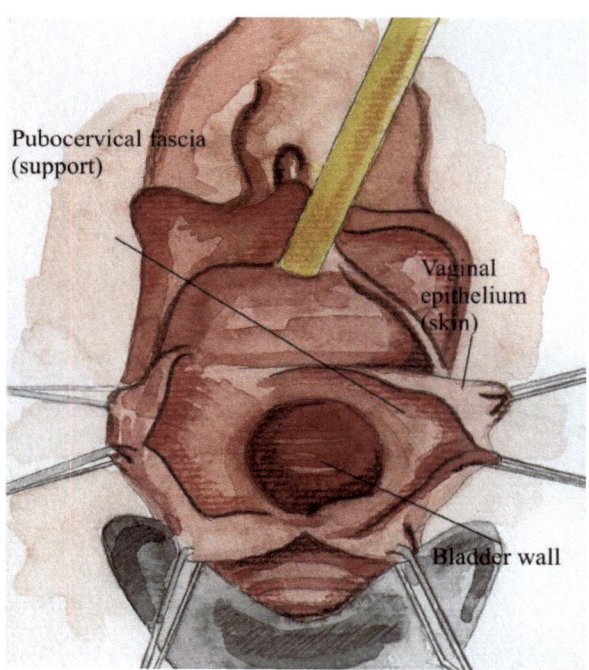

Fig. 7.36. Anatomical details after dissection
(*drawing by Vanessa Mureşan*)

7.3.1. Classical surgical procedures

Classic surgery, still widespread in many centers, proposes two techniques that address the middle compartment disorders. Their main disadvantage is the high rate of relapse, main element affected, and connective tissue, not being replaced, or surgically replaced with prosthesis.

7.3.1.1. Anterior colporrhaphy

It is currently also the most commonly used technique in cystocele surgery by central mechanism.

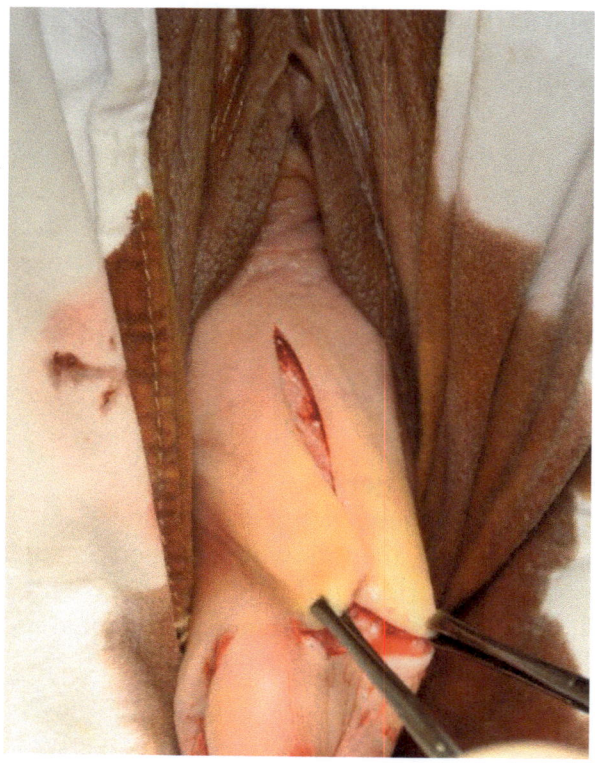

Fig. 7.38. Crossen incision longitudinal prolongation
(from the archive of **Moisa M.**)

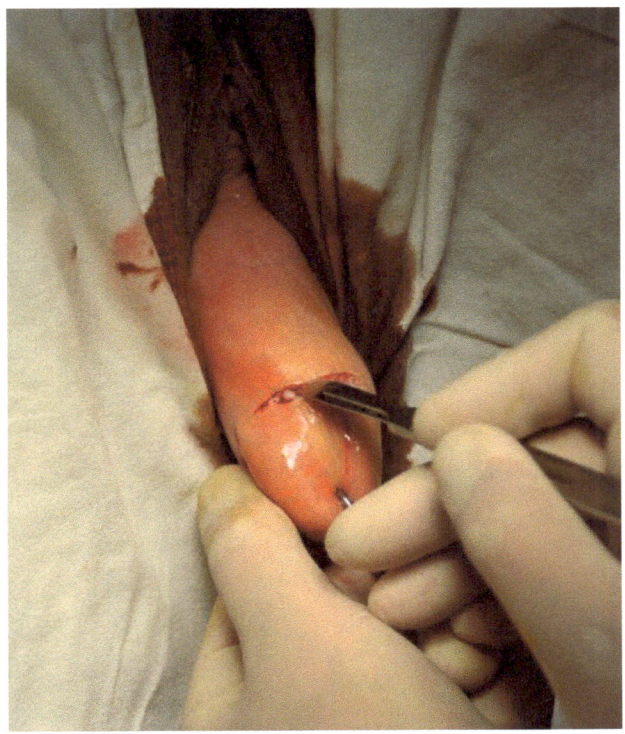

Fig. 7.37. Crossen Incision
(from the archive of **Moisa M.**)

This is mainly recognized by the fact that the vaginal mucosa corresponding to the cystocele has missing transverse vaginal sheaths as a result of pubocervical fascia overstretching.

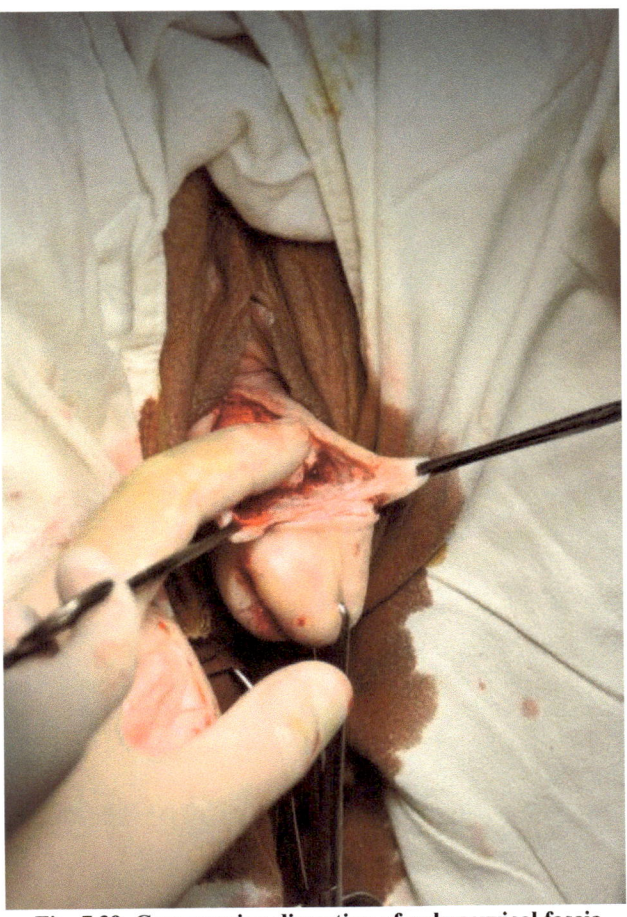

Fig. 7.39. Compression dissection of pubocervical fascia
(from the archive of **Moisa M.**)

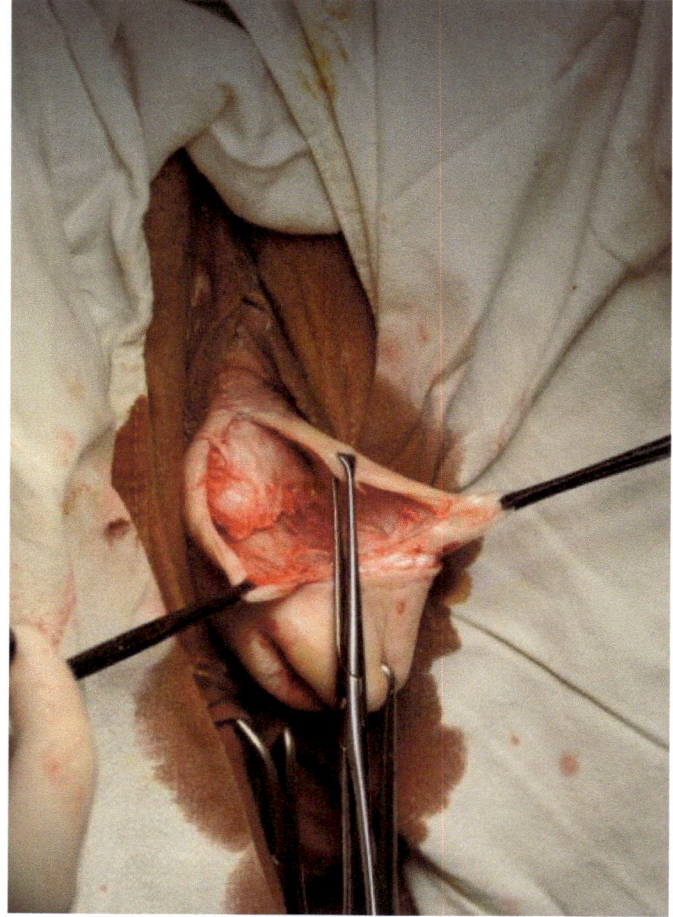

Fig. 7.40. Intraoperative detail after dissection
(from the archive of **Moisa M.**)

Diagnosis of cystocele through a central defect must be carefully established, because extensive MRI studies and careful anatomic measurements have shown that at least one-third of the patients with cystocele suffer from the loss of the apical support, so that the suspension of the vaginal apex is absolutely necessary in this category of patients (***., 2017).

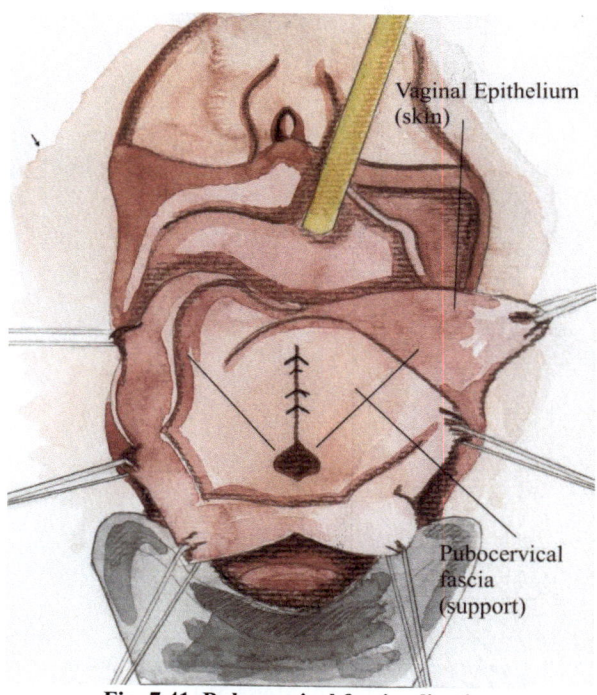

Fig. 7.41. Pubocervical fascia plication
(*drawing by Vanessa Mureşan*)

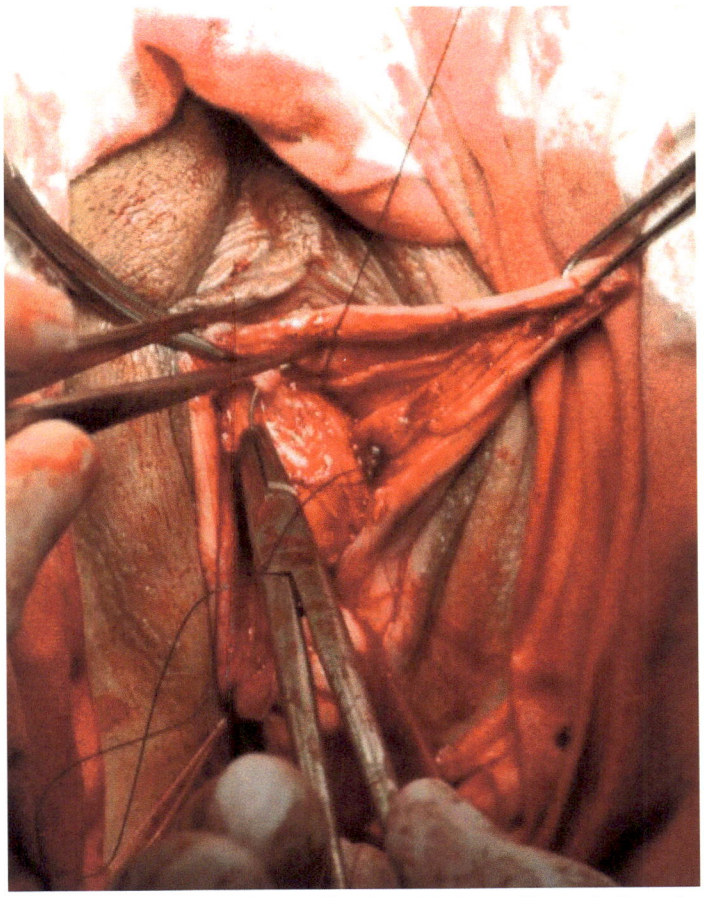

Fig. 7.42. Pubocervical fascia plication with bursa tissue closing wire
(from the archive of **Moisa M.**)

The intervention is mainly aimed at the pubocervical fascia plication in order to detect the central defect and to strengthen/ reinforce the overstretched fascia.

Surgical steps
1. The patient is placed in a gynecological position. The vulva, vagina, and perineum are prepared for the intervention while respecting the aseptic and antiseptic measures. A 16 French Foley catheter is introduced into the bladder. The incision trajectory is pointed on the anterior vaginal wall with two Chaput forceps. The incision is practiced sagittal, from 1.5-2 cm from the vaginal apex and close to the bladder neck, Fig. 7.35. Hydrolysis techniques may also be used. The surgery can be started with a Crossen incision, Fig. 7.37., and then, it can be continued with a longitudinal incision, Fig. 7.38.
2. After the incision, the edges are detected with Chaput forceps and the vaginal epithelium is dissected from the pubocervical fascia with a Metzenbaum scissors, which is inserted in closed position with the tip up and is retracted in an open position.

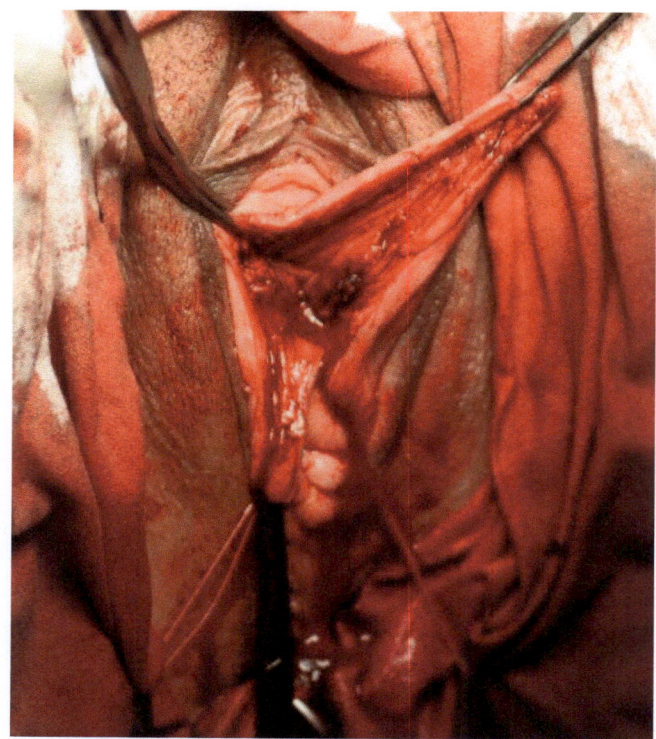

Fig. 7.43. Pubocervical fascia plication with bursa tissue wire, after wire tensioning
(from the archive of **Moisa M.**)

The lateral decollation of vaginal mucosa membranes can also be done with a compress on the finger and by sectioning, from time to time, the conjunctive joints thus emphasized (**Irvin W. & Hullfish K., 2005**), Fig. 7.3.6., 7.37., 7.38., 39. and 40.

The dissection continues laterally to the vaginal cul-de-sacs and proximally to the vaginal vault (if the patient had a hysterectomy in the medical history) or towards the cervix. At this level, haemostasis can usually be done by electrocautery.

3. The pubocervical fascia plication is usually performed with 0 or 2.0 slowly resorbable sutures approximating the fascia from one side to the other, or, with bursa tissue suture, Fig. 7.41., 42., 43.

Caution is recommended not to overfold the fascia, maneuver that could cause the wrinkling and obstruction of the ureters. Prior to suturing the vagina as a precautionary measure to check the integrity of the bladder mucosa and ureters function, a cystourethroscopy may be performed.

4. Suture of vaginal mucosa with continuous suture or separated of resorbable material. At the end of the intervention, a Foley catheter is mounted. The discharge of the patient can be done at 48-72 hours.

7.3.1.2. Paravaginal defect repair

The intervention addresses the correction of the vaginal vault prolapse and vaginal apex prolapse accompanied by lateral defect cystocele.

Less commonly used in Europe, the surgery can be performed both vaginally and abdominally – classically or laparoscopically. The goal is to reattach the pubocervical fascia to the arcus tendineus fasciae pelvis (ATFP). The vaginal approach is more difficult, involving the retropubic dissection until the ATFP is identified and the fascia is reattached with spotted wires. The abdominal approach (both classical and laparoscopic) is easier.

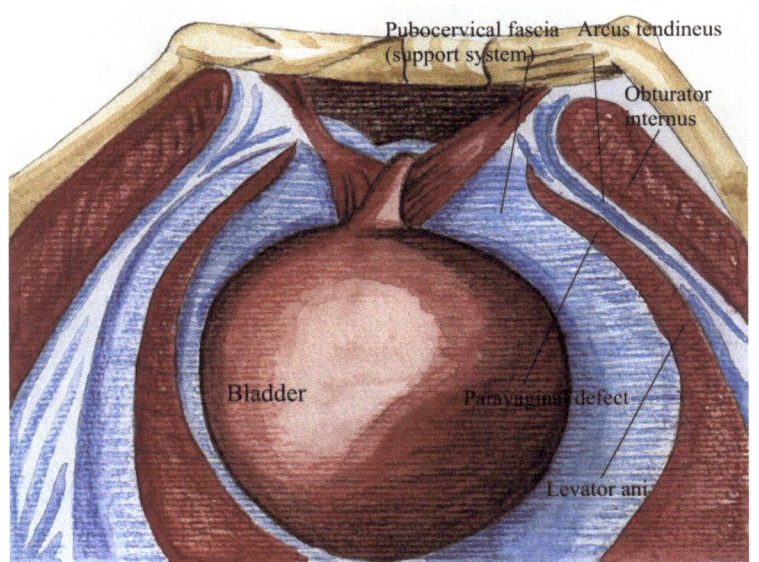

Fig. 7.44. Identification of paravaginal defect (*drawing by Vanessa Mureșan*)

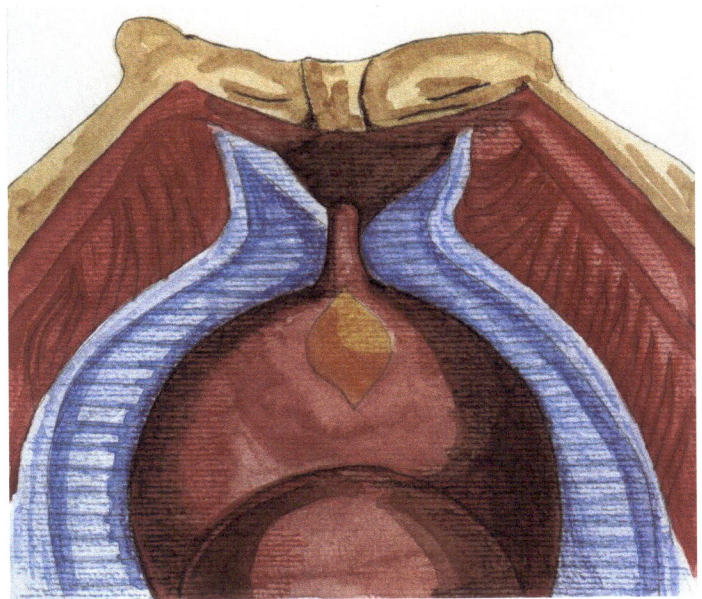

Fig. 7.45. Repairing the vaginal defect (*drawing by Vanessa Mureșan*)

The bladder base is closely attached to the anterior vaginal wall through the pubocervical fascia that is inserted laterally to the arcus tendineus fasciae pelvis (ATFP) bilaterally. When prolapse of the vaginal apex occurs, the bladder base is also detached from the ATFP and will tear through the vaginal introit together with the vagina.

This is by definition the mechanism of the bilateral paravaginal defect.

The aim of the intervention is to bilaterally reattach the lateral vaginal cul-de-sacs and the endopelvic fascia to the internal obturator muscles, pubococcygeus muscles and fascia at the ATPF level.

Surgical steps

1. A low Pfannenstiel incision is made with the identification of Retzius space, while being careful when intercepting the venous plexus of Santorini, located around the bladder.
2. The bladder is mobilized bilaterally, with the exposure of the retropubic space laterally, the identification of internal obturator muscle and bilateral pubococcygeus muscle and the internal obturator vasculonervous pedicle. The ischial spine is palpated and ATPF is identified as a fibrous tape located between the spine and the posterior side of the pubic symphysis, Fig.7.44.
3. The non-dominant hand is inserted intravaginally and lateral pouch of Douglas is identified. With the bladder medially removed, 2.0 non-resorbable sutures are passed through the

fibromuscular thickness of the vaginal wall, just above the finger inserted intravaginally, to the ATFP or the internal obturator muscle fascia, at about 1-2 cm from the ischial spine, Fig. 7.45. 3-5 sutures are passed over each side at a distance of about 1 cm. The most distal wire must be passed over as close to the pubic ramus as possible, towards the pubourethral ligament. A Foley catheter is mounted at the end of the intervention. Patient discharge can be done at 48-72 hours.

7.3.2. Surgical techniques using alloplastic material

The most common surgical technique addressing the middle compartment, which uses alloplastic materials, is the anterior compartment mesh in shape of letter "*H*". Pubocervical fascia is reconstructed this way, but also by its structure and the fact that it does not require lateral anchoring, the mesh functionally reconstructing the role of *"arcus tendineus fasciae pelvis"* (ATFP). The anatomical reconstruction of ATFP can only be done with the aid of the TFS proposed by Petros. The approach is vaginal in most of the cases, but laparoscopic techniques have also been proposed.

7.3.2.1. Transobturator four-arms mesh in surgical repair

This surgical technique is currently the most widely used method that uses alloplastic materials to correct anterior vaginal prolapse. Surgery is performed vaginally and it involves the replacement of pubocervical fascia with the polypropylene mesh. Arcus tendineus fasciae pelvis (ATFP) is not reconstituted as it is, because the lateral anchoring is done with the aid of the four arms, Fig. 7.46. (**Velemir L., et al., 2010**). Various technique variations involve the passing over of the 2 posterior arms, transobturator or laterocervical, with posterior anchoring, as far as a paracervix defect, high-grade cystocele and concomitant uterine prolapse is also associated. The medical technology industry has developed exponentially over the past 20 years, with several different types of prefabricated meshes. However, many authors prefer to make the piece of material individualized, according to the patient and the size of the defect (*****., 2011**).

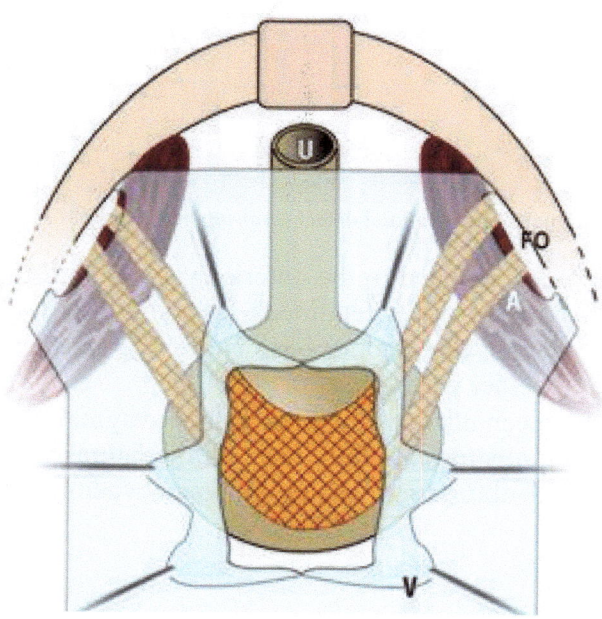

Fig. 7.46. **Final position of anterior mesh with 4 transobturatory arms**
(according to **Petros P.**)

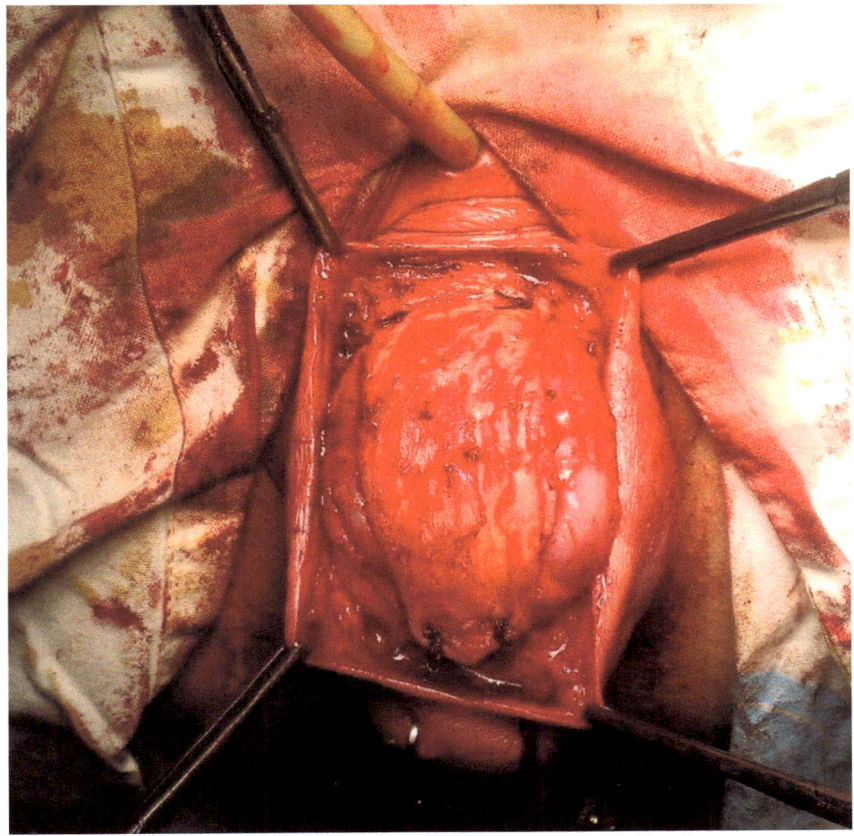

Fig. 7.47. Delimiting and fixing "the anterior bridge"
(from the archive of **T. Enache**)

Surgical steps

1. An elliptical incision is made at the level of the anterior vaginal wall, at 1.5 cm below the bladder neck and 1.5 cm above the cervix or the vaginal apex. Thus, a flap of about 3-4 cm long and 1 cm wide is done. This remains adherent to the submucosal layer of the anterior bladder wall. This first step was introduced by Prof. Klaus Goeschen as a bladder anti-erosion mechanism.

2. The paravesical space is dissected laterally and digitally, under the vesicovaginal fascia, which remains adherent to the vaginal mucosa to prevent vaginal erosions. The lateral dissection reaches the level of the endopelvic fascia that tapers the internal obturator muscle. At this level, ATFP can be palpated on the anterior side, and posteriorly, the dissection is made up to the ischial spine. Bleeding is generally minimal, being a sign of dissection in the cleavage plan.

3. The anterior vaginal mucosa flap, also called *"anterior bridge"*, is desepithelised with the electrocautery to prevent the occurrence of inclusion cysts postoperatory. The anterior bridge is fixed by 4 sutures to the bladder wall to prevent its further mobilization, Fig 7.47.

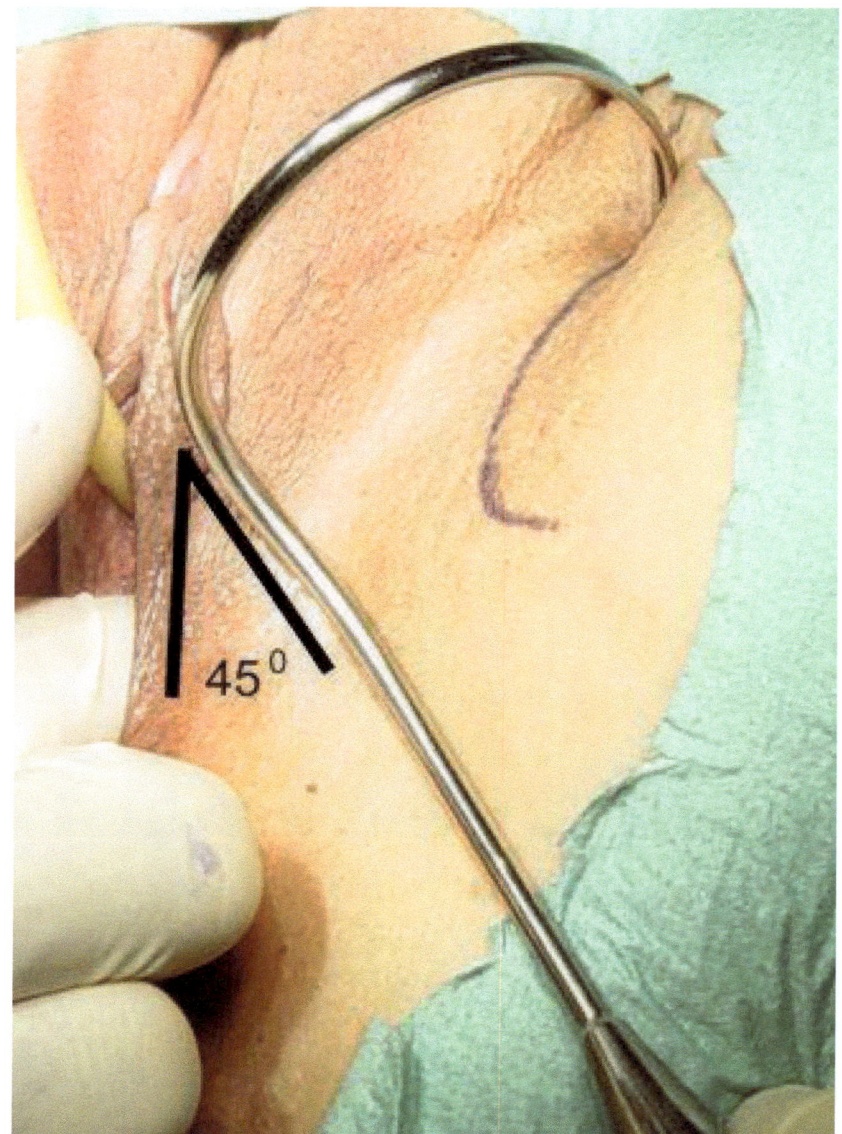

Fig. 7.48. **Passing over of the transobturator helix, at a 45° angle with the vertical axis**
(from the archive of **Mueller-Funogea I.A.**)

4. A bilateral incision is made to the skin, at 2-3 cm lateral from the clitoris knee and at 1.5 cm lower from the origin tendon of long adductor muscle. At this level, the helix penetrates transobturatorily at a 45° angle with the vertical, the tip of the instrument being intercepted by the index finger of the hand with the palm facing the inner side of the patient's thigh, Fig 7.48. The index finger is paravesical introduced, with the inner side in contact with the ischiopubic ramus and the internal side of the internal obturator muscle. Thus, the bladder is protected, avoiding its perforation during the helix passage.

The tip of the helix is pushed towards the index finger of the surgeon with the thumb of the same hand, while with the contralateral hand the angulation of 45° with the vertical is maintained. The instrument passes through the same layers as the suburethral mesh: subcutaneous adipose tissue, fascia and external obturator muscle, obturator membrane, fascia and internal obturator muscle. To the extent that the Surgical steps is accurately respected, the risk of damaging the main vascular sources in the region is practically null: the femoral vessels, the vasculonervous obturator bundle, and the corona mortis.

5. Once the tip of the helix has reached the index finger of the surgeon, it is pushed until it is exposed at the level of the vaginal incision.

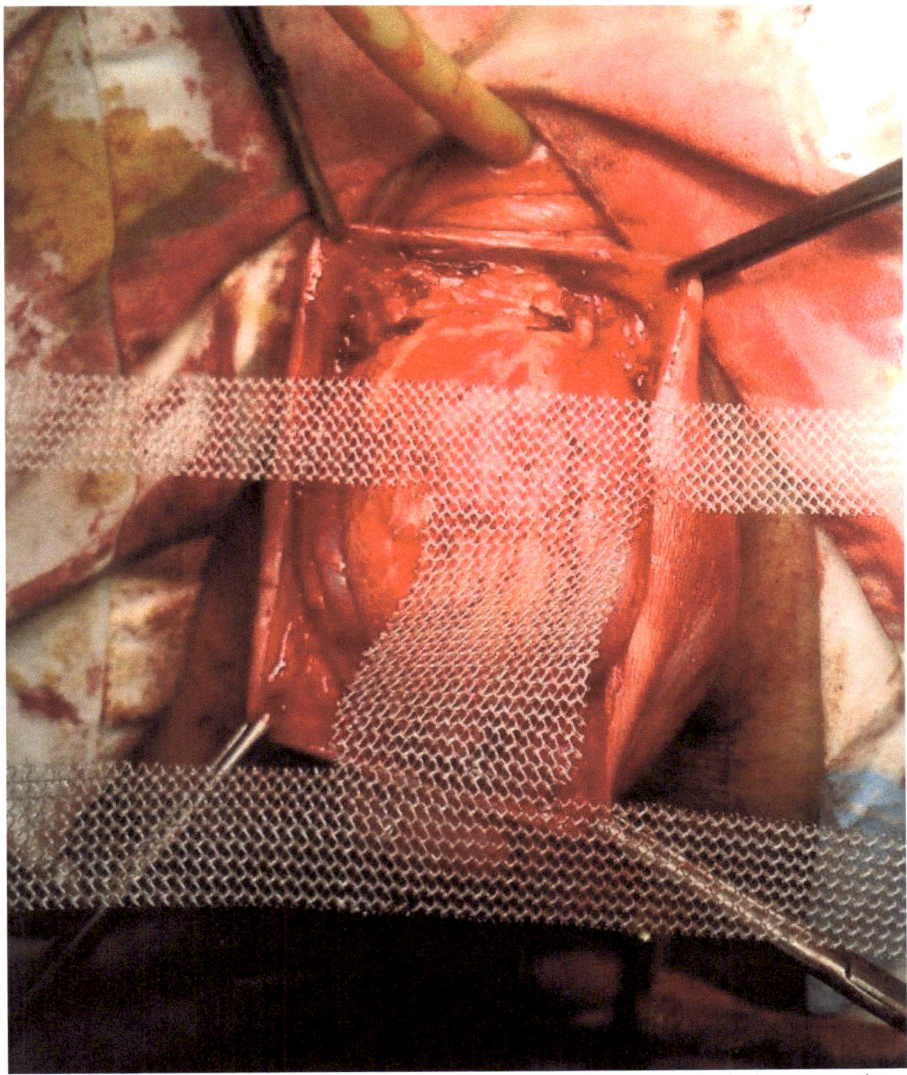

Fig. 7.49. Appearance of anterior mesh in the shape of the letter "*H*" before mounting
(from the archive of Enache **T.**)

The anterior arm of the mesh in shape of letter "*H*" is passed over through its ears and by extracting the helix in the opposite direction of its insertion, the fragment of mesh is passed over laterovesical and exteriorized at the level of the skin. Steps 4 and 5 are made bilaterally.

6. Posterior arms can be passed over in three ways, the determining factor being the coexistence or the non-coexistence of uterine prolapse or vaginal apex.

6.1. As long as there is no prolapse, the posterior arms are passed over transobturator with the help of the helixes, but following a slightly different technique. With the index finger of the hand facing the inner side of the thigh, a dissection is made laterovesical, towards the posterior side, with the inner side of the finger in contact with the inner side of the internal obturator muscle up to the proximity of the ischial spine. An incision is then made at 1 cm lower and 1 cm lateral than for the ones for the passage of anterior arms.

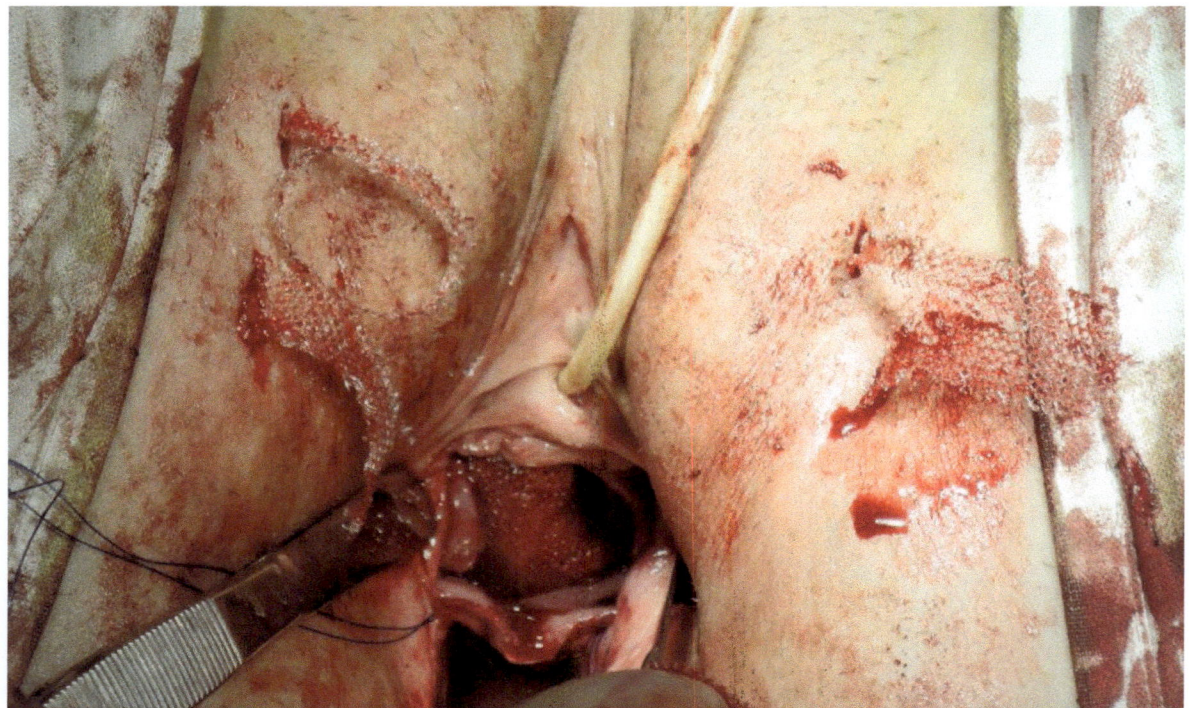

Fig. 7.50. Anterior mesh in the shape of the letter "H" with 4 arms passed over transobturatorily
(from the archive of **Enache T.**)

The helix is inserted with the tip at the incisions mentioned, but with the handle in a 90° angle with the vertical.

The instrument is pushed perpendicularly on the tissue until it meets the external obturator muscle, then it is rotated to 90° until the handle reaches a vertical position. Under the control of the index finger of the hand with the palm facing the inner side of the patient's thigh, the tip of the helix is pushed with the thumb of the same hand, the contralateral hand maintaining the vertical position of the instrument handle.

The layers crossed by the instrument are the following: subcutaneous adipose tissue, fascia and external obturator muscle, obturator membrane, fascia and the internal obturator muscle. The posterior arms of the mesh are passed through the ears of the helix and the fragments of mesh are exposed to the tegument through the extraction of the instrument in the opposite direction of its insertion. The maneuver is executed bilaterally. Fig. 7.49. and 7.50.

6.2. If there is a uterine prolapse that must also be corrected, the anchoring of the posterior arms is done by suspending the sacrospinous ligaments, after passing them over laterocervical.

This Surgical steps is performed by introducing an Overholt forceps, from downwards to backwards, from the incision made on the posterior vaginal mucosa and exposing the tip at the level of the anterior vaginal incision.

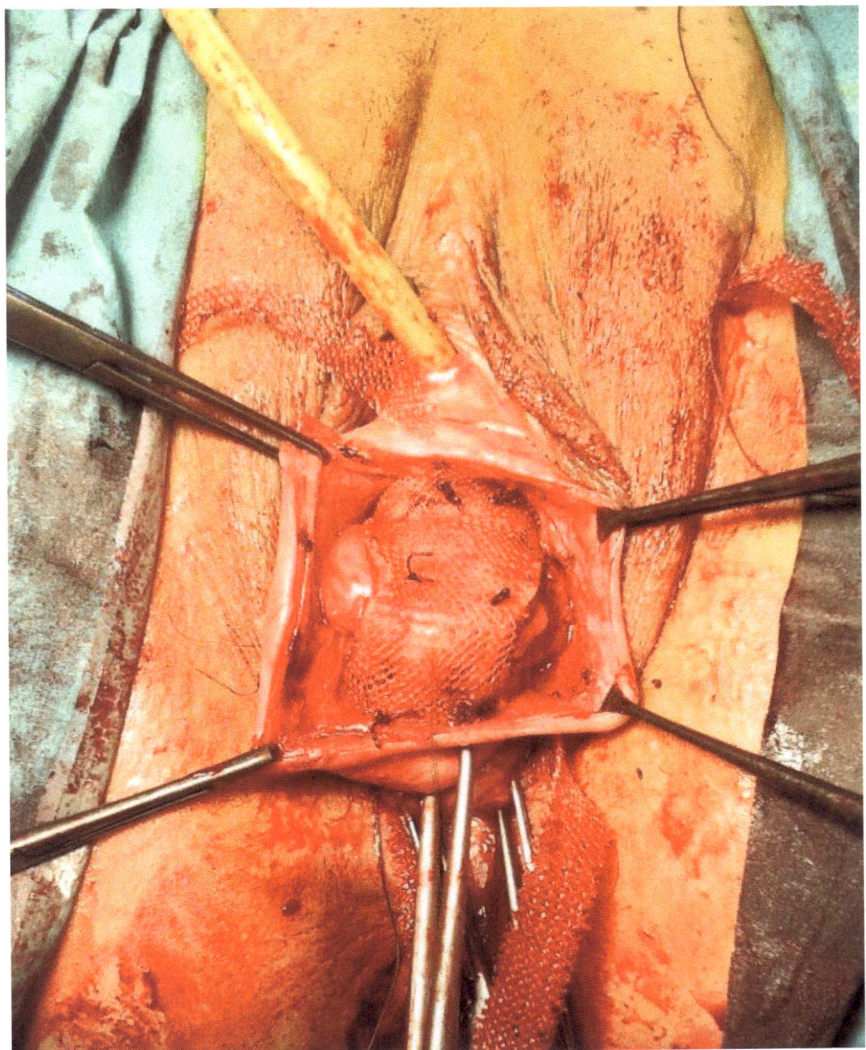

Fig. 7.51. Anterior "*H*"-mesh with the posterior arms passed over laterocervical and sacrospinous fixed
(from the archive of **Enache T.**)

Thus, a bilateral laterocervical tunnel is obtained, which the repeated opening of the forceps will enlarge, until a channel with the approximate dimensions of the posterior arm is achieved.

With the opening of the forceps, the end of this arm is grabbed and by extracting the forceps, the fragment of mesh appears at the level of the posterior vaginal incision. The posterior arms of the mesh are anchored to the sacrospinous wires that have already been passed at that level. The sacrospinous wires can be either one or two bilaterally, depending on the size of the anatomical defect. If there is a 3rd of 4th degree Baden-Walken prolapse, 2 wires are preferred bilaterally, one for the posterior arms of the anterior mesh and one for the correction of DeLancey level I correction (with posterior mesh or "patch", according to the therapeutic option). Thus, a more solid anchoring is obtained. Sacrospinous wires are connected at the end, before the last surgical step – closing the posterior vaginal mucosa, Fig. 7.51.

In this case, by passing over the posterior arms laterocervical and their anchoring to the sacrospinous ligaments, the paracolpos is recreated with its important role of vector interconnection of all mechanisms of support of the pelvic organs. Through this technical artifice, the anterior "*H*" mesh with 4 arms also helps in the correction of the uterine prolapse. For the posterior compartment, depending on the associated defects, appropriate surgical techniques will be approached.

6.3. If anterior vaginal prolapse is associated with a vaginal vault prolapse, the sacrospinous anchoring of the posterior arms of the anterior mesh is preferred, with the aim of recreating the vector disposition of the affected ligament structures. The absence of the cervix associated with an atrophy of sacrouterine and cardinal ligaments leads to a different technical approach proposed by P. Petros. Finger dissection technique is practiced as in step 6.1. up to the ischial spine, then it continues posteriorly by palpating the sacrospinous ligaments bilaterally.

With the *"viper"*, each 2.0 non-resorbable monofilament suture is passed over, one at the time, bilaterally, at 2 cm lower than the ischial spine. This maneuver is possible due to the absence of the cervix and the lax ligament structures. Posterior arms are anchored to the wires passed over sacrospinous. Thus, the physiological vector disposition is reconstructed, thus obtaining the interconnection of the middle and the posterior compartment. Additionally, their correction is applied depending on the associated defects of the posterior compartment.

7. The mesh is positioned slack, without subvesical plications, and immobilized by a few sutures to the bladder wall, laterally from the *"anterior bridge"*. The final disposition of the mesh, seen from cranial, through abdominal dissection in a cadaver, after being mounted vaginally, is observed in Fig. 7.52.

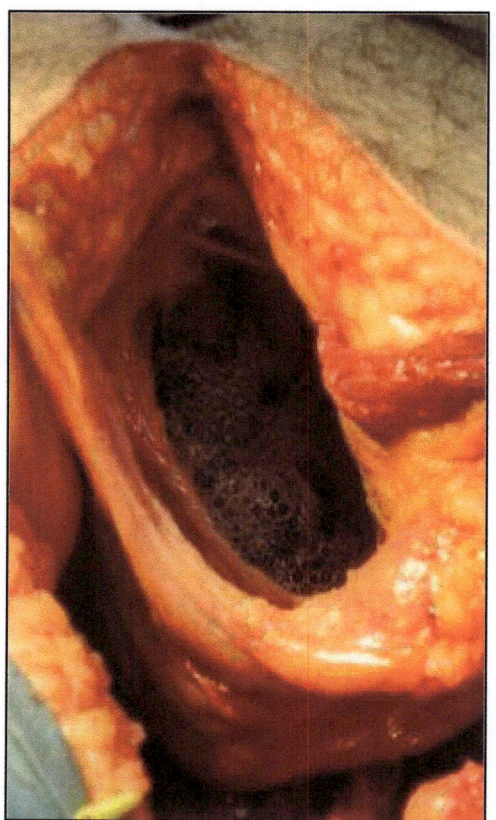

Fig. 7.52. 4 arms anterior mesh – "in situ" aspect in a cadaver after abdominal dissection
(from the archive of **Enache T.**)

After the hemostasis control, a diagnostic cystoscopy is performed to observe a possible bladder perforation.

To the extent that such a complication is observed, the instrument is extracted and repositioned more laterally, trying to avoid a new accident.

8. The vaginal incision is closed in a double layer with separate resorbable multifilament sutures for the suture of vesicourethral fascia and continuous suture for vaginal mucosa.

A vaginal mesh and a vaginal catheter are mounted to the patient. Both are maintained for 24 hours. The patient can be discharged 48 hours after surgery to the extent that no complications, hematoma, urinary retention, etc., occur. The patient can be discharged 48 hours after surgery to the extent that no complications, hematoma, urinary retention, etc., occur.

7.3.2.2. Tissue fixation system for the middle compartment

The surgical procedure involves the same reconstruction system that has been described in the tissue fixation system for the treatment of stress urinary incontinence. In the case of median compartment, the theoretical principle underlying the surgical correction is borrowed from the constructions field. The reconstruction is of type of ceiling beams supporting a gypsum-board ceiling. In other words, the reconstruction of the cardinal ligaments and the arcus tendineus fasciae pelvis (ATFP) will lead to the correction of the cystocele, regardless of the mechanism of appearance.

Surgical steps

1. An incision is performed on the anterior vaginal mucosa after its prior tensioning to 1-1.5 cm from the cervix or the post hysterectomy scar, practically at the level of the vesicocervical junction. The incision can be transverse or longitudinal, depending on the surgeon's preference.

2. The bladder is dissected from the cervix or the post hysterectomy scar. The dissection continues laterally with care to detach the bladder from the lateral vaginal fornices. This maneuver is a mechanism of protection against erosion. Using a smooth and curved Mayo dissecting scissors, the lateral dissection continues with the tip directed towards the vaginal mucosa up to the lateral wall of the pelvic excavation. Then the finger will be inserted to create a tunnel with a satisfying diameter.

3. The insertion of the TFS applicator onto the scissors guide until it encounters the pelvic wall. The tip of the anchor then perforates the fascia, then the extraction of the anchor remains encased in the tissue. The traction of the mesh verifies the anchor fixing quality.

4. The same steps are also made contralateral. At this point, the mesh is tensioned until a resistance is encountered, which signals the recovery of the muscular tone. At this moment of intervention, the reconstruction of the cardinal ligaments was performed.

5. A second vertical incision of about 5 cm in length, which starts at about 1 cm distal from the vesical trigone area, is practiced.

6. The bladder is dissected from the vaginal mucosa to create a channel wide enough to be able to insert the mesh. The tunnel is made with the dissecting scissors, and its orientation is from the internal side of the ischiopubic ramus to the ATFP insertion on the pubis.

7. The TFS applicator is inserted through this channel until resistance is encountered. At that level, the fascia is perforated with the tip of the anchor, and then the applicator is removed. The procedure is also repeated contralateral. The tape is stretched until resistance is encountered, then the applicator is extracted, the tape remaining fixed.

8. The vaginal cuts are sutured with separate wires.

The patient is discharged no later than 24 hours postoperatory. The final aspect is schematically represented in Fig 7.53. Horizontal mesh offers structural support to the proximal half of anterior vaginal wall, recreates paracervix, crosses ATFP in the proximity of ischial spine, and re-anchors ATFP to the excavation walls. *"U"* mesh reinforces the ATFP structure proximally thus offering support to the distal half of the vagina, compensating the central defect and reattaching the pubocervical muscle to the symphysis.

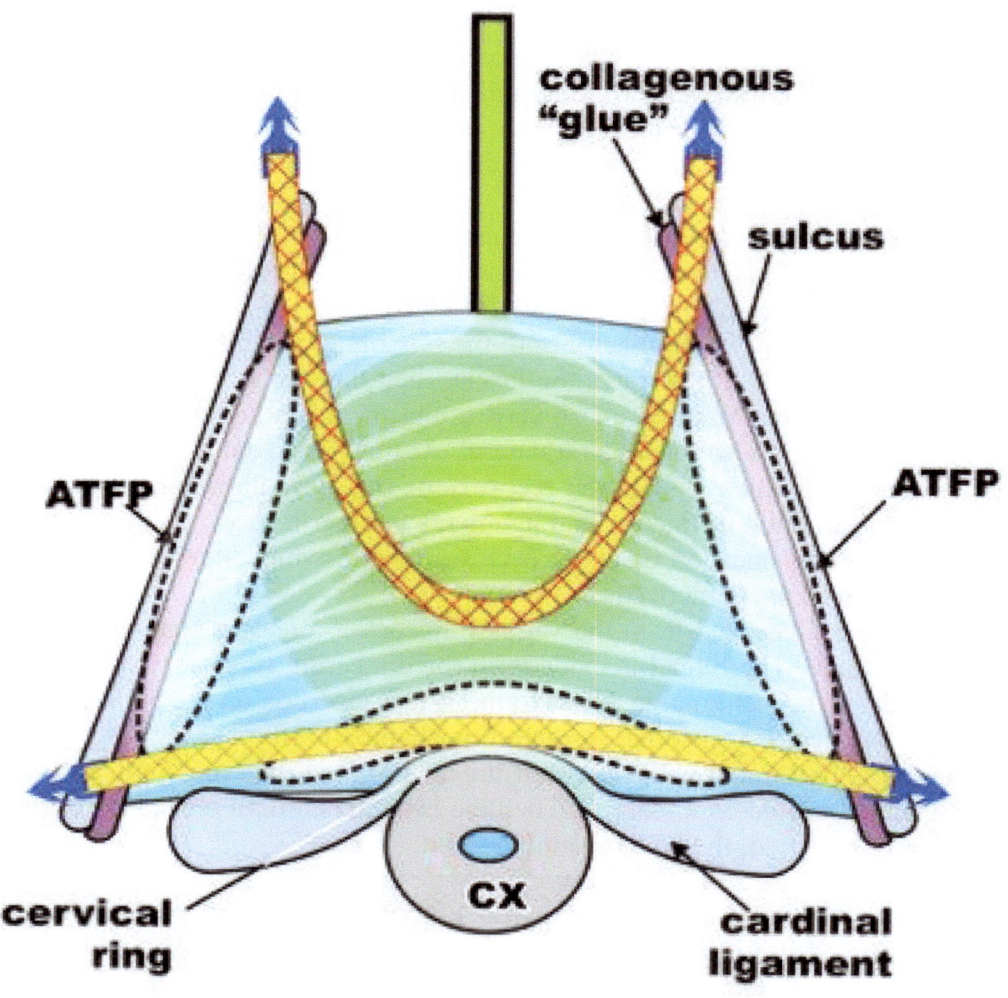

Fig. 7.53. **Correction of middle compartment defects by TFS** (according to. **Petros P., 2010**)
ATFP – arcus tendineus fasciae pelvis, cardinal ligament – cardinal ligaments; CX – cervix; cervical ring – paracervix; collagenous "*glue*" – collagenous "glue"

7.3.2.3. Anterior pelvic organ prolapse repair using a six tension-free strap, low-weight transvaginal mesh: OPUR® kit

With OPUR mesh and technique, we propose to mimic the anteroposterior fascia and the uterosacral ligaments that support the bladder and the uterus or vaginal vault after hysterectomy (**Delorme E., 2011**). The technique represents vaginal surgery by an anterior route.

OPUR® mesh (Fig.7.54.)

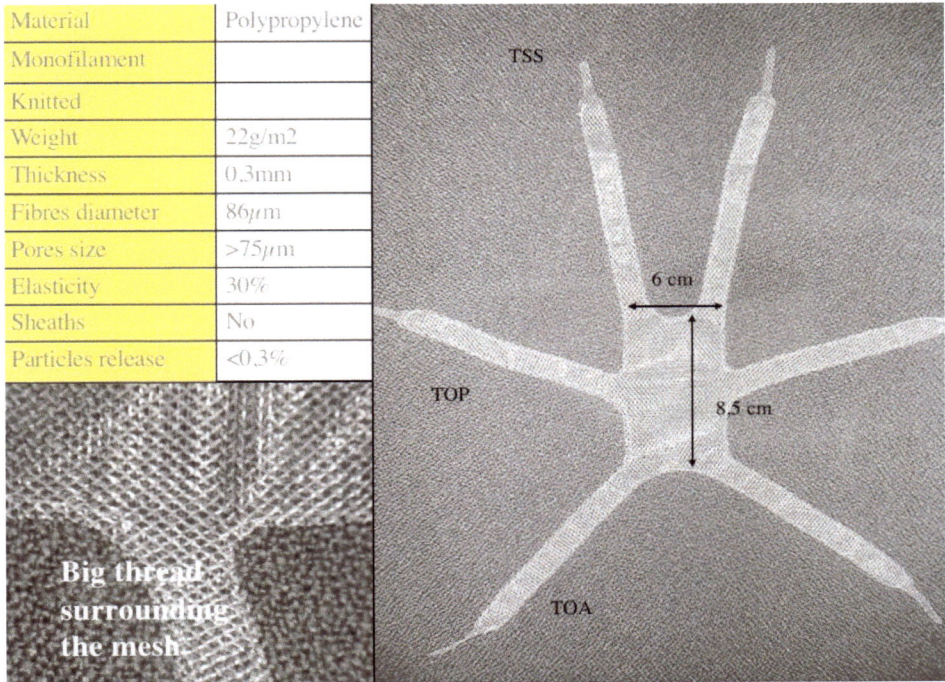

Fig. 7.54. Mesh six straps (OPUR®)

Design of the OPUR mesh

Since 2005, we have used a thin polypropylene subvesical mesh fixed by six tension-free straps (ABISS) (Fig. 7.54.). It is a large-pore, knitted mesh made of monofilament polypropylene thread, with a diameter of 80μ. This gives a lightweight implant of 22 mg/m².

The mesh must be spread wide enough to cover the defect between the two levator ani muscles. However, it seems that implants placed by the vaginal route should not be too wide to leave the pelvic muscles supple and not to stiffen the dynamic pelvic floor.

It is difficult to evaluate how much the implant will shrink after surgery. Based on an empirical approach, we decided that the mesh should be 15% larger than the defect to be covered. The mesh is 9 cm long because the average distance between the cervix and the bladder neck is 7 cm. It is 6 cm wide, because the average distance between the levator ani muscles is about 4.5 cm.

The mesh is fixed by six straps: two anterior transobturator straps (ATO), two posterior transobturator straps (PTO), which support the mesh laterally, and two posterior arms, which are trans-sacrospinous.

The implant is reinforced by a big thread (150 microns) surrounding the mesh to reduce the straps elasticity when the surgeon pulls the arm through the vaginal wall.

Why 6 straps?

The distance between the ATO and the PTO is maximum 4.5 cm, whereas the base of the bladder from the bladder neck to the cervix is about 7 cm. This is why the TO arms cannot support the entire bladder base.

The suture attaching the implant to the cervix seems not to be strong enough to resist the contraction of the implant, which is why we opted for a superior, posterior suspension of the implant by two posterior trans-sacrospinous straps. It seemed more secure to have a strap opposite a strap rather than a suture.

The natural suspension of the pelvic organs is anterior/ posterior, and transversal. The six straps mimic the natural fascia: the ATO mimic the pubovesical ligaments, the PTO the arcus tendineus fascia pelvis ligaments (ATFP) and the posterior trans-sacrospinous straps (TSS) the uterosacral ligaments. The implant aims to mimic the bladder fascia described by P. Petros in the integral theory and by J. Delancey (**Petros P., 2004; Wei J.T., De Lancey J.O.L., 2004**).

The OPUR mesh can support the bladder and uterus or treat vaginal vault prolapse.

Dissection

1/ With the uterus in place (Fig. 7.55.)

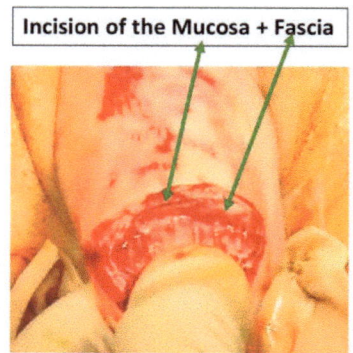 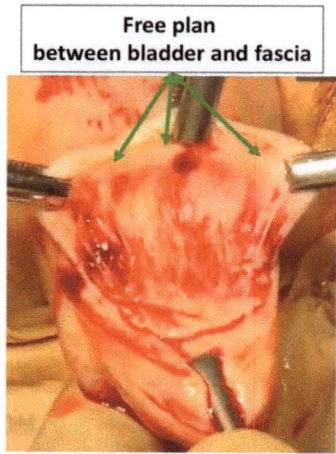 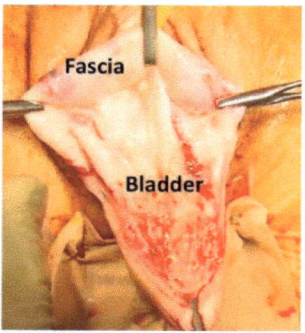

Fig. 7.55. Dissection with the uterus in place (according to **Delorme, E.**)

Vaginal dissection is simplified by an extensive infiltration of the surgical site. This consists in injecting 100 ml of saline solution with 2.5 mg of adrenaline. It is injected with a long thin needle (20 G).

The incision is anterior and transversal, 2 cm before the tip of the cervix. This incision must be deep and open the mucosa and fascia.

A strong pull on the cervix will show the right dissection plane, between the bladder and the vaginal fascia.

The vaginal wall is rolled out on itself, like the lid of a can. Rolling the vaginal wall and pulling on the uterus exposes the line of dissection, which is perfectly bloodless.

The dissection stops above the bladder neck, which must remain intact; the anterior, lower edge of the implant must remain above the bladder neck.

Sideways of the bladder neck the traction on, exposes the ATFP (Fig. 7.56.). This is the door to the paravesical and pararectal fossa, just behind the obturator foramen. The ATFP must be opened very carefully using scissors, with the scissors lateral to the urethra, where the fascia is the widest. Opening the ATFP against the bladder would be dangerous, with a risk of damaging the bladder or ureter.

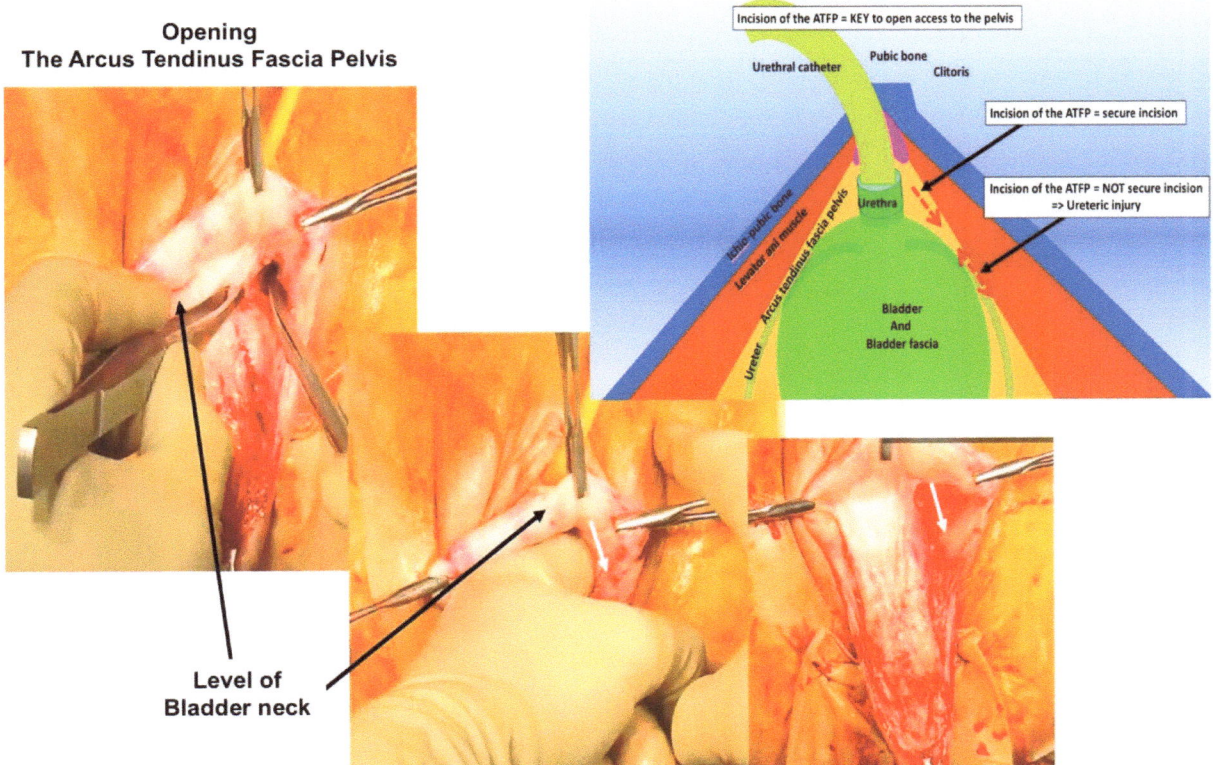

Fig. 7.56. **To open the arcus tendineus fascia pelvis: the key to go inside the pelvis area** (according to **Delorme, E.**)

The finger inserted laterally to the bladder frees the posterior face of the obturator muscle from the fat. Then it follows the lateral pelvic wall from front to back before reaching the ischial spine, an essential endopelvic landmark. Inside the ischial spine, the finger frees the anterior face of the sacrospinous ligament from the outside in and from top to bottom. Perirectal fat often adheres to the anterior section of the sacrospinous ligament. Inside, most often, the finger will find the outer edge of the sacrum where the sacrospinous ligament is attached. Sometimes, while freeing the SSL from the rectal fat, a rigidity corresponding to the middle rectal artery can be felt on the inside of the finger. Great care must be taken with the dissection here, and it is usually possible to pass the finger behind the artery to reach the edge of the sacrum.

2/ Cystocele after hysterectomy

More often than not, after hysterectomy, the cystocele is accompanied by an anterior enterocele.

After infiltration of the vaginal wall, a sagittal vaginal incision, about 4 cm long, is made, 3 cm above the bladder neck. It is a full thickness incision of the vaginal wall, and dissection will be made between the bladder and the fascia. It is possible to roll the vaginal wall out on itself, as this exposes the dissection plane very well, but it is not always necessary.

The opening of the ATFP and the dissection are the same as previously described for surgery with the uterus in place.

The enterocele must be resected via the vaginal route and its peritoneal entrance closed with a resorbable suture.

Technique for inserting the straps

The OPUR® kit contains three needles specifically for the implant straps: the blue one is for the ATO, the green one for the PTO and the white one for the TSS.

The needles are used for the first step, which is to introduce nitinol wire loops inside the routes of the mesh straps.

The second step is to use these nitinol loops to pull the mesh straps through the pelvic wall.

1 - The route for the ATO is the anterior trans-obturator route (Fig. 7.57.).

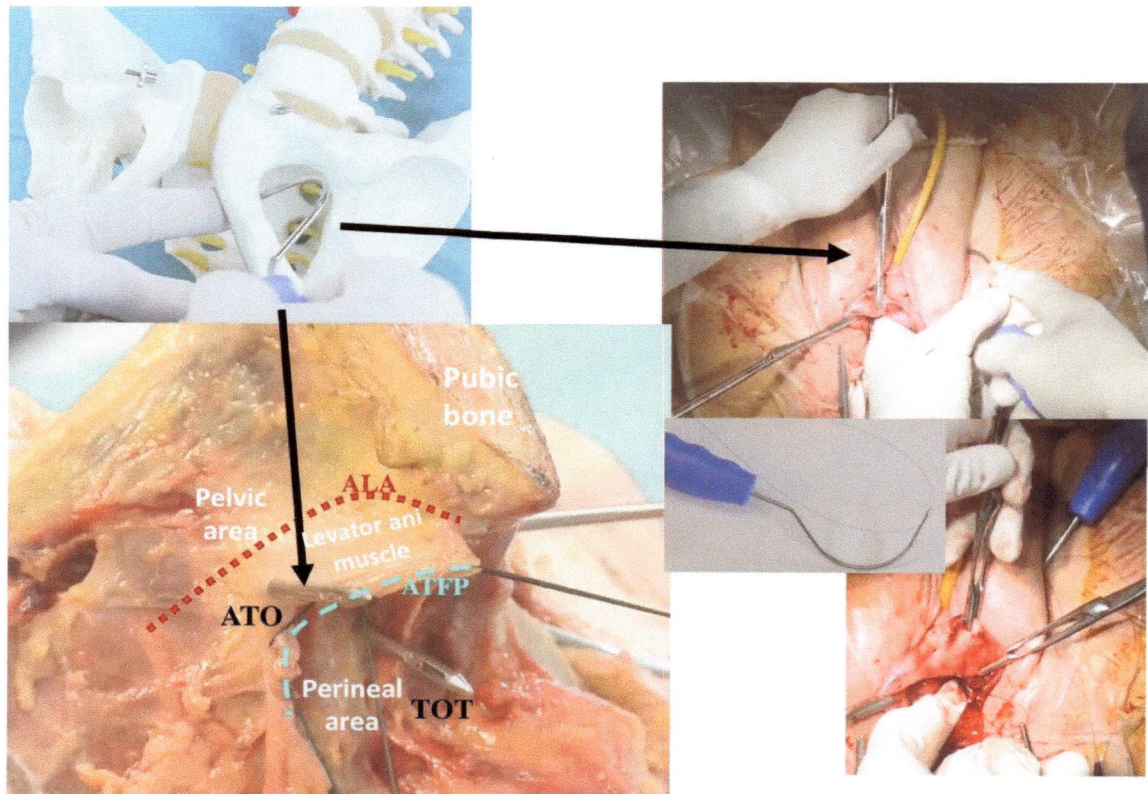

Fig. 7.57. The anterior arm way is anterior to the trans-obturator route (according to **Delorme, E.**)

The route of the blue needle is out-in. It is an oblique route from the corner between the pubic bone and the ischiopubic ramus, through the obturator muscles, into the pelvis, arriving opposite the trigone, just above the bladder neck. This route is rather different from the TOT route because it is a pelvic and not a perineal route (the perineal route is horizontal).

2 – The medial and lateral straps are the PTO (Fig. 7.58.)

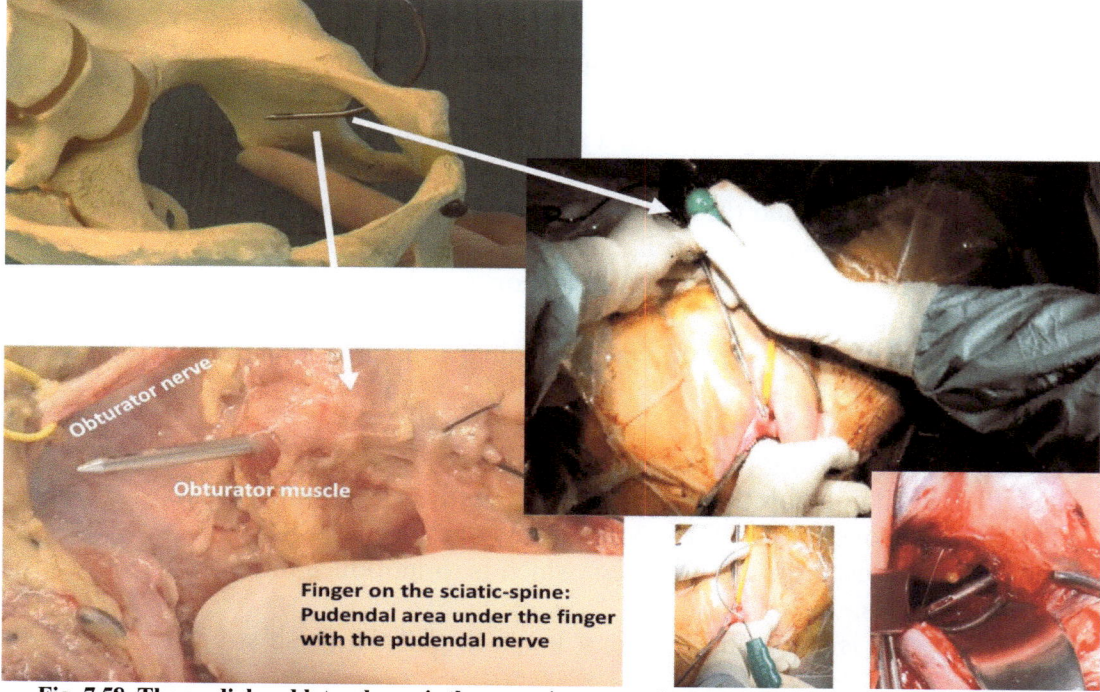

Fig. 7.58. The medial and lateral arm is the posterior trans-obturator arm (according to **Delorme, E.**)

The route is out-in. The needle entry point is in the ischiatic corner of the obturator foramen (between the ilio-ischial ramus and the ischiopubic ramus).

We have described the pudendal line. The finger covers this line when its tip is placed on the ischial spine. The pudendal nerve is under the finger on same axis as the finger. The green needle in the kit is used via the out-in route to introduce the PTO.

The needle insertion point on the skin is just in front of the mid-point of the ilio-ischial side of the obturator foramen. The needle way is parallel to the finger, outside the pudendal line, two centimeters above and lateral to the ischial spine, following an anterior-posterior trajectory through the thickness of the internal obturator muscle. It passes inside the pelvis and leaves the obturator muscle at the ischial spine level. The needle must go beyond this point, as there would be a risk of injuring the sciatic nerve roots.

The needle must not be turned to bring it into the vaginal incision, as this would tear the internal obturator muscle. The Nitinol loop is easily caught with a pair of forceps inside the pelvis so that it can be left in standby position until the implant is inserted.

This technique for the insertion of the PTO straps and their location is from the lateral side of the mesh to two centimeters outside the ischial spine. This prevents any damage to the pudendal nerve and keeps the strap away from the lateral sulcus of the vaginal vault, reducing the risk of shrinking and painful adherence to the vaginal wall.

3/ The posterior, trans-sacrospinous strap (Fig. 7.59.)

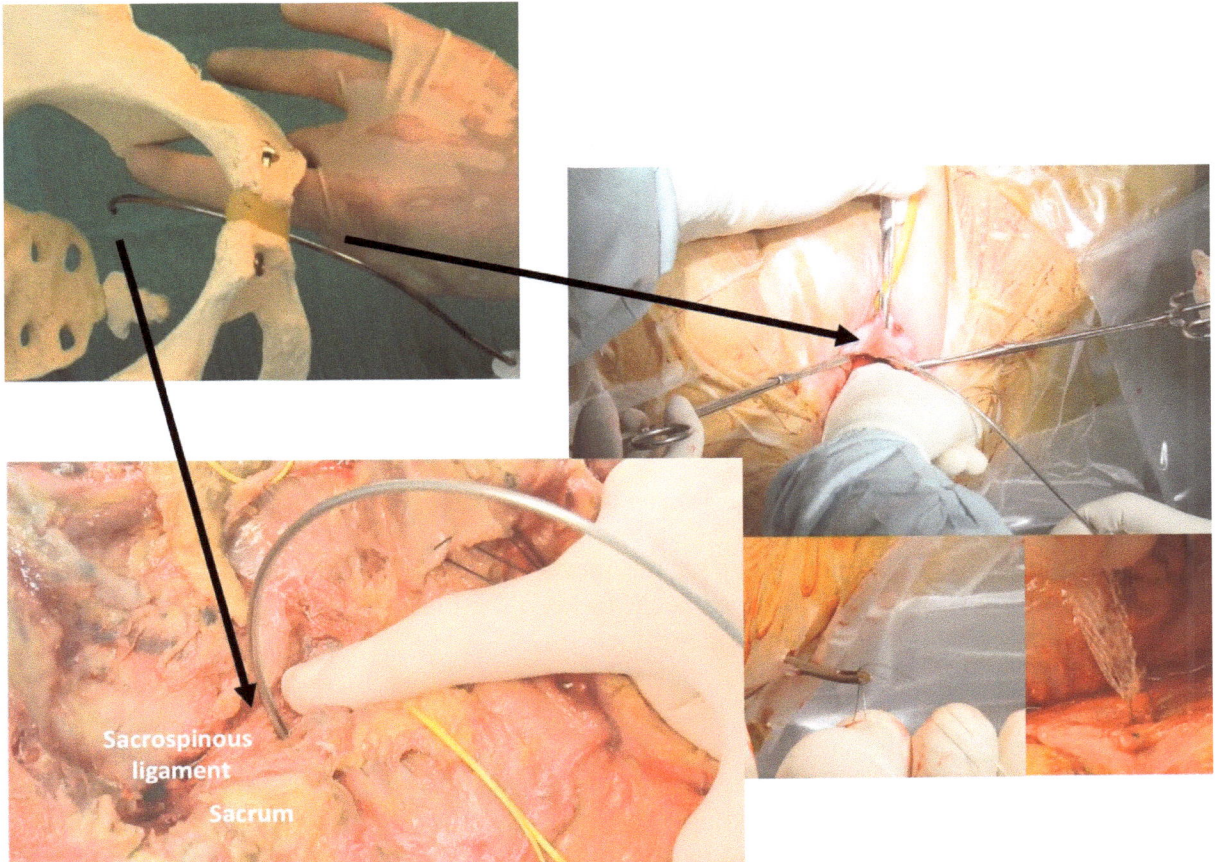

Fig. 7.59. **The posterior arm: trans-sacrospinous arm** (according to **Delorme, E.**)

The route for the TSS is in out. We have been using this technique since 2008 and it is performed with a specific long needle (white needle in the OPUR® kit).

The tip of the finger is placed on the ischial spine and the needle is slid along the inside of the finger until contact is made with the ischial spine. The finger pushes the needle onto the ligament as close as possible to the edge of the sacrum (1 cm from it). The end of the needle is placed close to the sacrum mid-height on the ligament. The needle is then pushed vertically through the ligament so that the gluteal muscle arrives at the buttock skin about 8 cm above and outside the anus. This is why the buttocks must be off the operating table during the procedure and the area up to the sacrum must be sterile. A nitinol loop is placed in the eye of the needle and the needle is drawn inside the pelvis through the sacrospinous ligament and caught at the vaginal incision.

The in-out route seems less dangerous than the out-in route, for several reasons:
- the needle can be placed directly on the sacrospinous ligament, away from the dangerous surrounding structures, and its trajectory is away from this dangerous area (pudendal nerve outside and sciatic nerve roots above the sacrospinous ligament);
- it is a short way through the pelvic wall;
- the NITINOL loop is fixed onto the needle outside the buttock, thereby avoiding any difficult endopelvic procedure and reducing the dissection area;
- finally, the fact that the needle trajectory passes very close to the sacrum allows the posterior strap to be positioned very close to the uterosacral ligament.

Implantation of the mesh (Fig. 7.60.)

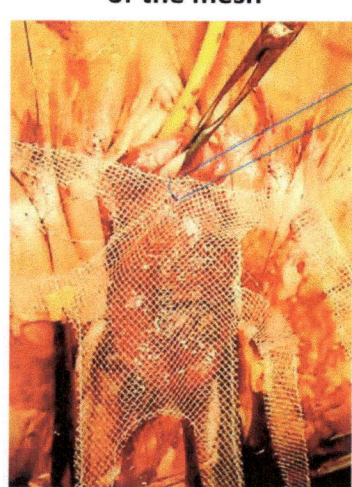
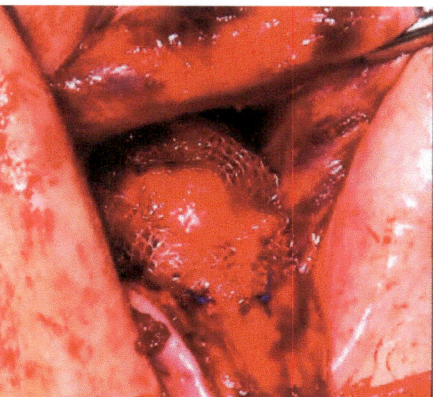
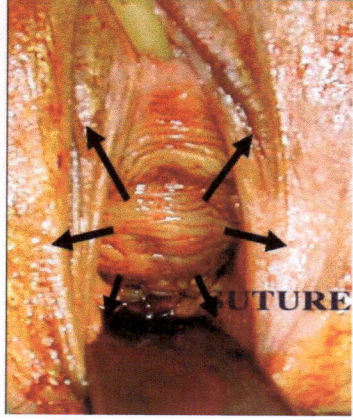

Fig. 7.60. **Implantation of the mesh** (according to **Delorme, E.**)

The middle of the anterior edge of the mesh is attached to the vaginal fascia with one resorbable suture, just above the bladder neck, to keep the bladder neck and the urethra mobile during effort and prevent stress urinary incontinence.

The ATO and PTO are pulled through the vaginal wall.

The posterior, upper edge of the mesh is attached to the uterine isthmus with two resorbable sutures when the uterus is present. After hysterectomy, the vaginal insertion of the uterosacral ligaments is identified. The upper corners of the implant are attached by one non-resorbable suture to the vaginal insertions of the uterosacral ligaments. This enables the mesh to spread wide and cover the entire base of the bladder.

The TSSs are pulled through the vaginal wall.

Once the implant is in place, the vaginal wall is unrolled and then sutured by a continuous suture with resorbable thread in two planes (fascia and mucosa).

The straps are then pulled in a particular order: the TSSs are pulled hard, which raises the vaginal apex, and then the ATOs are pulled gently without excessive tension. Finally, the PTOs are adjusted without any tension at all, as their role is only hold the mesh in place laterally when it contracts. In addition, pulling hard on the posterior transobturator straps would run the risk of tearing the fragile obturator muscles.

Conclusion

One first prospective study with 3 years' follow-up confirmed the low morbidity of the OPUR® procedure and the good anatomical and functional outcomes (**Guyomard A., Delorme E., 2016**).

A retrospective study of a series of 311 patients, with 3 to 6 years' follow-up had the same outcomes as the first publication (Tables 7.1.-7.3.).

Table 7.1. Per and postoperative complications (nb %), retrospective study monocentric, 311 patients, median follow-up 3 years

Complications	Total nb (%)
No complication	194 (62,4)
Urinary infection	35 (11,3)
PMR >100ml Less 15 days	69 (22,2)
Haematoma (puborectal, vaginal, labia majora, pelvic)	23 (7,4)
Repeat surgery under GA	4 (1.3)
Repeat surgery under LA	6 (1.9)
Neuropathic pain	2 (0.6)
Abscess (pararectal, vaginal)	4 (1.3)
Peroperative bladder trauma	2 (0.6)
Prosthesis erosion	4 (1.3)
Complications	Total nb (%)
No complication	194 (62,4)
Urinary infection	35 (11,3)
PMR >100ml Less 15 days	69 (22,2)
Haematoma (puborectal, vaginal, labia majora, pelvic)	23 (7,4)
Repeat surgery under GA	4 (1.3)
Repeat surgery under LA	6 (1.9)
Neuropathic pain	2 (0.6)
Abscess (pararectal, vaginal)	4 (1.3)
Peroperative bladder trauma	2 (0.6)
Prosthesis erosion	4 (1.3)

PMR: post mictional residue, GA: general anaesthesia LA: local anaesthesi

Table 7.2. Anatomical results of the surgical procedure, retrospective study monocentric, 311 patients, median follow-up 3 years

	Preoperative	Immediate postoperative	p value	Last consultation	p value
Cystocele			<.0001		<.0001
≤ I	3 (1.0)	309 (99.4)		302 (97.1)	
II	18 (5.8)	2 (0.6)		8 (2.6)	
III	261 (83.9)	0 (0)		1 (0.3)	
IV	29 (9.3)	0 (0)		0 (0)	
Hysterocele			<.0001		<.0001
≤ I	156 (50,2)	310 (99.7)		306 (98.4)	
II	74 (23.8)	0 (0)		4 (1.3)	
III	55 (17,7)	1 (0.3)		1 (0.3)	
IV	26 (8.4)	0 (0)		0 (0)	
Rectocele			<.0001		0,1885
≤ I	279 (89.7)	304 (97.7)		279 (89,7)	
II	13 (4.2)	3 (1)		25 (8.0)	
III	15 (4,8)	4 (1.3)		7 (2.3)	
IV	4 (1.3)	0 (0)		0 (0)	
TVL (cm)	9,5 ± 1,6	10,1 ± 2,6	0,0024		

All values shown are n (%).
TVL: total vaginal length. (Mean ± Std)

Table 7.3. Functional results at the last consultation. Retrospective study monocentric, 311 patients, median follow-up 3 years

	Preoperative	Last consultation			
		Cured	Improved	Same	Worse
No SUI	206 (66,4)			160 (78)	46 (22)
Slight SUI	88 (28,4)	55 (62,5)	11 (12,5)	11 (12,5)	11 (12,5)
Severe SUI	16 (5,2)	12 (75)	4 (25)	0 (0)	
No OB	66 (21,3)			28 (42)	38 (58)
OB without incontinence	203 (65,5)	61 (30)	88 (43)	20 (10)	34 (17)
OB with incontinence	41 (13,2)	7 (17)	29 (71)	1 (2)	4 (10)
No dysuria	80 (25,8)			70 (87,5)	10 (12,5)
Slight dysuria	194 (62,6)	150 (77)	19 (10)	24 (12)	1 (1)
Severe dysuria	36 (11,6)	30 (83)	6 (17)	0 (0)	
Good vaginal comfort	53 (17,1)			50 (94,3)	3 (5,7)
Poor vaginal comfort	257 (82,9)		235 (91,4)	22 (8,6)	

All values shown are n (%).
SUI: stress urinary incontinence; OB: overactive bladder
Vaginal confort: no shrinking, no vaginal pain spontaneously or during examination, if there is sexual intercourse

For us, vaginal mesh with six straps is probably a good option to cure anterior prolapse alone or with hysterocele or vaginal vault prolapse.

7.4. Posterior compartment surgery

The surgical approach of posterior compartment represents the ultimate test bridge of perineal surgery. Narrow anatomic spaces, occupied by important organs and highly vascularized predispose to high risks and need both sophisticated instruments and special surgical abilities. Ligament defects imply all the three DeLancey levels, cardinal and uterosacral ligaments, rectovaginal fascia, and perineal body. Regarding posterior compartment defects, there are two types of pathologies, often associated: uterine prolapse and posterior vaginal prolapse (**Petros P., 2010**). Classical surgery offers few pathogenic solutions for these disorders, often choosing excisional surgery. Principles of Integral Theory, of specific restoration of affected structures are difficult to accomplish by classical surgery (**Miller D.,** *et al.,* **2011**). At present, there is a strong tendency of giving up excisional therapy, taking into account that it does not treat the causes but the effect of pelvic floor disorders. For this reason, we consider that vaginal hysterectomy, as treatment of uterine prolapse does not represent a viable solution anymore (**Petros P., 2010**). Uterine prolapse can be conceptually assimilated to an inferior hernia, a weak area at the inferior limit of abdominal cavity. By analogy with hernias of anterior abdominal wall, treatment cannot imply the excision of herniated organ in the absence of complications, enterectomies, omentectomies, etc., but by the restoration of parietal defect.

7.4.1. Classical surgical procedures

Although they have an important rate of complications and relapses, the classical techniques are still widespread.

7.4.1.1. Posterior colpoperineorrhaphy

Posterior colpoperineorrhaphy is a surgical technique for rectocele. This can or cannot accompany utero-vaginal prolapse and can or cannot be asymptomatic. Constipation or disorders of gastrointestinal motility can be some of the symptoms. It is important to remember that surgical treatment must be applied only to symptomatic patients.

Surgical steps

1. Patient is placed in a gynecological position. The vulva, vagina, and perineum are prepared while respecting the asepsis and antisepsis rules. We consider that the dissection of vagina can be performed better by using hydrodissection techniques. Vasoconstriction solutions with epinephrine or adrenaline can be used to facilitate hemostasis and according to the associated pathology of the patient.

Two Chaput forceps are placed at the cutaneo-mucous junction of the vaginal introit, not too far one from the other, so that by bringing them together to easily allow the vaginal tact. Another forceps is placed towards the vaginal apex delimiting the rectocele, above its superior edge. A transverse incision between the two forceps is performed at the level of cutaneo-mucous junction and subsequently the rectovaginal space is dissected towards the vaginal apex, behind the rectocele, Fig. 7.61.A. In the classical technique, the excess of vaginal mucosa is sectioned; however, we believe that this is not necessary, as postoperatory the vaginal mucosa has the tendency to adapt to the new sizes. In order to help the dissection, as it advances, some Chaput forceps can be placed also on the two lateral edges of the triangle of vaginal mucosa that was previously delimited, thus tensioning the vaginal wall, Fig. 7.61.B.

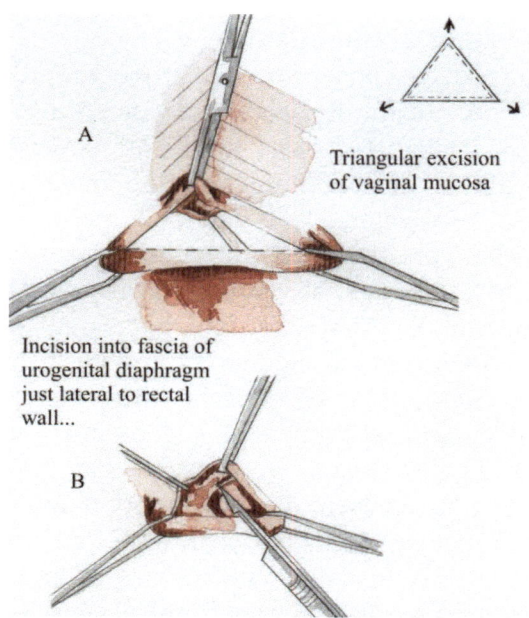

Fig. 7.61. Incision and dissection of posterior vaginal mucosa (*drawing by Vanessa Mureşan*)
A – dissection and excision of vaginal mucosa; B – lateral dissection

2. Pulling the Chaput forceps and tensioning the posterior vaginal wall, the rectum is carefully dissected thus evidencing the rectovaginal fascia, Fig. 7.62. Then the edges of the fascia are approximated on medial line with slowly resorbable sutures passed separately or "*in burse*". At this surgical moment, the approximation of levator ani muscles can be done, a procedure that must be applied selectively to patients because it can produce severe dyspareunia, Fig. 7.63. A, B, C.

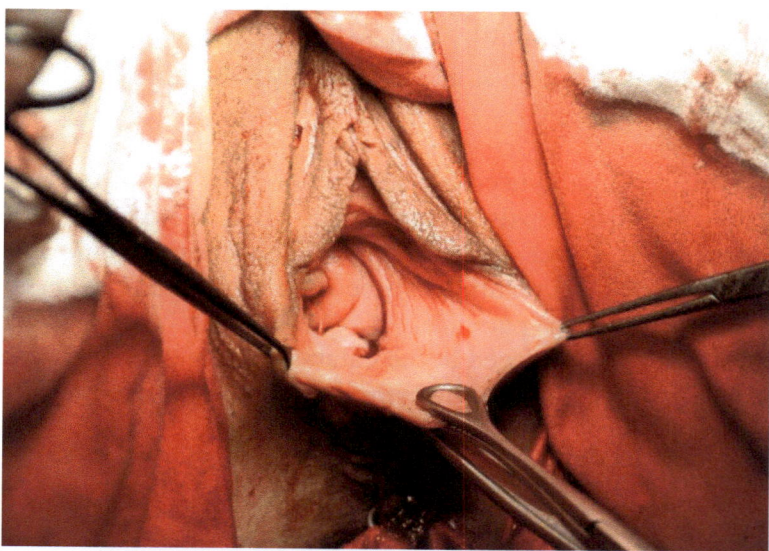

Fig. 7.62. Dissection of rectovaginal fascia with Metzenbaum scissors
(from the archive of **Moisa M.**)

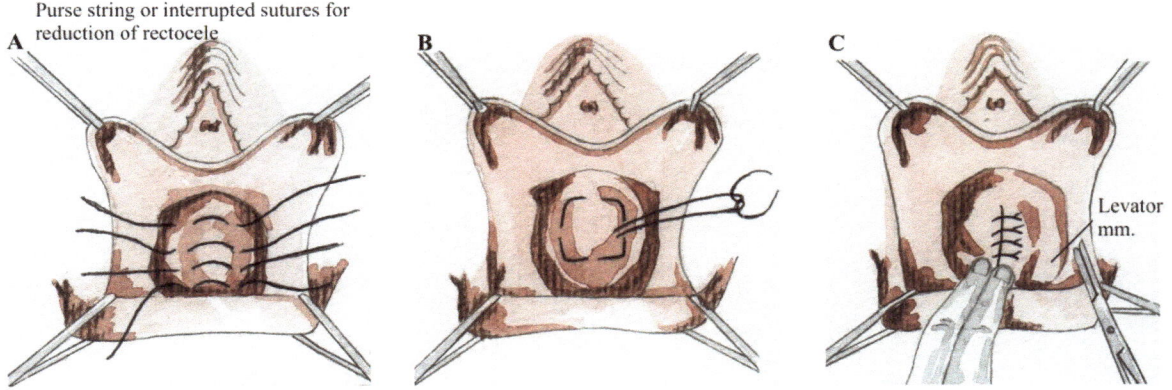

Fig. 7.63. Myorrhaphy of levator ani muscles (*drawing by Vanessa Mureşan*)
A- separate wires; B - ; C – levator ani muscle

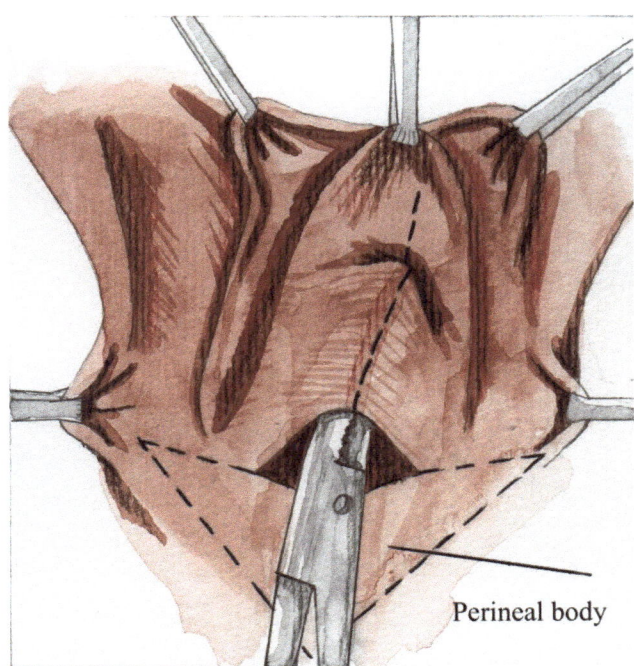

Fig. 7.64. "*V*" incision at the level of perineal skin (*drawing by Vanessa Mureşan*)

3. If the intervention also implies posterior perineorrhaphy, which happens most often due to perineal body's dehiscence, a "*V*" incision is practiced at the level of perineal skin, which is possible if perineum is at least 2 cm height, Fig. 7.64. Skin at this level is dissected thus evidencing the superficial transverse muscle and the bulbocavernosus muscles and the skin excess is excised, Fig. 7.65 and 7.66.

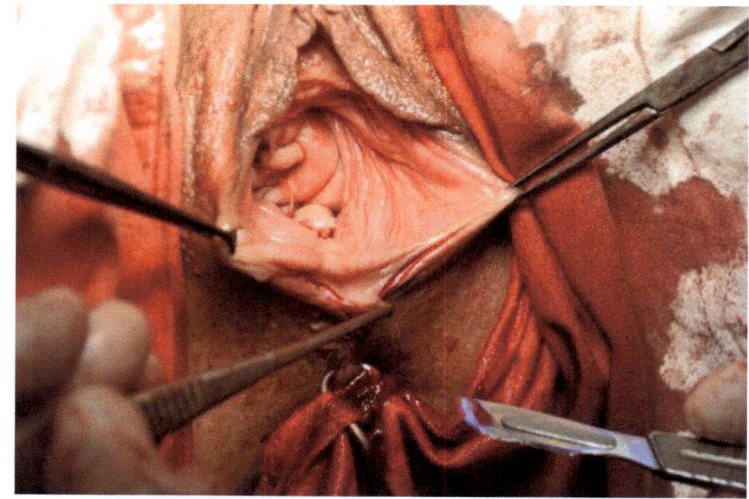
Fig. 7.65. "V" incision at the level of perineal skin
(from the archive of **Moisa M.**)

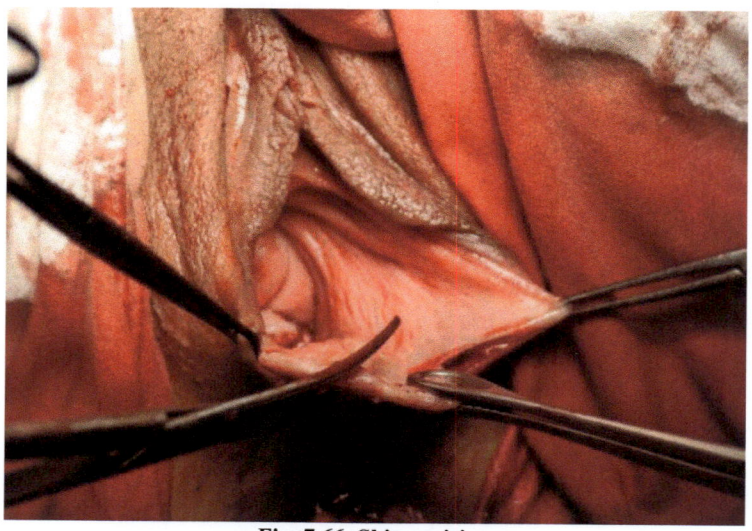
Fig. 7.66. Skin excision
(from the archive of **Moisa M.**)

4. Perineorrhaphy implies the approximation of superficial transverse and bulbocavernosus muscles on median line with separate wires of dilacerate edges, Fig. 7.67.A and B. This should be done carefully so as not to tension the muscles too much, which could lead to their tearing and the aggravation of symptoms or creating some vicious scars that could lead to severe dyspareunia. An intraoperative aspect is presented in Fig 7.68.

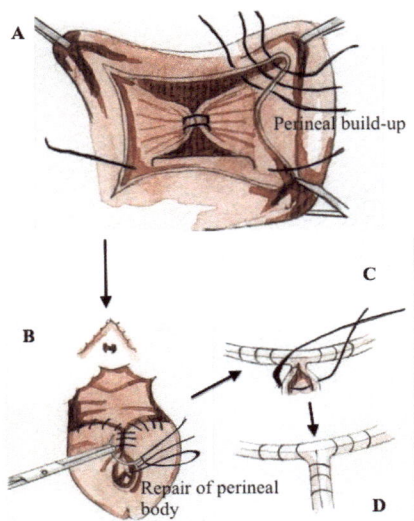

Fig. 7.67. Perineorrhaphy (*drawing by Vanessa Mureșan*)
A – perineal body; B - reconstruction ; C – suture of vagina; D – suture of perineum

The suture of vagina and perineum is done on the incision lines with slowly resorbable sutures passed separately or interrupted suture, Fig. 7.67.C and D.

Postoperatory aspect is presented in fig. 7.68. The patient is mounted a Foley catheter and is usually released in 48 hours.

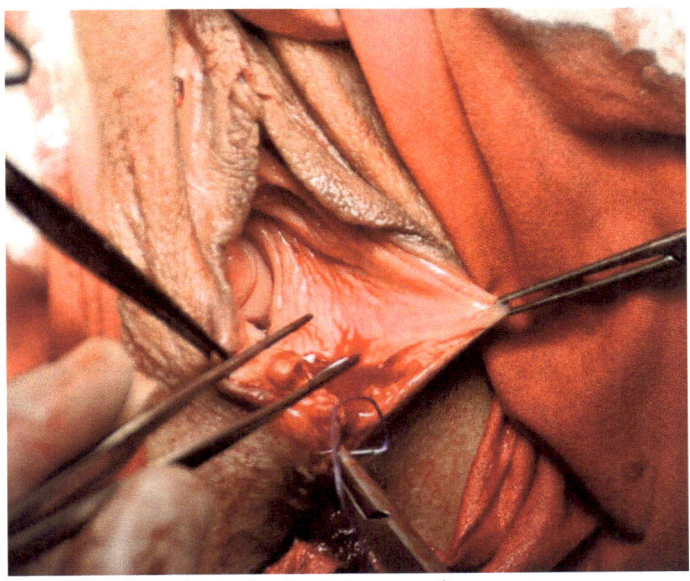

Fig. 7.68. Myorrhaphy, intraoperative aspect
(from the archive of **Moisa M.**)

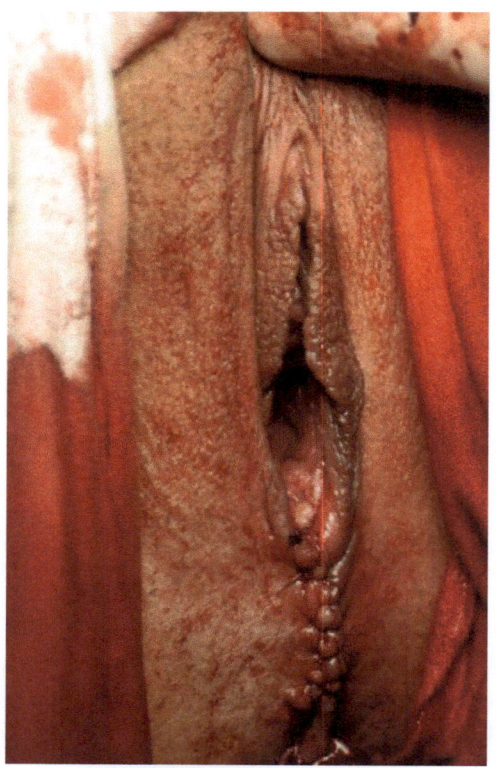

Fig. 7.69. Postoperatory aspect
(from the archive of **Moisa M.**)

7.4.1.2. Surgical treatment of vaginal vault prolapse

The most commonly used method of treatment of vaginal vault prolapse in hysterectomised patients is the Amreich-Richter operation, especially used in the Anglo-Saxon countries (**Bradley C.S.** & **Nygaard I.E., 2006**).

Even if it did not have an adequate spreading in Romania, in the USA it is the elective surgery for this pathology. It is considered a right procedure for sexually active women with total prolapse of vaginal canal. Total prolapse interferes with the function of bladder, defecation, and sexual intercourse.

Usually, the patients with this pathology also suffer from urinary incontinence, after the suspension of vagina it is possible that this phenomenon appears.

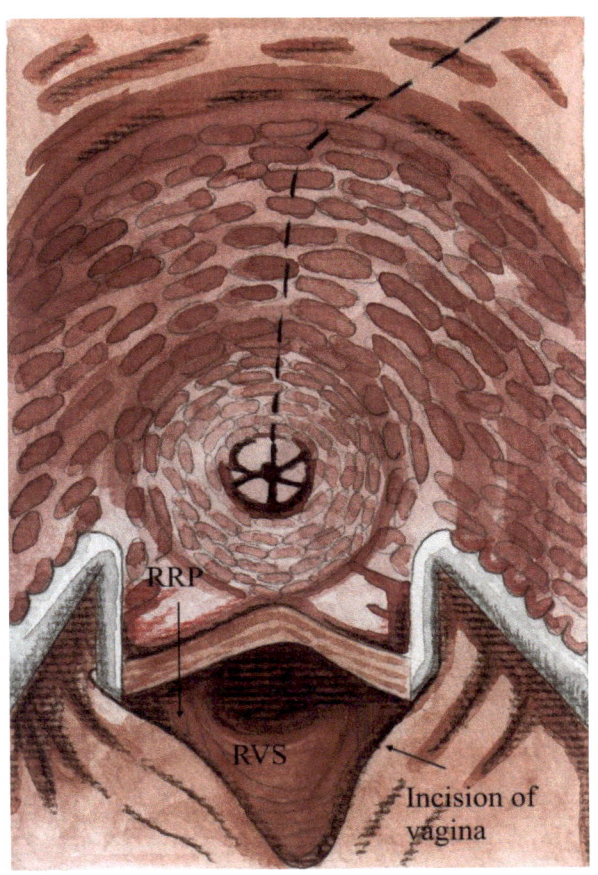

Fig. 7.70. Incision and dissection of right pararectal space
(*drawing by Vanessa Mureşan*)
RPF – right pararectal fascia; RVF – rectovaginal fascia

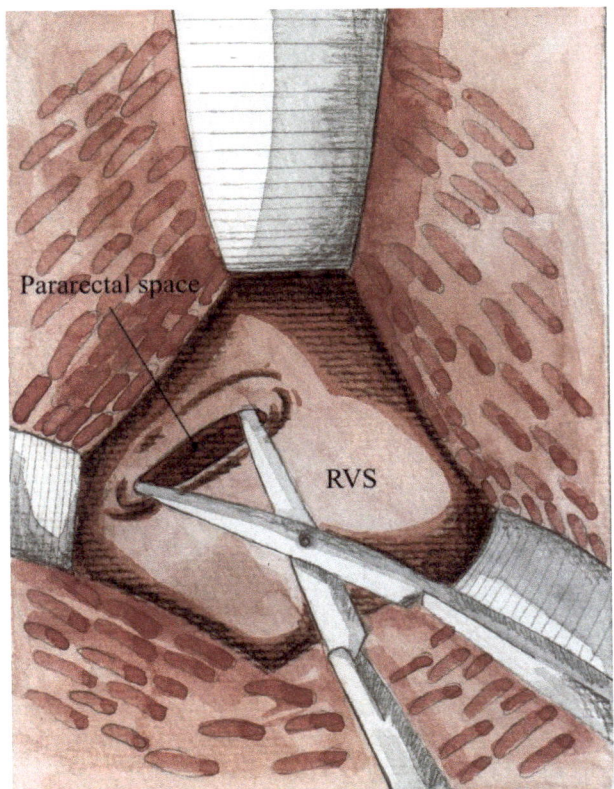

Fig. 7.71. Dissection of right pararectal space
(*drawing by Vanessa Mureşan*)

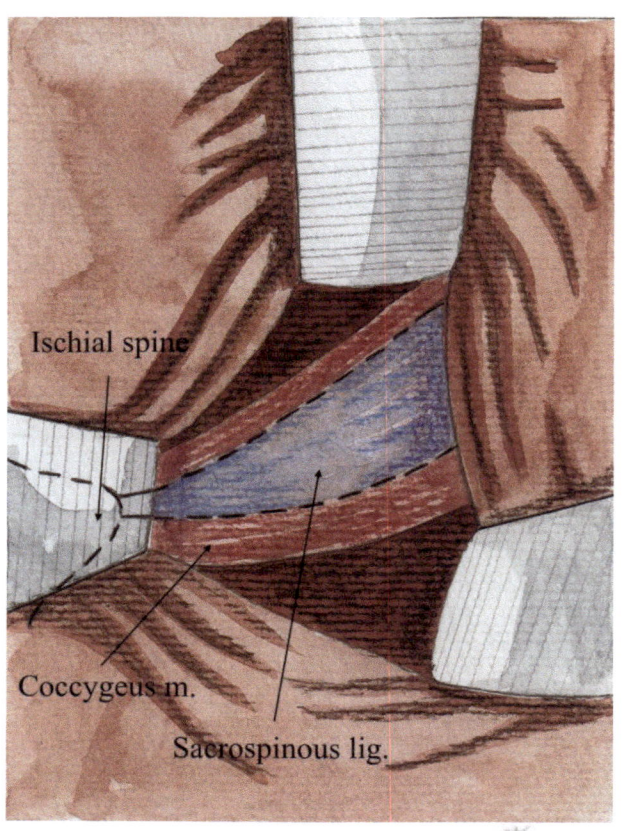

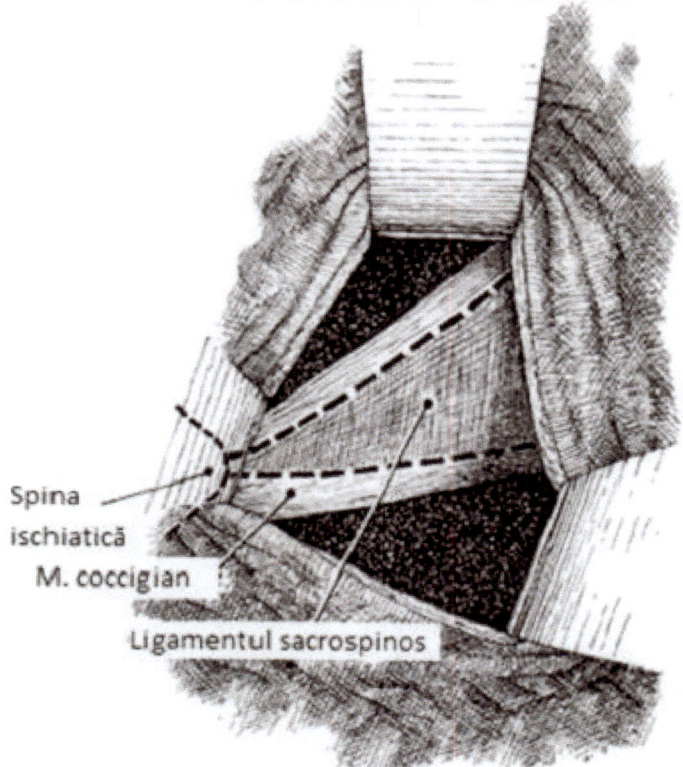

Fig. 7.72. Dissection of sacrospinous ligament
(*drawing by Vanessa Mureșan*)

If solving this new pathology must be performed at the same surgical time or afterwards, at 6 months postoperatory, remains questionable. In the USA, where the procedure is the most common, it is usually advisable to be performed at the same surgical time (**Wheeless C.R.Jr. & Roenneburg M.L., 2017**).

Surgical steps

1. The patient is placed in a gynecological position. The vulva, the vagina, and the perineum are prepared according to the aseptic and antiseptic measures. The anterior suture line of vaginal mucosa and vaginal vault is identified. The posterior vaginal mucosa is dissected at the rectovaginal septum (RVS) similar to posterior colporrhaphy.

Rectal pillars are identified on each side, and the right rectal pilar (RRP) is perforated blindly digitally or with a forceps, Fig. 7.70.

2. The right side of pararectal space is afterwards exposed ideally using Breisky-Navratil spacers because they are long and have the right curvature. Using the spacers, the rectum is pushed to the left, and the cardinal ligament and the urethra, anteriorly. Thus, the pelvic diaphragm is penetrated towards the right sacrospinous ligament, palpating the ischial spine, Fig. 7.71.

3. The dissection of the sacrospinous ligament with the removal of the areolar tissue around should be done carefully because of its important connections with vascular, nervous and muscle structures, Fig. 7.72., and by also taking into account the low visibility at this level.

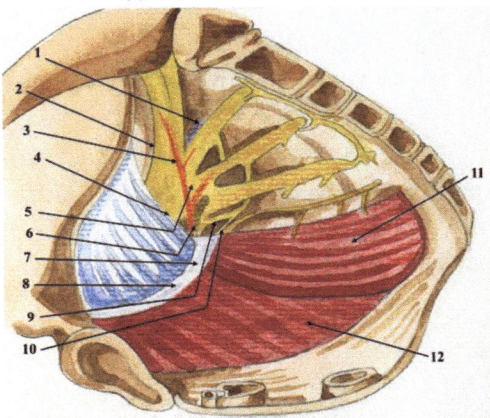

1. Superior Gluteal Artery; 2. Sciatic Nerve; 3. Nerve to Quadratus Femoris Muscle; 4. Internal Pudendal Artery; 5. Nerve to Obturator Internus Muscle; 6. Inferior Gluteal Artery; 7. Ischial Spine; 8. Tendinous Arch of Levator Ani Muscle; 9. Posterior Femoral Cutaneous Nerve; 10. Pudendal Nerve; 11. Coccygeus Muscle; 12. Levator Ani Muscle.

Fig. 7.73. Anatomical relations of sacrospinous ligament
(*drawing by Vanessa Mureșan*)

A particular attention should be paid to the connections with the superior gluteal artery, internal pudendal artery, and sciatic nerve. The dissection should not exceed the coccygeus muscle superiorly and the ischial spine laterally. The spacers should never reach behind the sacrospinous ligament and the ligature should not pass behind the ligament, because there is a risk of injury of inferior gluteal artery at this level, Fig. 7.73.

4. The ischial spine is palpated and a 2.0 non-resorbable suture is passed with the Deschamps needle holder at approximately 1.5 – 2 cm medially to the spine through the sacrospinous ligament, Fig. 7.74. If the wire is passed too close to the spine, it can intercept the internal pudendal artery. The passed wire is anchored on the forceps until a second one is passed in a similar manner.

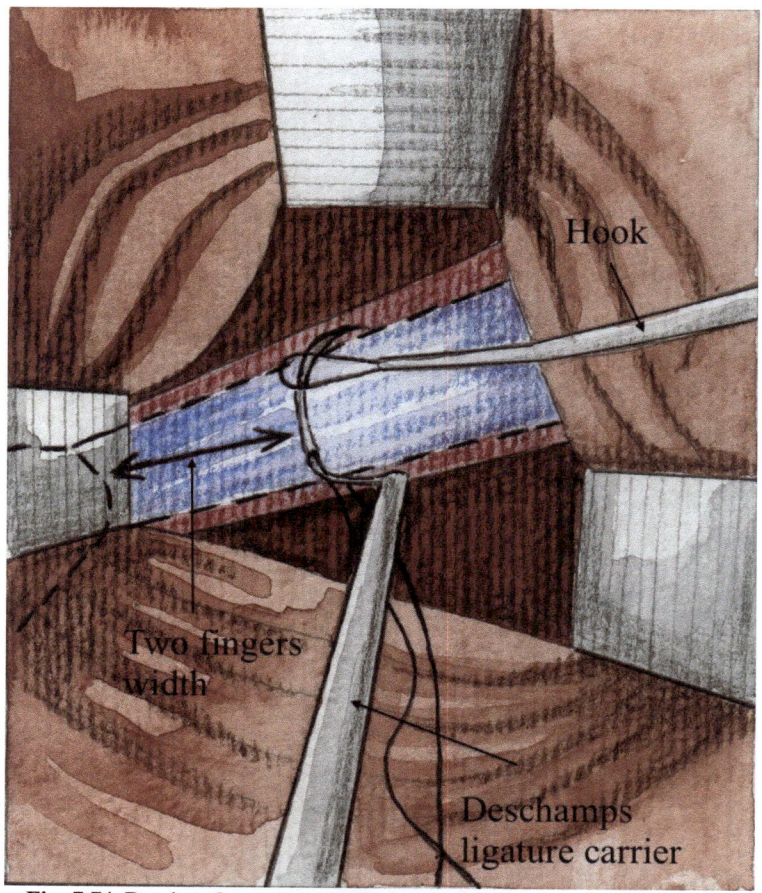

Fig. 7.74. Passing the sutures at the level of the sacrospinous ligament
(*drawing by Vanessa Mureşan*)

One of the ends of the wires passed through the sacrospinous ligament is afterwards passed through the muscular layer of the vagina incorporating the rectovaginal fascia, but without passing through the vaginal mucosa due to the high risk of suture granuloma. By tying the wires, the vaginal apex is anchored to the sacrospinous ligament, Fig. 7.75.

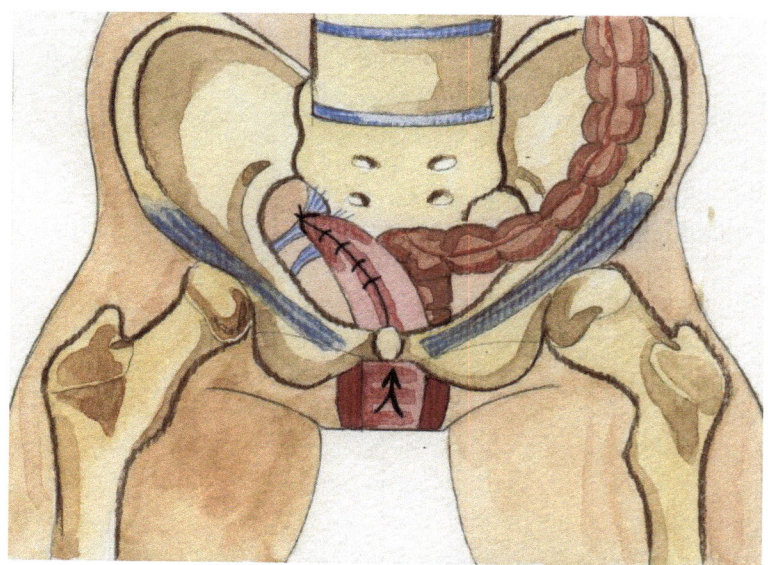

Fig. 7.75. Amreich – Richter procedure
(*drawing by Vanessa Mureşan*)

5. The procedure ends with a classic posterior colporrhaphy. The vaginal mucosa is sutured with a slowly resorbable suture in an interrupted suture or separately.

7.4.1.3. Surgical treatment of elitrocele

The elitrocele is the rupture of the high posterior vaginal wall consisting of peritoneum and usually small intestine loops in the rectovaginal space between the back of the vagina and the anterior side of the rectum.

Procedures for prevention and/ or solving enterocele on vaginal or abdominal hysterectomy are known and described. Among them, the following should be mentioned: McCall, Halban, Moschowitz culdoplasty, and procedures for vaginal reduction of elitrocele in patients with a history of hysterectomy.

Among the methods of prevention and/ or solving elitrocele on hysterectomy is the McCall culdoplasty, a procedure known to have the best results.

The procedure involves the incorporation of uterosacral and cardinal ligaments at the surface of peritoneum and implies the attachment of these ligaments to the vaginal apex. Squeezing the wires (1 or 2) passed through the above-mentioned structures leads to the orientation of the respective ligaments towards the median line, a maneuver that leads to elitrocele obliteration, Fig. 7.79.

The only important incident of this procedure is the kinking of ureters due to their proximity to the uterosacral ligaments.

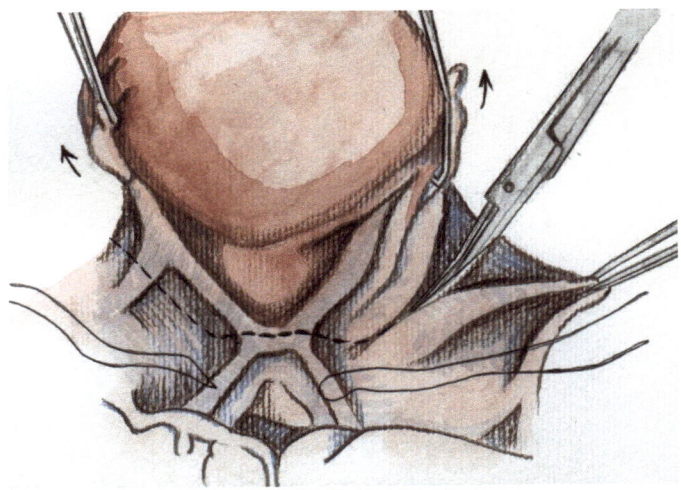

Fig. 7.76. McCall culdoplasty
(*drawing by Vanessa Mureşan*)

There are also variants of the technique, in the sense of incorporating the uterosacral and cardinal ligaments in the lateral angle of the vaginal layers on each side.

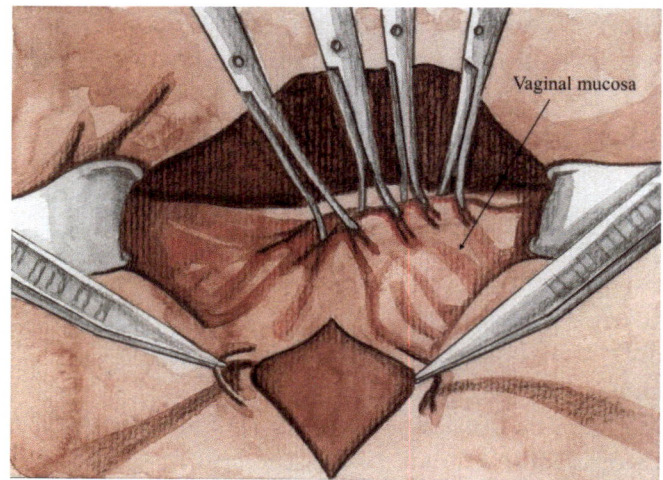

Fig. 7.76. "V" shaped incision at the dorsal commissure of the vulva
(*drawing by Vanessa Mureşan*)

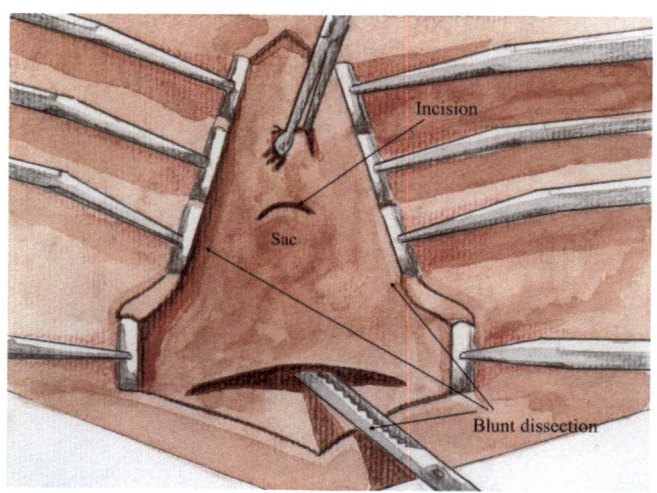

Fig. 7.77. Incision of hernial sac after its dissection
(*drawing by Vanessa Mureşan*)

Vaginal solving of elitrocele in patients with a history of hysterectomy is a special technique.

Surgical steps

1. The patient is placed in a gynecological position. The vulva, vagina, and perineum are prepared according to the aseptic and antiseptic measures.

The first surgical steps are identical to those described in posterior colporrhaphy. A "V" shaped incision is performed at the perineal body surface and dissection is continued towards the posterior vaginal mucosa, Fig. 7.76. Chaput tissue grasping forceps are placed on the medial line of the posterior vaginal mucosa above the rectocele, almost invariably associated to the elitrocele, in order to tension the vaginal wall, thus facilitating the dissection.

2. The vagina is dissected with a thin curved scissors that is inserted in closed position and is retracted in open position, thus enabling dissection in avascular spaces. Dissection is continued towards the vaginal apex with the highlighting of the elitrocele. The hernial sac of the elitrocele is evidenced with a Chaput tissue grasping forceps, is kept in tension and the perirectal fascia is carefully removed with a finger-mounted compress so that the elitrocele is visible. A small incision is then practiced in the hernial sac, Fig. 7.77.

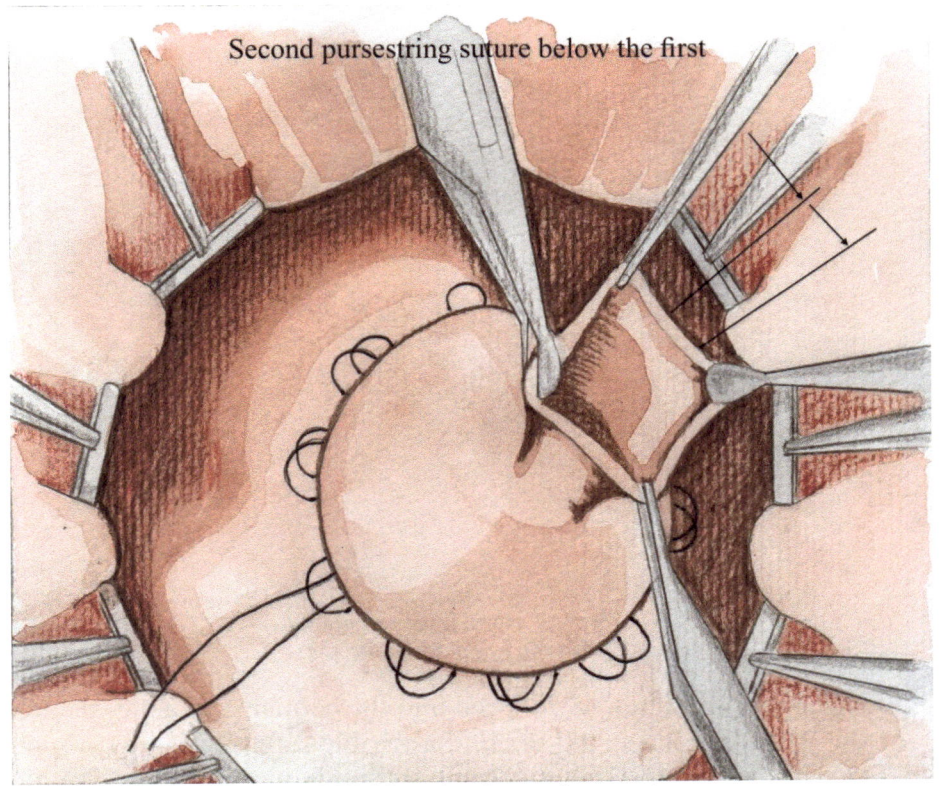

Fig. 7.78. Mounting the two bursa sutures
(*drawing by Vanessa Mureşan*)

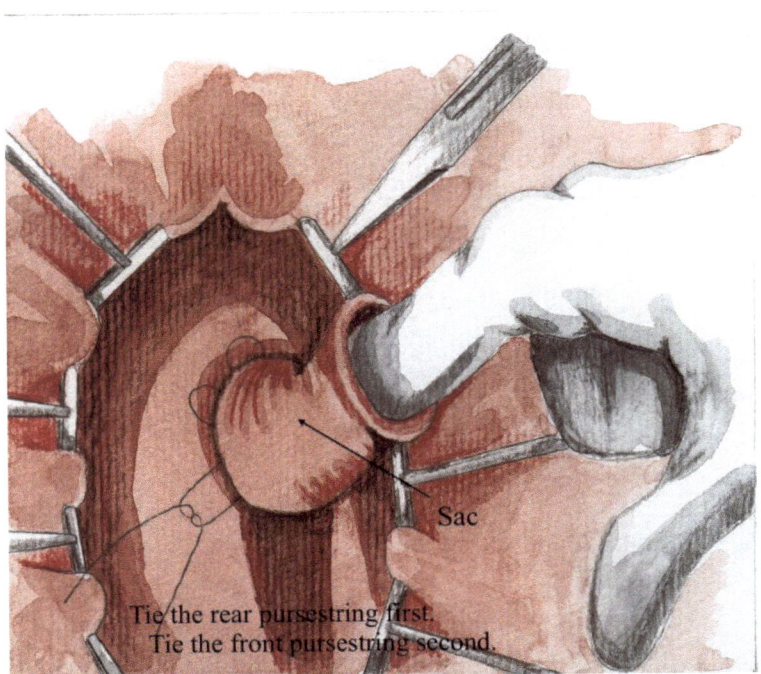

Fig. 7.79. Removing the hernial content from the finger before tying the sutures
(*drawing by Vanessa Mureşan*)

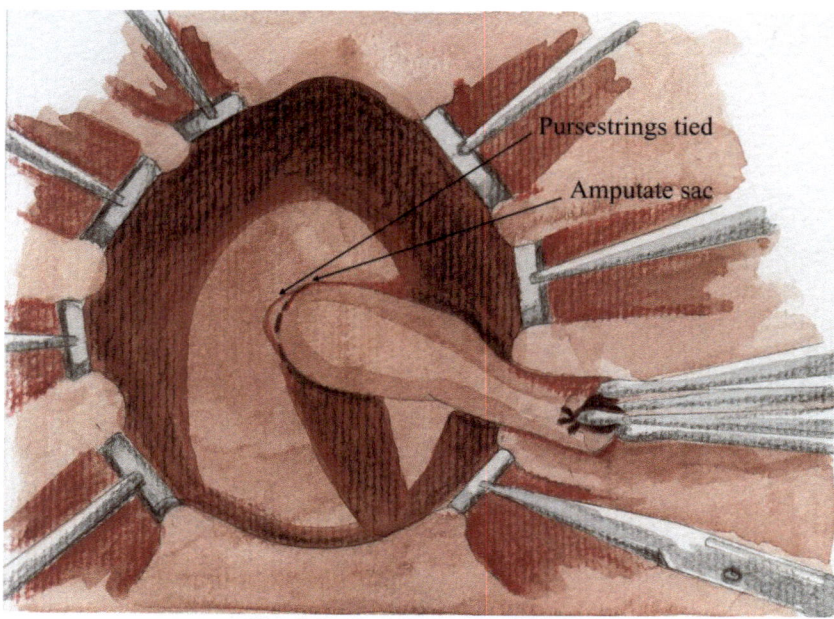

Fig. 7.80. Hernial sac amputation
(*drawing by Vanessa Mureşan*)

3. A finger is immediately introduced into the hernial sac and all the intraabdominal intestinal content is pushed. Then, a 0 slowly resorbable suture is passed around the neck of the hernial sac, without being tied; a second suture is passed below the first one, also without being tied, Fig. 7.78. Before binding the wires, the finger is inserted again into the hernial sac to remove the contents, Fig. 7.79.

4. After binding the sutures, the hernial sac can be removed, Fig. 7.80.

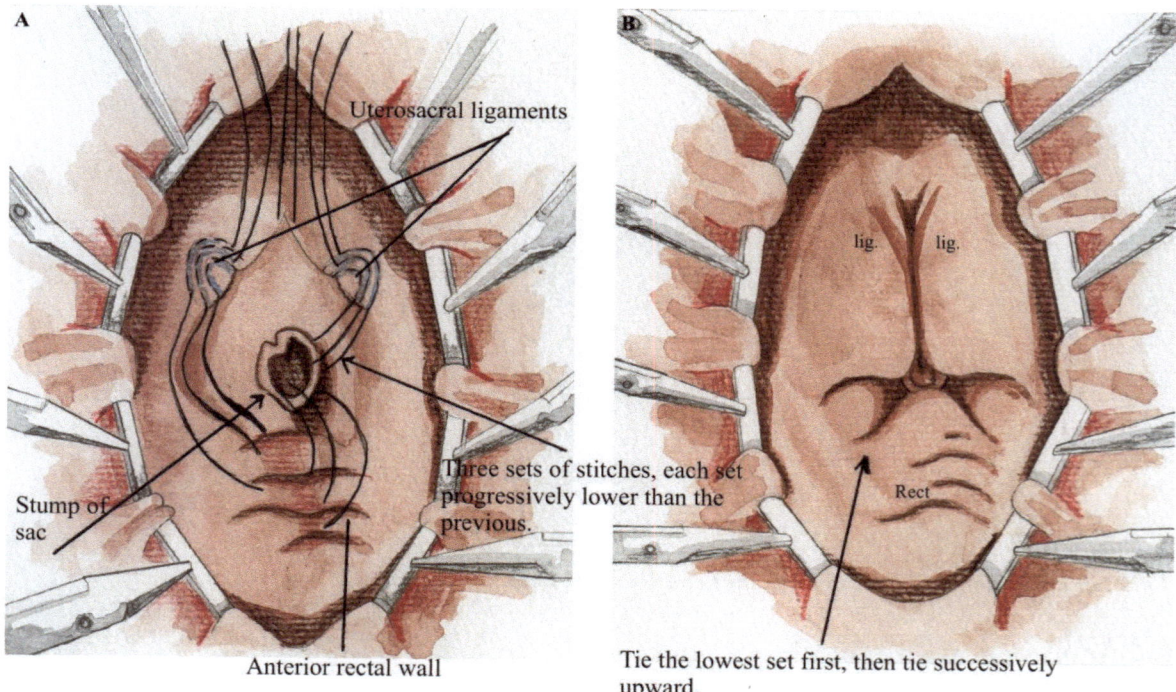

Fig. 7.81. Elitrocele reduction (*drawing by Vanessa Mureşan*)
A) Placement of sutures;
B) Plication of resistance structures

5. Afterwards, the hernial sac blunt is sutured with a 0 slowly resorbable suture to the anterior side of the rectum and to the two uterosacral ligaments. The maneuver is repeated 2-3 times. Each suture is placed deeper into the genital canal than the previous one, Fig. 7.81.A. The passed wires are kept on forceps until all are passed and then they are bind reverse to the way they were passed (the first wire is bind with the last wire passed). This way, the uterosacral ligaments, the hernial sac blunt and the anterior rectal wall are plicated, Fig. 7.81.B. In addition, the appearance of a new elitrocele becomes unlikely.

6. The last step is the rectocele reduction by using the technique described above. We propose to avoid the excision of vaginal mucosa. The vaginal layer is sutured with a 0 slowly resorbable suture passed separately or in interrupted suture. Further, the perineal body is restored by techniques described above, which imply the plication of superficial transverse muscles and bulbocavernosus muscles, with great attention to sexually active women, Fig. 7.82.

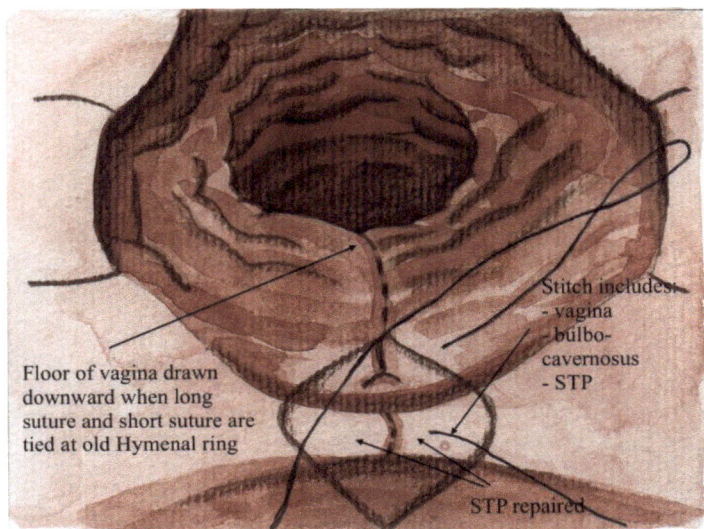

Fig. 7.82. Rectocele reduction
(*drawing by Vanessa Mureşan*)

7.4.1.4. Colpocleisis

It is a solution for patients with congenital physical or moral defects, elder patients and patients who, for various reasons, do not have or consent not have a sexual life. Recurrent prolapse after this intervention is extremely rare. The procedure practically obliterates the vagina except for two small lateral canals, which are theoretically useful for eliminating vaginal discharges. Resuming sexual life is however impossible after this intervention. Mueller total colpocleisis is not practiced today anymore. The most common procedure is Neugebauer-Le Fort partial colpocleisis, which implies the attachment of anterior vaginal wall to the posterior one after the detachment of a mucosa quadrangle from the two vaginal walls (**Sîrbu P., 1981**).

Surgical steps

1. The patient is placed in a gynecological position. The vulva, vagina, and perineum are prepared according to the aseptic and antiseptic measures. The labia minora can be anchored laterally with two 2.0 resorbable sutures.

The cervix is pulled with a cervix forceps and an anterior vaginal mucosa quadrangle to be excised is marked with the scalpel, Fig. 7.83.A. The same is done for posterior vaginal mucosa, Fig. 7.83.B.

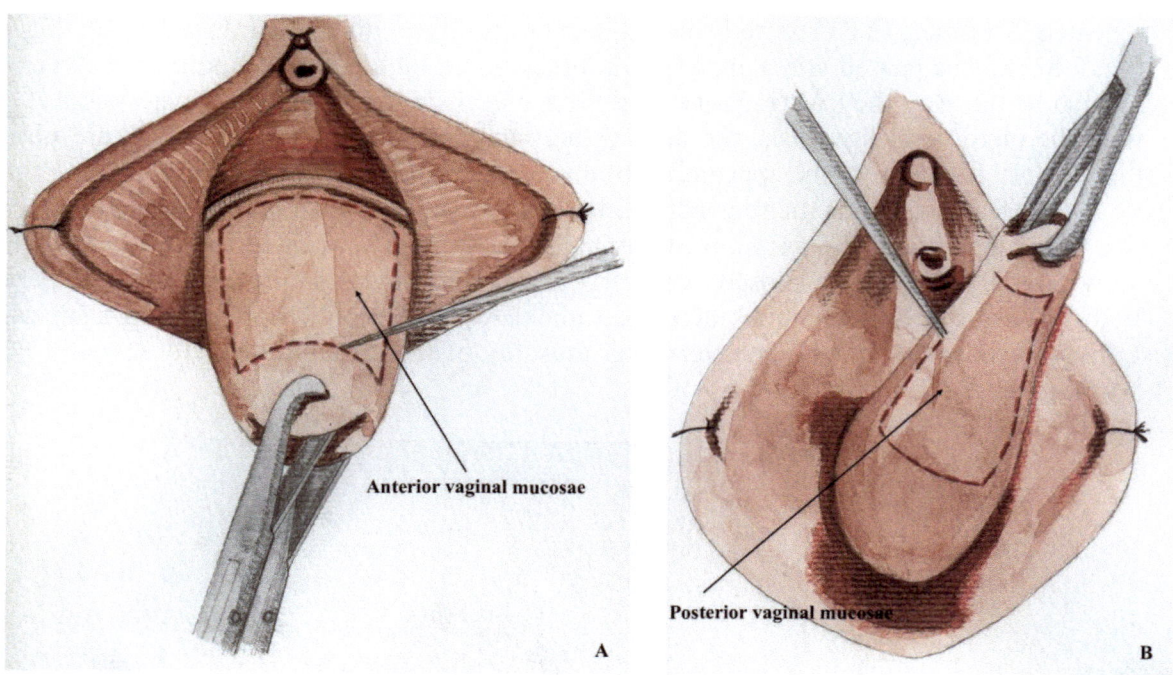

Fig. 7.83. Quadrangle spotting (*drawing by Vanessa Mureşan*)
A) Anterior quadrangle spotting; B) Posterior quadrangle spotting

The posterior vaginal mucosa quadrangle is dissected starting from the vaginal mucosa to the cervix. The same technique is used to dissect the vaginal mucosa from the perirectal fascia using the curved thin scissors inserted into closed position and retracted into open position.

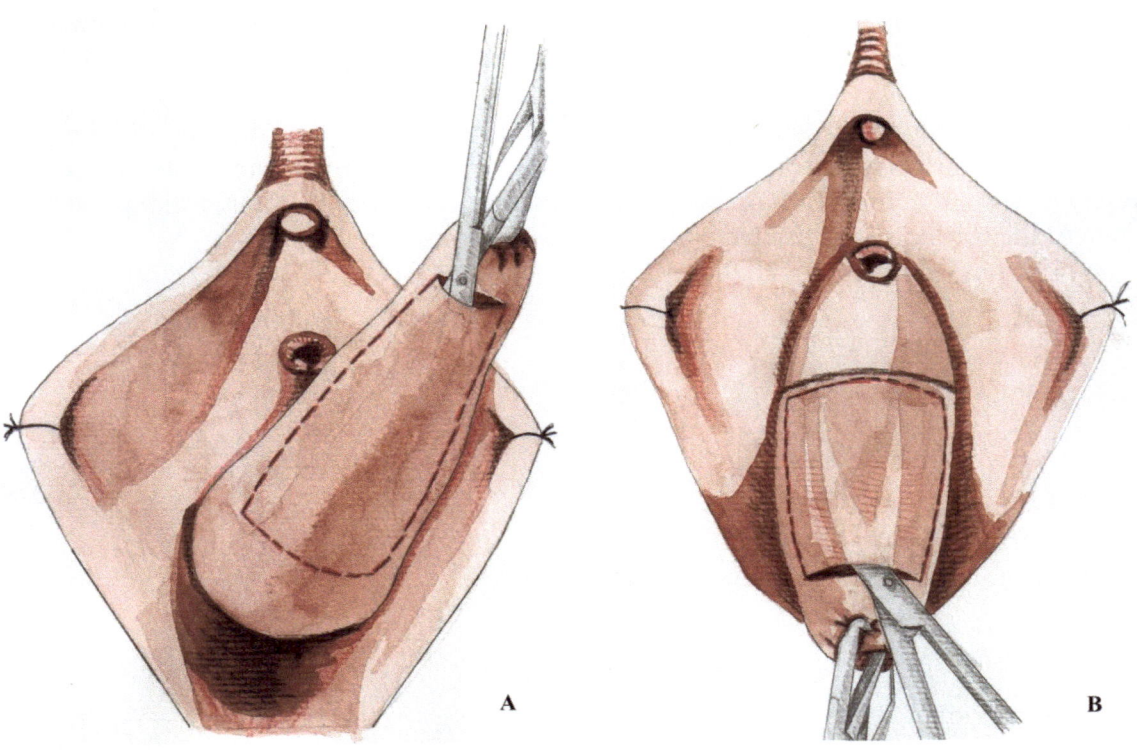

Fig. 7.84. Dissection and excision of quadrangle (*drawing by Vanessa Mureșan*)
A) of posterior mucosa; B) of anterior mucosa

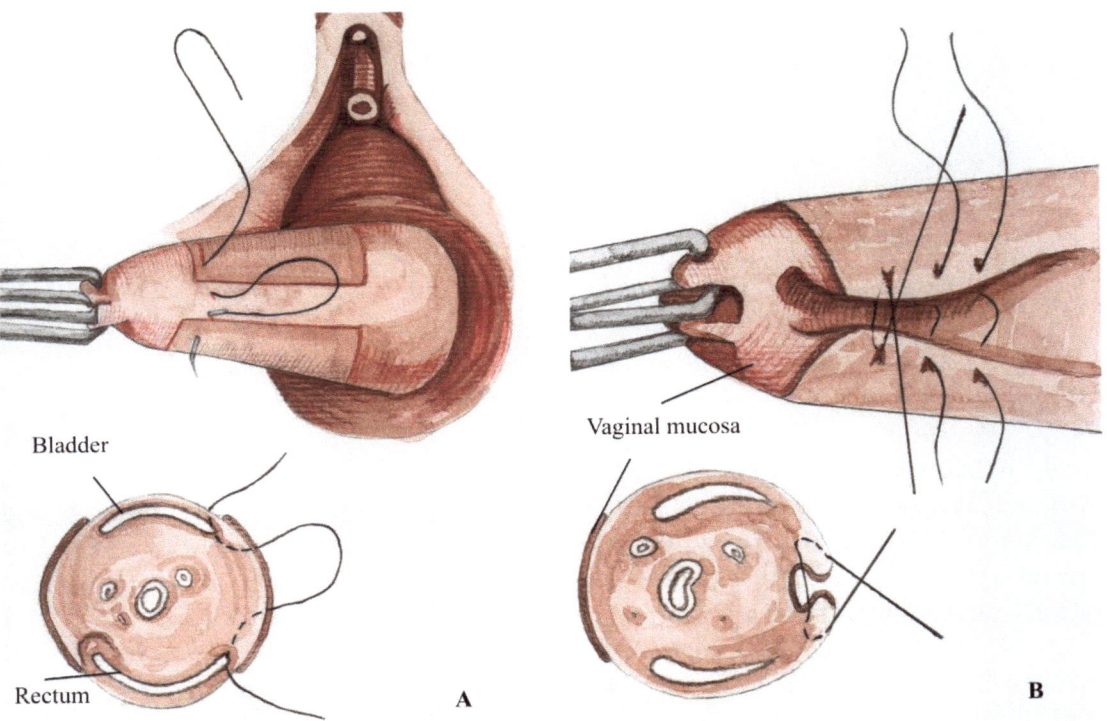

Fig. 7.85. Performing the Lembert suture pattern
(*drawing by Vanessa Mureșan*)
A) Subsequently, slowly resorbable sutures are successively passed, which approximate the pubocervical fascia anteriorly and the perirectal one posteriorly;
B) When the sutures are passed, a tunnel is created along each lateral edge of the cervix for the drainage of cervical secretions

2. The previously marked mucosa quadrangle is excised, Fig. 7.84.A and the same is done for the anterior vaginal mucosa quadrangle up to approximately 1.5 – 2 cm from the urethral meatus, Fig. 7.84.B. Thus, the perirectal fascia is exposed posteriorly and the pubocervical fascia, anteriorly.

3. Subsequently, slowly resorbable sutures are passed, which approximate the pubocervical fascia anteriorly and Lembert suture pattern is performed for the perirectal fascia posteriorly, Fig. 7.85.A. As the sutures pass, a tunnel is created along each lateral edge of the cervix for the drainage of cervical secretions, Fig. 7.85.B.

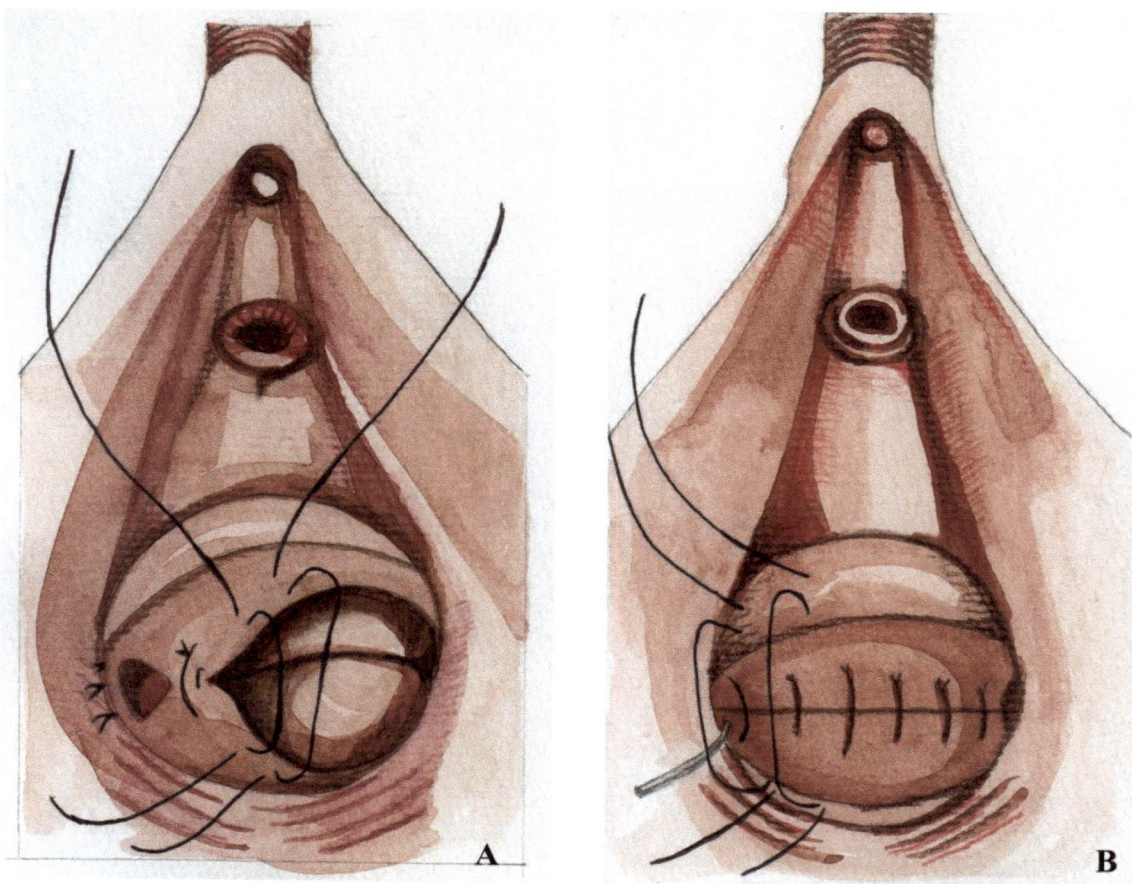

Fig. 7.86. Suture of pubocervical fascia to the rectovaginal fascia
(*drawing by Vanessa Mureşan*)
A) Above the cervix; b) sutures are passed between the anterior and posterior vaginal mucosa

4. 0 slowly resorbable sutures are afterwards passed between the anterior pubocervical fascia and the posterior perirectal fascia, above the cervix, Fig. 7.86.A, and, at the end, sutures are passed between the anterior and posterior vaginal mucosa, Fig. 7.86.B. The result is that the anterior pubocervical fascia and the posterior perirectal fascia are completely plicated and the cervix is invaginated.

5. At the end of the intervention, a test can be done regarding how a bundle of thin sutures can be passed on each side of the cervix, laterally, demonstrating that leakage of cervical secretions can occur. The final picture, Fig. 7.87., shows the completely sutured vaginal mucosa. It is worth mentioning, as in the case of other procedures that address the complete utero-vaginal prolapse, that the cystourethral angle modifies as a result of the intervention, which can lead to effort urinary incontinence.

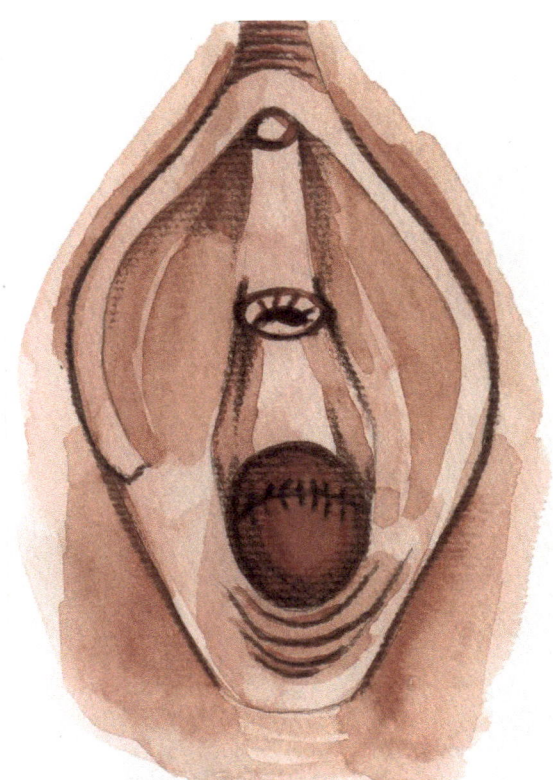

Fig. 7.87. Final postoperatory aspect
(*drawing by Vanessa Mureşan*)

A widespread variant is also Goodell – Power – Le Fort colpocleisis. The main difference compared to the technique described above is the dissection of a triangular part of vaginal mucosa both from the anterior and the posterior vaginal wall, with a side facing the cervix and the tip towards the vaginal introit. The rest of the technique is similar.

7.4.1.5. Vaginal recalibration

The raise of the vaginal caliber is one of the most frequent causes of decrease of the quality of life of women over 40 years old, as well as their partners'. In many cases, this change is not associated with other pelvic floor disorders, thus not being accompanied by a certain symptomatology, which usually makes the patient go to the doctor. This type of pathology is more and more prevalent in the women population, primarily due to the changes in the social perception of sexuality.

From a pathophysiological point of view, the circumferential connective-elastic tissue of the vaginal wall is affected, practically being only an affection of the vaginal canal. However, the changes are potentiated by the decrease in muscle tone and the estrogenic component that manifests at menopause. The caliber disorders can be associated with various ligament lesions at different compartment levels, in which case specific symptoms may be present. The most common association is with the lesions of the perineal body, in which case the vaginal cuff appears. In all these situations, the first step is the correction of each ligament defect according to "*Integral Theory*". Correction of vaginal caliber should be the last step in restoring pelvic anatomy.

We believe that restoration of the normal vaginal caliber must follow one of the principles of vaginal reconstructive surgery, namely the avoidance of mucosa excision. This may become essential in so far the main symptom is a sexual dysfunction, because excising a part of the vagina also leads to the decrease in the number of nervous receptors at this level. A second undesirable effect is a greater possibility of tethered vagina induced by the scar, which can have as main consequence dyspareunia. Indirectly, however, loss of elasticity may result in various, multi-compartment symptoms.

Surgery aims at reconstruction of an optimal caliber for a satisfactory sexual life. This optimal caliber can vary from one patient to another and should be discussed in detail preoperatively. A commonly used reference is the easy intromission of the index and medius fingers at the end of the surgery.

It seems that a similar surgical technique was used in Romania in the interwar period in the houses of tolerance in order to increase sexual activity.

Surgical steps

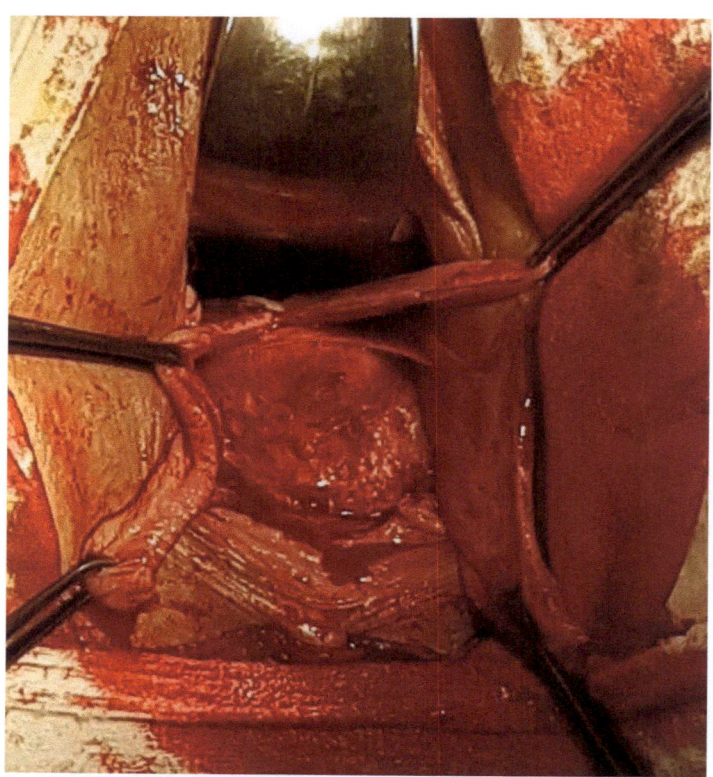

Fig. 7.88. **Intraoperative aspect after mucosa incision and under vaginal tissue dissection**
(from the archive of **M. Moisa**)

1. A physiological saline solution with adrenaline (1ml adrenaline 1 ‰ diluted in 200ml of serum) is injected for both hemostatic and hydrodissection purposes in the future incision.

2. A longitudinal incision is made to the posterior vaginal wall, starting cranially from the cutaneous-mucosal edge of the posterior commissure towards half of the cervicovaginal distance.

3. The under vaginal tissue is dissected with a surgical scissors on a variable distance depending on the extent of the defect and the desired caliber, Fig. 7.88.

4. After hemostasis control, the continuity of the mucosa is restored by making a suture, starting from the cranial angle of the vaginal incision to the posterior vaginal commissure. The sutures are passed more through the vagina's edges so that a quite prominent median channel results, Fig. 7.89. The vaginal caliber will be reduced by lifting this mucosa layer. The final postoperatory aspect can be seen in Fig. 7.90.

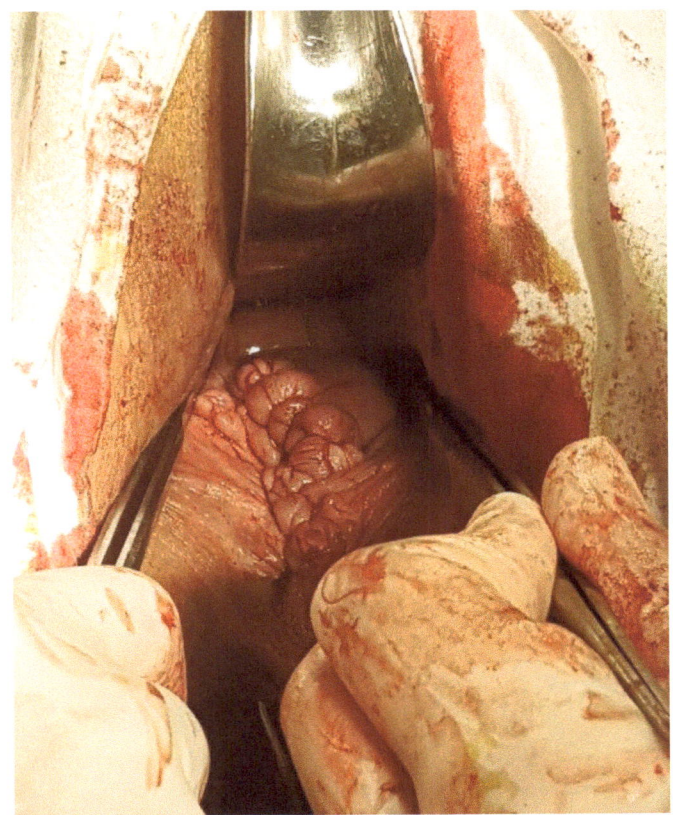
Fig. 7.89. Median channel at the level of posterior vaginal mucosa
(from the archive of **M. Moisa**)

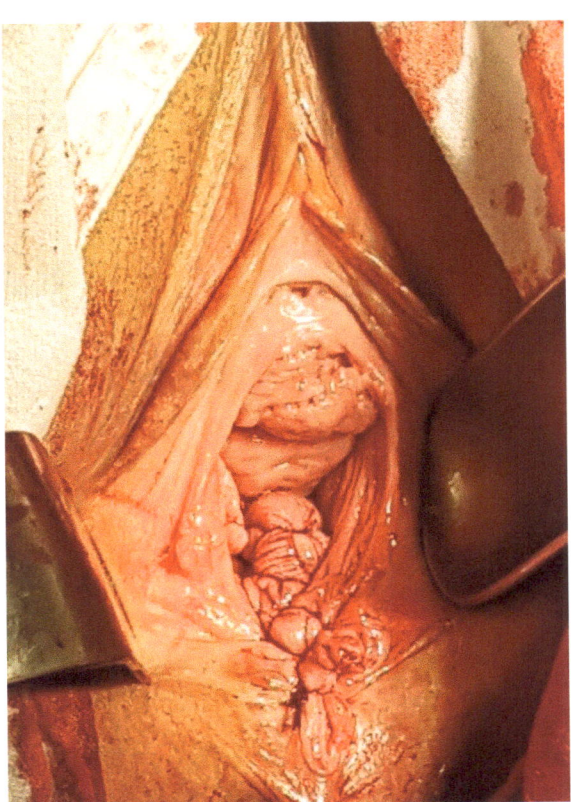
Fig. 7.90. Final postoperatory aspect
(from the archive of **M. Moisa**)

The patient is mesh-covered for 24 hours postoperatory, the discharge being made at 48 hours at the latest, if no complications occur.

7.4.1.6. Bilateral plication of the puborectal muscles: a new surgical concept for treating gaping genital hiatus

Introduction

Vulvo-perineoplasty is a surgical repair procedure that aims to reconstitute the introitus anatomy as well as possible and correct the gaping genital hiatus. The original purpose of the first vulvo-perineoplasty procedure, described by Musset in 1978 (**Musset R., 1997**), was to repair obstetrical tearing, mainly in the treatment of rectovaginal fistulas. Since then, the indications have been extended and the number of different techniques multiplied. Currently, the most frequent procedures used to correct a gaping genital hiatus are levator myorrhaphy and perineal myorrhaphy or perineoplasty (Fig. 7.91).

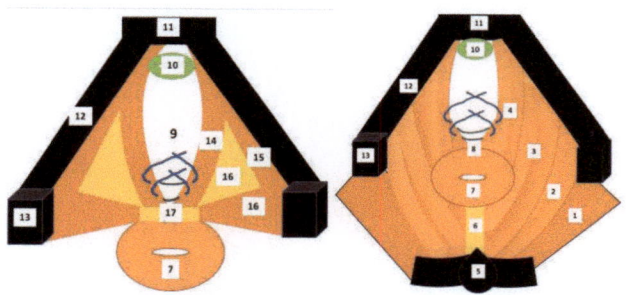

Perineorrhaphy   Levator myorrhaphy

Fig. 7.91. Perineorrhaphy and levator myorrhaphy (according to **Delorme, E.**)

Transverse myorrhaphy of the levator muscles is being reassessed due to the non-negligible risk of residual perineal pain, in particular de novo dyspareunia (**Le Normand L., et al.**).

This is the description of an innovative technique for repairing a gaping genital hiatus: the sagittal myorrhaphy technique by lateral plication of the puborectal bundles of the levator ani muscle to treat a gaping genital hiatus (Fig. 7.92). This technique has only been the subject of one retrospective publication so far (**Serrand M., 2017**).

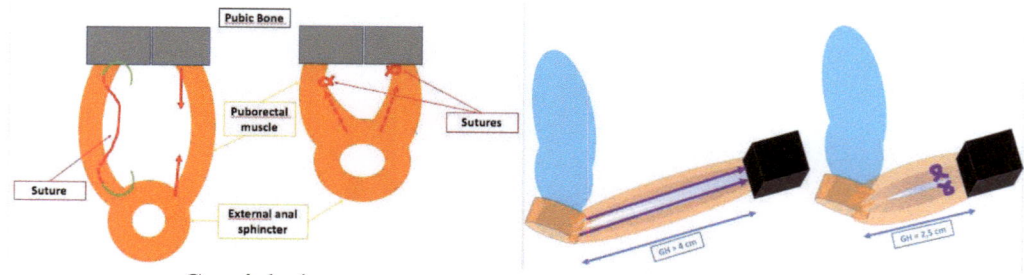

Cranial view   Lateral view

Fig. 7.92. Puborectal plication (PRP) (according to **Delorme, E.**)

Anatomical reminder (Fig. 7.93)

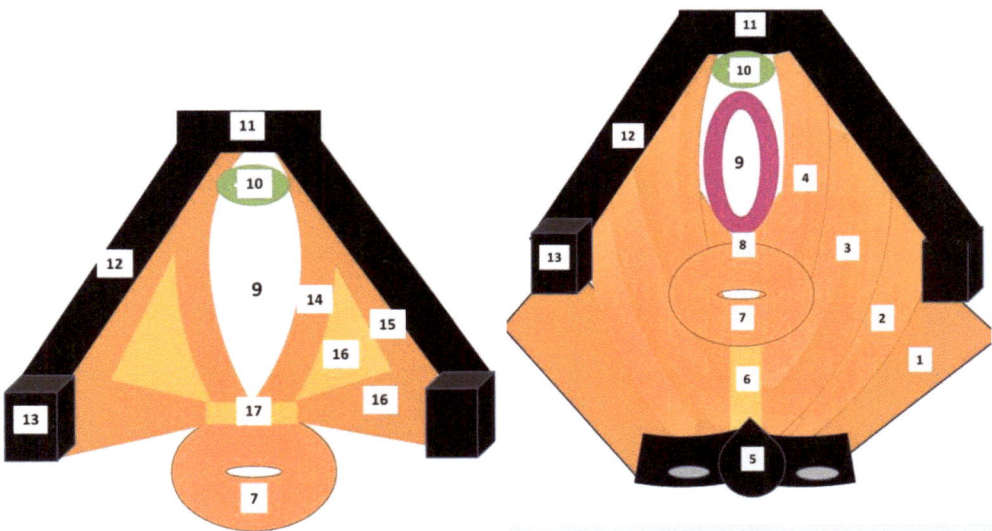

Superficial plane: perineal   **Deep plane:** levator ani muscles

1 - gluteal muscle, 2 - iliococcygeus muscle, 3 - ischiococcygeus muscle, 4 - puborectalis muscle, 5 - sacrum and coccyx, 6 - anococcygeal ligament, 7 - anal canal, 8 – perineal body,
9 – vagina, 10 – urethra, 11- pubic bone, 12 – ischiopubic ramus, 13 - ischium,
14 – bulbospongiosus muscle, 15 – ischiocavernosus muscle, 16 – perineal membrane,
17 – perineal body

Fig. 7.93. Anatomy of the genital hiatus (according to **Delorme, E.**)

The perineum is a diamond-shaped anatomical structure oriented from the back to the front with the pubic symphysis in front of it and the coccyx behind. It consists of a set of muscles, fasciae, vessels, and nerves forming two parts: the urogenital triangle at the front and the anal triangle at the back. The lower segment of the vagina or genital hiatus has a sagittal orientation, consisting of two lateral surfaces that correspond bottom to top to the perineal muscles (vaginal compressor, bulbospongiosus) and above to the internal side of the puborectal muscles. At this level, the vaginal wall consists only of the mucosa and the vaginal submucosa, which rest directly on the layer of muscles described above. The genital hiatus is bordered anteriorly by the urethra and laterally by the lateral urethral sulci, which join the lateral wall. At this level, the vaginal wall consists of the mucosa resting on the submucosa and on the pubocervical fascia consisting of collagen fibers and smooth muscle fibers. The perineal body (PB) borders the genital hiatus posteriorly. The PB is a dense fibromuscular mass shaped like a pyramid in the median plane between the internal anal sphincter and the lower third of the posterior vaginal wall. According to the Shafik study (**Shafik A. et al., 2007**), which concerned 46 cadaver dissections, including 17 nulliparous patients, the PB consists, in its upper part, of the external anal sphincter into which most internal fibers of the puborectal muscles are inserted. The lower plane of the PB consists of the central insertion of the superficial and deep transverse muscles, which makes them "digastrics" type muscles.

The puborectalis muscle forms the largest part of the lateral muscle wall of the vagina. It consists of three bundles: puborectal, pubovaginal, and puboanal. The posterior fibers of the pubovisceral bundle are common to the external anal sphincter (**Terminologica Anatomica de Kearney, 2004**).

Physiopathology of the genital hiatus

According to Pardo et al. (**Pardo J.S., Sola V.D., Ricci P.A., et al., 2006**), 96% of the women report anatomical changes such as the widening of the genital hiatus after giving birth 1 or more times. According to Woodward et al. (**Woodward A.P., Matthews C.A., 2010**), 38% of the women report deterioration in the quality of their sex life after giving birth and only 15% of the women with a postpartum sexual problem talk to a health professional about it (**Barret et al., 2000**). The resulting sexual discomfort is due to anatomical trauma, to a large extent, and, in some cases, with a gaping genital hiatus and reduced vaginal sensitivity or periorificial dyspareunia. This causes psychological trauma and impaired self-image (**CNGOF, 2009**).

Finally, it is possible that puborectal reconstruction will restore Delancey's (**Wei J.T., De Lancey J.O., 2004**) level III, which could have a positive impact on stress urinary incontinence (**De Lancey J.O., 1994**).

Indications for sagittal plication of the puborectal muscles

Puborectal plication (PRP) is classically indicated in genito-urinary prolapse surgery, in addition to supporting the prolapsed organs. PRP may also be proposed on its own to treat a symptomatic gaping genital hiatus.

- Prolapse repair and PRP: This may be proposed if the genital hiatus (GH) (POP-Q classification) is 4 cm or more. However, in certain cases after prolapse repair, spontaneous normalization of the genital hiatus is observed. Clinical observation has tended to show that there are two situations in which a gaping genital hiatus would require surgical repair: when it is associated with a lateral cystocele and when perineal contraction in the gynaecological position does not significantly alter the GH (over 3 cm).
- Isolated surgical repair of widened vulva: this can only be justified if the GH is 4 cm or over and the patient has a complaint such as poor self-image, loss of femininity, vaginal hypersensitivity adversely affecting her sex life or certain types of dyspareunia (puborectal pain).

Surgical procedure

The operation is performed under a spinal anaesthetic or a general anaesthetic. The patient is in the gynaecological position. The surgical procedure is bilateral. After submucosal infiltration, the operation begins with an incision using the cold scalpel technique along the right or left hymeneal line (Fig. 7.94).

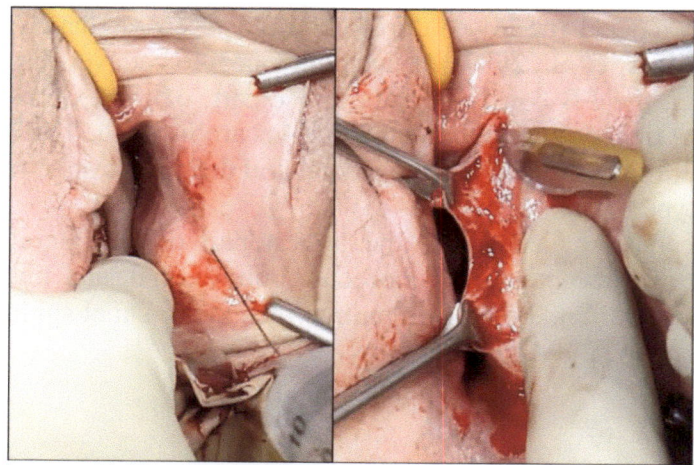

Fig. 7.94. **PRP: Submucosal infiltration, incision, and dissection of the mucosa** (according to **Delorme, E.**)

A fine subcutaneous dissection (cold scalpel or Metzenbaum scissors) moves the vaginal mucosa inwards, outwardly exposing the superficial muscle fascia (vaginal compressor muscle and the bulbospongiosus muscle) then the deep muscle fascia consisting of the visceral fibers of the puborectalis muscle. The PRP is performed with 2 U-sutures (preferably 0 or 1 dissolvable sutures using a 40 mm 5/ 8 circle needle) (Fig. 7.95).

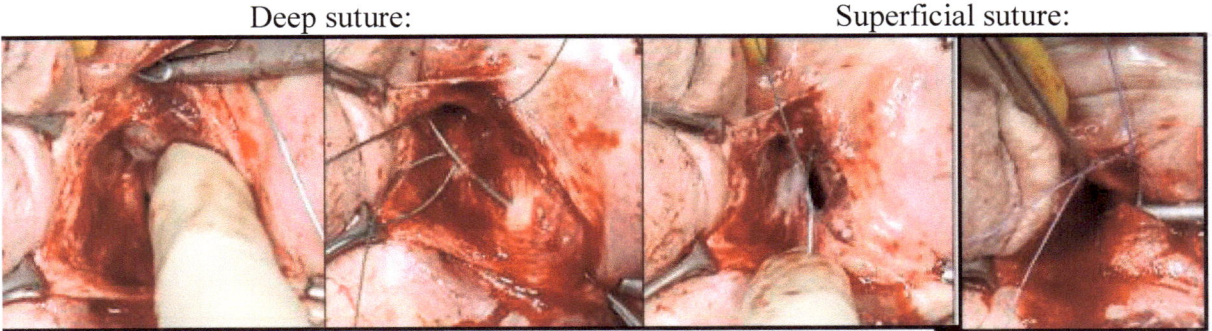

Fig. 7.95. PRP: sagittal puborectal suturing: deep suture and superficial suture (according to **Delorme, E.**)

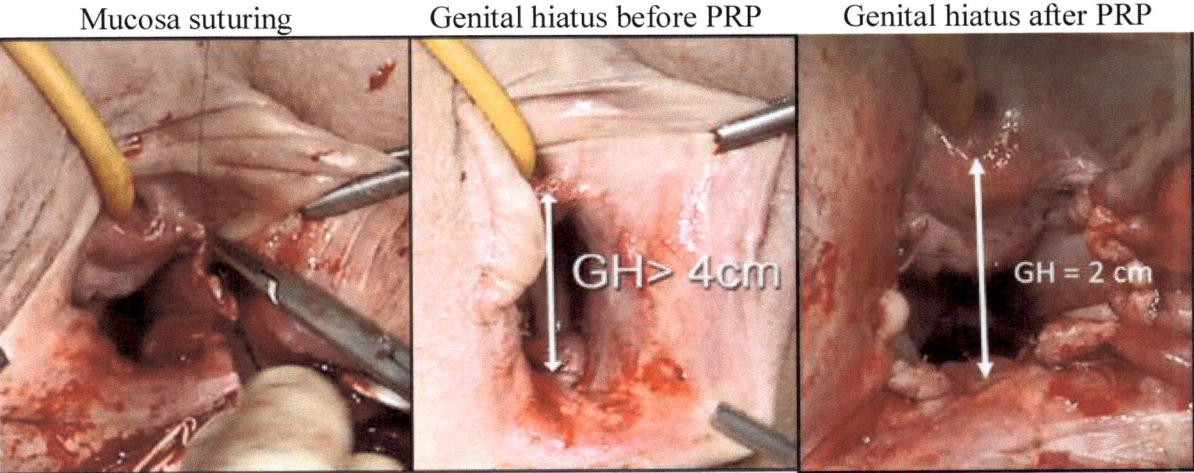

Fig. 7.96. Mucosa suturing, comparison at the beginning and end of the procedure (according to **Delorme, E.**)

At the front, the first suture is passed through the solid retropubic insertion of the puborectalis muscle. At the back, the same thread takes in, very largely, the puborectalis muscle at the point where it inserts into the external sphincter of the anal canal (using a Reverdin right needle or more simply the 40 mm 5/ 8 swaged needle). This suture ligature plicates the puborectalis muscle whilst bringing the external anal sphincter closer to the pubic insertion of the puborectalis muscle. The second suture doubles the first one to consolidate the PRP. The vulvar incision is closed by a continuous suture using absorbable monofilament thread, caliber 4.0. The procedure is the same on each side.

Postoperative outcomes

Our conclusions are based on the only retrospective study evaluating longitudinal plication of the puborectal muscles. The only postoperative morbidity we observed was a local haematoma in 2/ 69 patients who underwent the surgery and one case of de novo dyspareunia.

Table 7.4. Postoperative outcomes

OUTCOMES	Prior to surgery	After surgery			p
		6 weeks	6 months	12 months	
GH (mm)	65.0 ± 5.0 (n=69)	31.0 ± 0.7 (n=67)	35.0 ± 0.6 (n=55)	35.0 ± 0.5 (n=40)	< 0.00001
Satisfactory sex life	5/(n=27) (18.52%)		24/(n=25) (96.00%)	24/(n=27) (88.89%)	< 0.00001
Dyspareunia	6/(n=27) (22.22%)		1/(n=25) (4.00%)	1/(n=27) (3.70%)	0.220

n = number of patients; p < 0.05 is significant.

Conclusion

PRP has a low immediate and medium term postoperative morbidity rate compared to conventional myorrhaphy and perineorrhaphy of the levator ani muscles. The anatomical outcomes, evaluated by measuring the GH, confirm the stability of the results in the medium term. Reconstruction of the genital hiatus has a positive impact on the quality of sexual intercourse and on self-image. This remains to be confirmed by further studies.

7.4.2. Surgical techniques using alloplastic material

The use of synthetic prostheses has been through an accelerated development, and a variety of procedures has been proposed for the reconstruction of *posterior compartment* (**Feiner B., et al., 2009**). However, the technical difficulties have not succeeded imposing a steady procedure, as there are currently several techniques and some kind of skepticism related to their efficiency, due to many complications that have occurred over time (**Rardin C.R. & Washington B.B., 2009**).

This compartment includes uterine prolapse, subtotal posthysterectomy cervical prolapse, and total posthysterectomy prolapse of vaginal vault prolapse. All three entities, however, represent a single disease, whose etiology consists in the affection of cardinal and uterosacral ligaments. For this reason, the surgical correction is unitary and aims at their restoring, ideally reconstructing the vector disposition. The differences that occur during the interventions, and which relate to the presence or absence of the cervix are rather particularities of each case.

The lesions of rectovaginal fascia and of perineal body, as well as the modifications of vaginal caliber are also in the category of posterior compartment defects. Their correction can be done separately or along with other procedures aimed at repairing some concomitant defects.

Thus, in the following, we will present surgical techniques for the correction of affected connective structures, preferring not to discuss the treatment of certain diseases. We believe that this approach has a practical value in that each patient can associate defects of various ligaments and fascia in various degrees, so that the surgical techniques can be combined in several ways.

7.4.2.1. Posterior intravaginal mesh

The method implies the insertion of a polypropylene mesh at the level of posterior vaginal fornix, and its pathogenic aim is the reconstruction of level I DeLancey, cardinal and uterosacral ligaments. It is a technique that has been developed in the last years, the mesh being inserted with a instrument called *"tunneller"* that passes through the ischioanal fossa, pararectal and translevator, so that its final position is approximately transversal, parallel with the interspinous line and located at approximately 1 cm posterior to it. On the median line, it attaches to the posterior side of the cervix, to the uterosacral ligaments on the cervix or on the posterior side of the vaginal apex. The mesh vectorally substitutes the cardinal ligaments and, to a small extent, the uterosacral ligaments, Fig. 7.99 (**Farnsworth B., 2007**).

The tunneller is made up of two components, a curved sheath at one end and an inner rod having a tip at one end, and at the other end some loops with which it can be fixed at the end of the mesh, Fig. 7.97.

Surgical steps
1. A transverse incision is made at the level of posterior vaginal mucosa, at 2 cm below its insertion on the cervix.
2. Digital dissection is performed with the index finger of the same hand posterolateral to the ischial spine and bilaterally.

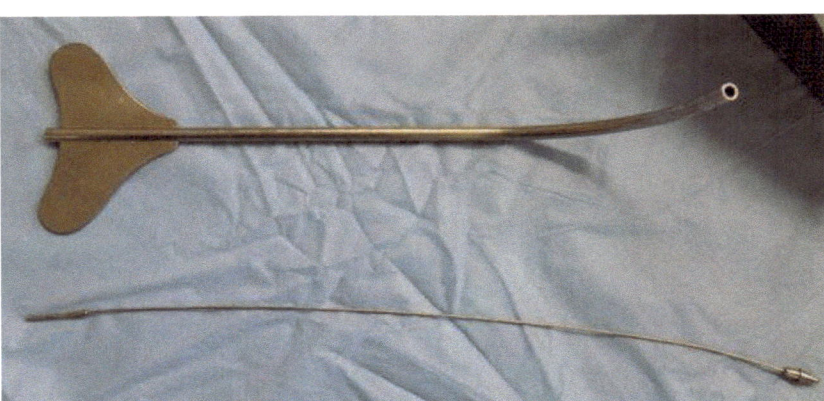

Fig. 7.97. Tunneller

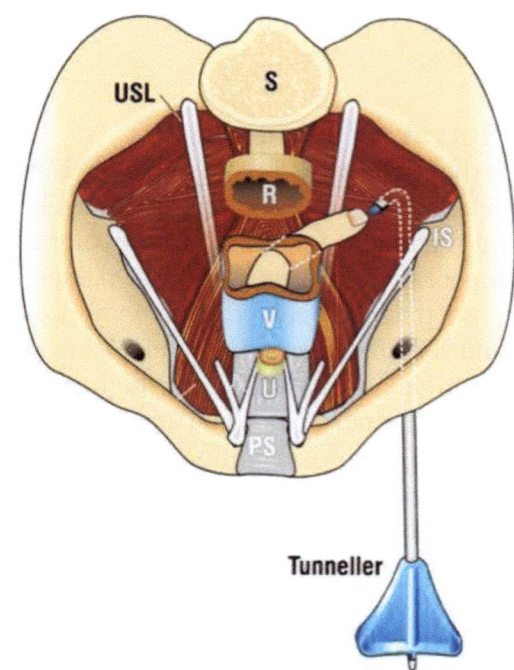

Fig. 7.98. Mounting the posterior mesh with the tunneller
(according to **Petros P., 2010**)

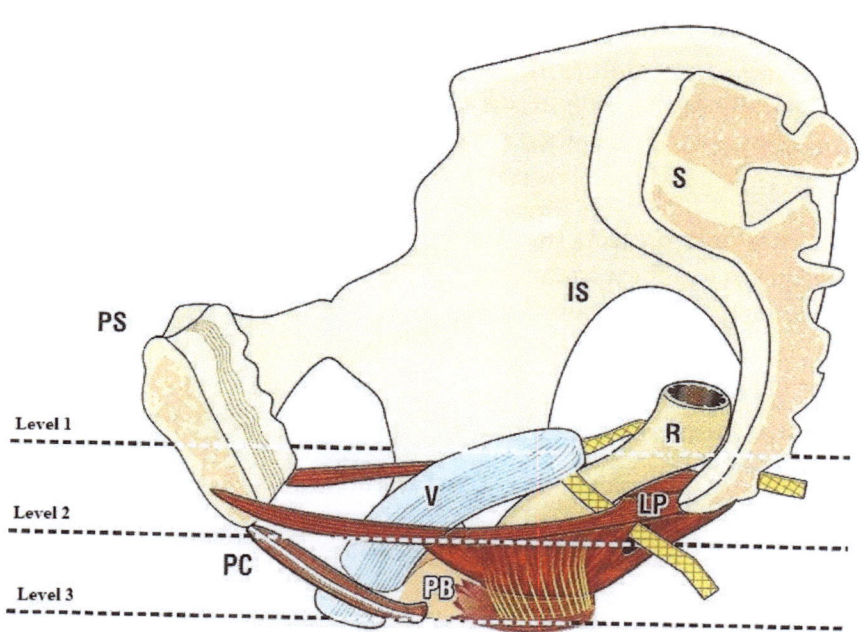

Fig. 7.99. Placement of posterior mesh – postoperatory aspect
(according to **Petros P., 2010**)

3. Performing an incision at the level of each buttock, bilaterally, 2 cm lateral to the middle of the anococcygeal line, Fig 7.100.

4. Insertion of the tunneller through these incisions through the ischioanal fossa in the direction of the ischial spine, while the same hand of the side approached is placed at the level of the vaginal incision, removing the rectum from the instrument medially and guiding its tip.

5. Near the ischial spine, at 1-2 cm posterior and medial to it, the direction of the instrument is changed cranially, anteriorly and medially to the vaginal incision. The levator plate perforation is undergone at the level of the trajectory, Fig. 7.98.

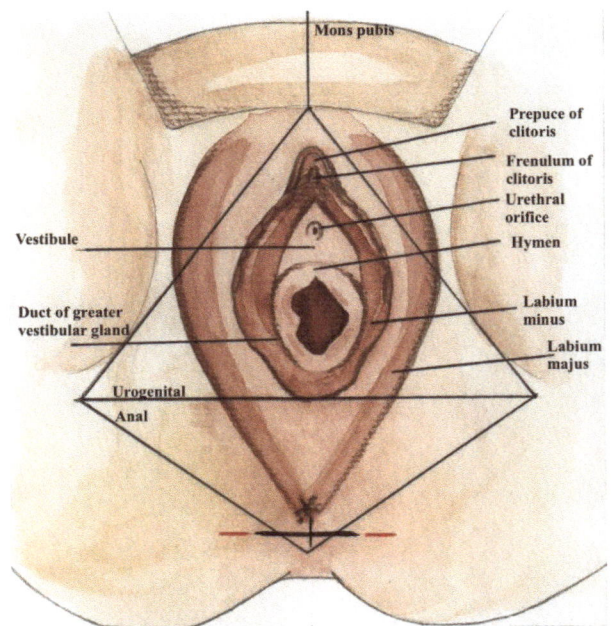

Fig. 7.100. Incisions at the level of the buttocks (*drawing by Vanessa Mureşan*)

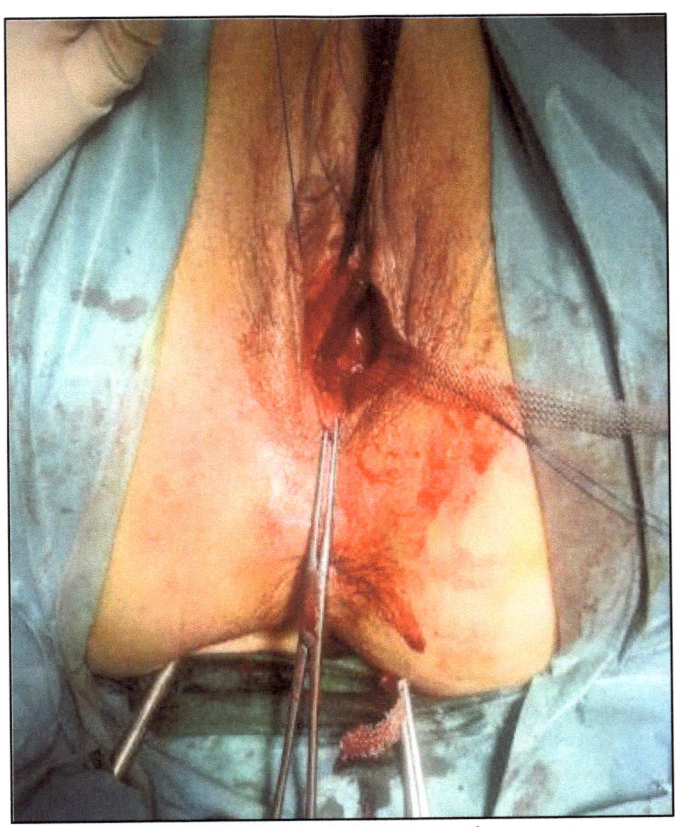

Fig. 7.101. Posterior mesh. Intraoperative aspect
(from the archive of **Enache T**.)

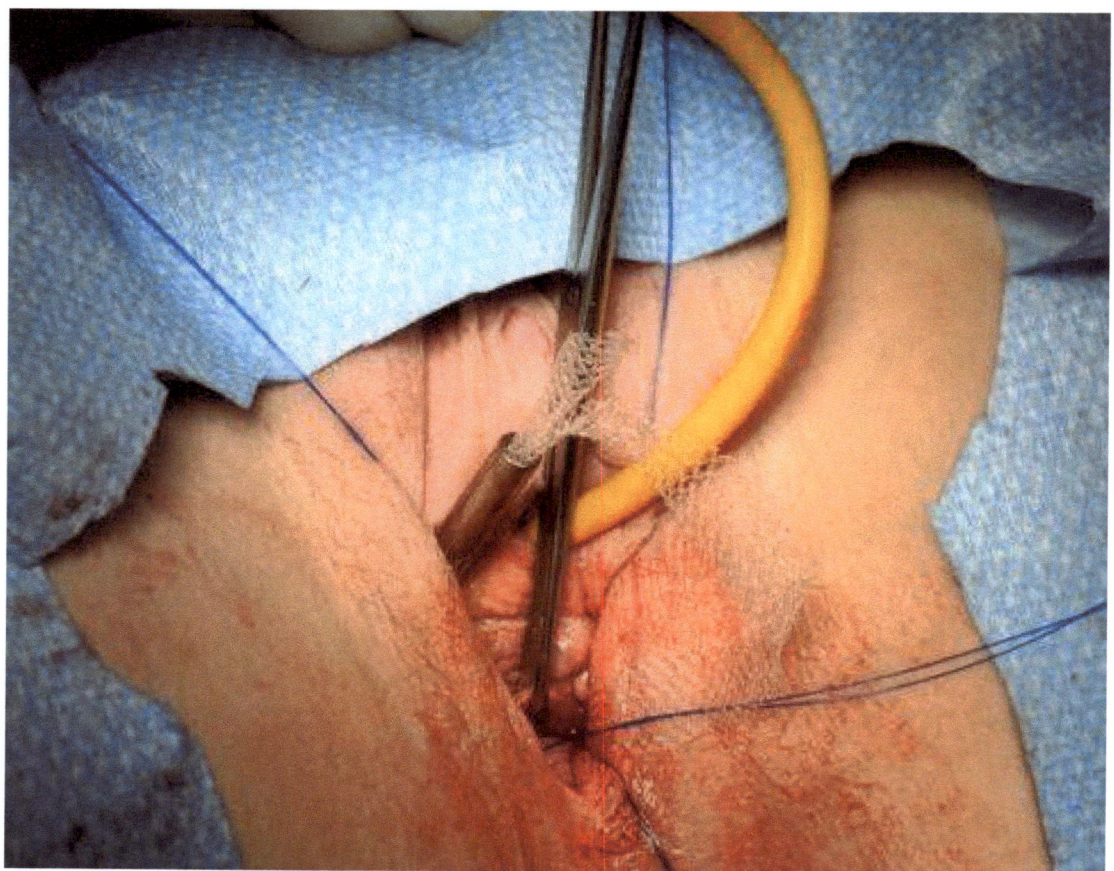

Fig. 7.102. Fixing the free end of the mesh to the "*tunneller*"
(from the archive of **Funogea A.** & **Goeschen K.**)

6. The detachment of the tip and the inner rod and its opposite mounting with anchoring the end of the mesh to the vaginal incision. After passing the end of the mesh through the anchoring end of the "tunneller", the instrument is extracted in the opposite direction to the insertion with the mesh externalization at the level of the buttock injury, Fig 7.101. and 7.102. The maneuver is executed bilaterally, the mesh finally having an almost horizontal trajectory, parallel to the interspinous line and passing to the posterior side of the cervix. The ends, distal to the levator plate, pass through the ischioanal fossa to the level of the buttock tegument.

7. Fixing the mesh at the level of the cervix insertions of uterosacral ligaments with one resorbable multifilament suture, bilaterally.

8. Suture of incisions at the level of vaginal mucosae with separate sutures.

The patient is mesh-covered for 24 hours postoperatory, the discharge being made at 48 hours at the latest, if complications do not occur.

The main drawback of this technique is that it does not correct the posterior vector component, but only the lateral one. The lack of a pathophysiological correction is also reflected in modest post-surgical results. The most common cause was the anterior movement of the mesh, by dilaceration of levator ani muscles fibers.

7.4.2.2. Posterior intravaginal mesh with bilateral sacrospinous fixation

The intravaginal posterior mesh successfully substitutes the lateral support means of the uterus, but does not achieve an efficient posterior pulling, which is physiologically realized by uterosacral ligaments, Prof. Dr. Klaus Goeschen's method. One method of reconstituting their function is the bilateral fixation of the mesh to the sacrospinous ligaments. It is in fact a reevaluation of the Amreich-Richter surgery. However, the anchoring is only achieved by digital marking of ligaments, bilaterally and without the wide dissection specific to classical surgery. The passing of the suture is done with a instrument invented by Prof. Klaus Goeschen – „*vaginal viper*", Fig. 7.103. and 104 (**Farnsworth B.,** *et al.,* **2008**). At present, there are other similar instruments, but we will continue to use it as an example.

From a biophysical point of view, it reconstructs the main ligament support elements of posterior vaginal fornix and cervix: cardinal and uterosacral ligaments. The vector result is ideal because it respects the principles of Integral Theory of Petros and Ulmsten (**Amrute K.V.,** *et al.,* **2007**). The lateral vector is reconstituted by the lateral disposition of the mesh and the posterior component is done by the sacrospinous anchoring. This technique provides an effective support and restores "*ad integrum*" the anatomical position of the cervix and the posterior vaginal fornix.

Surgical steps

1. A transverse incision is made at the level of posterior vaginal mucosa, at 2 cm below its insertion on the cervix.

2. Digital dissection is performed with the index finger of the same hand posterolateral to the ischial spine and bilaterally.

3. The marking of sacrospinous ligaments with the index finger, bilateral, that start from the level of ischial spine and have a posterior, cranial, and medial trajectory.

4. Passing of a 2/0 non-resorbable monofilament suture through each sacrospinous ligament using the "*Viper*", as close to its posteromedial end and marking the ends of the suture with an autostatic spreading-forceps. The maneuver is achieved by positioning the instrument's handle (M) in the opposite hand of the side of the patient being operated. The grip is in such a way that the thumb is in contact with the piston that actions the sliding needle (P), Fig. 7.103. The instrument is inserted with the same hand of the same side of the patient being operated on, the index finger being in contact with the sacrospinous ligament in its posterior side. The tip of the instrument is positioned so that in the lower concavity (C) at this level it penetrates when in contact with the ligament. The tip of the "Viper" will be pressed on the ligament with the index finger which it was initially spotted with. At this point, with the thumb of contralateral hand, the plunger is activated to the top with the mobilization of the sliding needle that will pierce the ligament and will meet the suture passed over the end of the instrument, Fig. 7.104. The retraction of the plunger follows and thus of the needle, this way realizing the anchoring of the suture to the sacrospinous ligaments. By retracting the instrument, both ends of the sutures are located at the level of the vaginal incision.

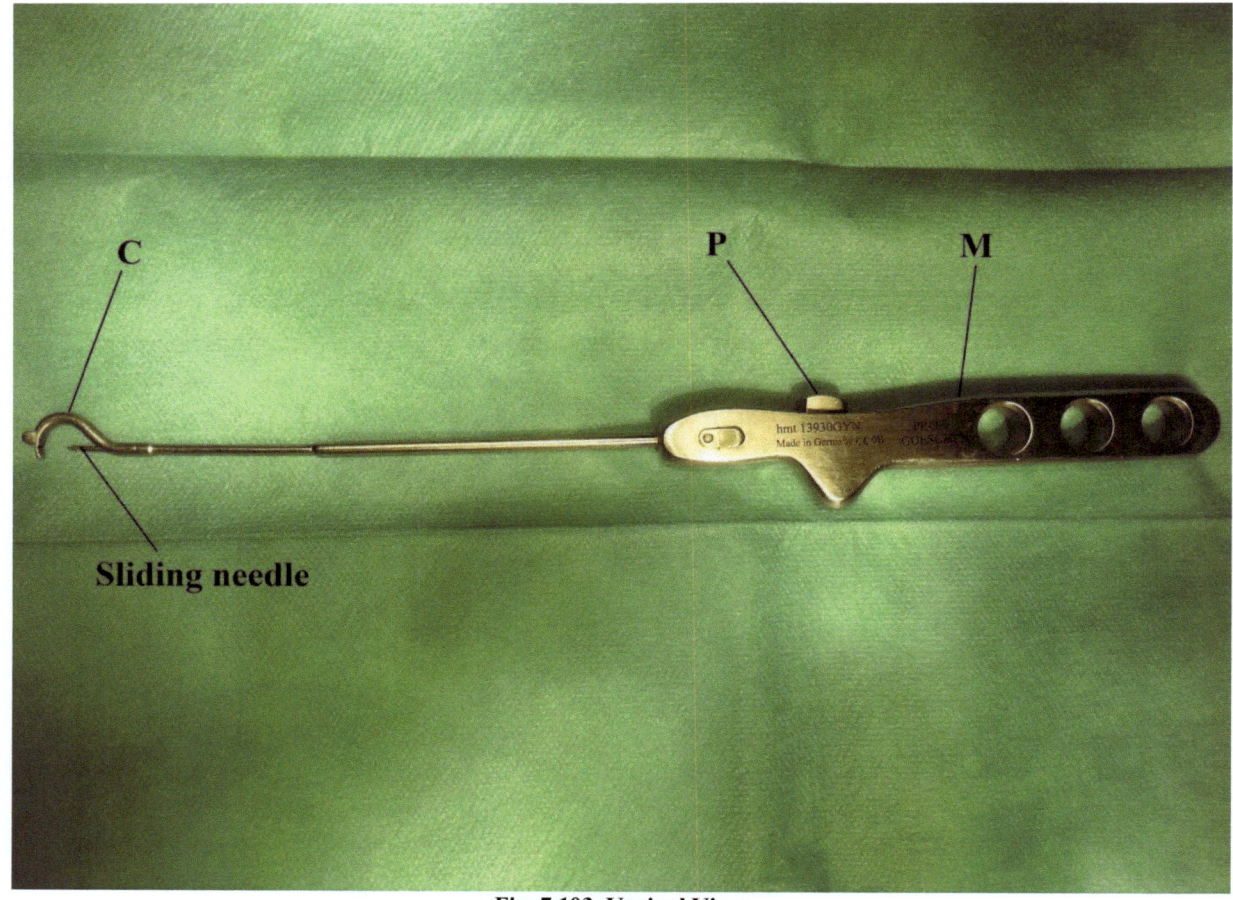

Fig. 7.103. Vaginal Viper
M – handle; P – plunger; C – concavity oriented downwards from the tip of the instrument

5. Realizing an incision at the level of each buttock, bilaterally, at 2 cm lateral to the middle anococcygeal line.

6. Insertion of the tunneller through these incisions through the ischioanal fossa towards the ischial spine, while the hand correspondent to the side approached is placed on the vaginal incision, moving the rectum from the instrument's way, medially, and guiding its tip.

7. Near the ischial spine, at 1-2 cm posterior and medial, the instrument's direction is changed cranially, anteriorly and medially towards the vaginal incision, after perforating the levator plate, similar to the above-mentioned description.

8. Detachment of the tip and the internal rod, and its mounting inversely, with the anchoring tip of the mesh towards the vaginal incision. After passing the end of the mesh through the anchoring end of the "tunneller", the instrument is extracted in the opposite direction to its insertion while externalizing the mesh at the level of the buttock incision, Fig. 7.105.

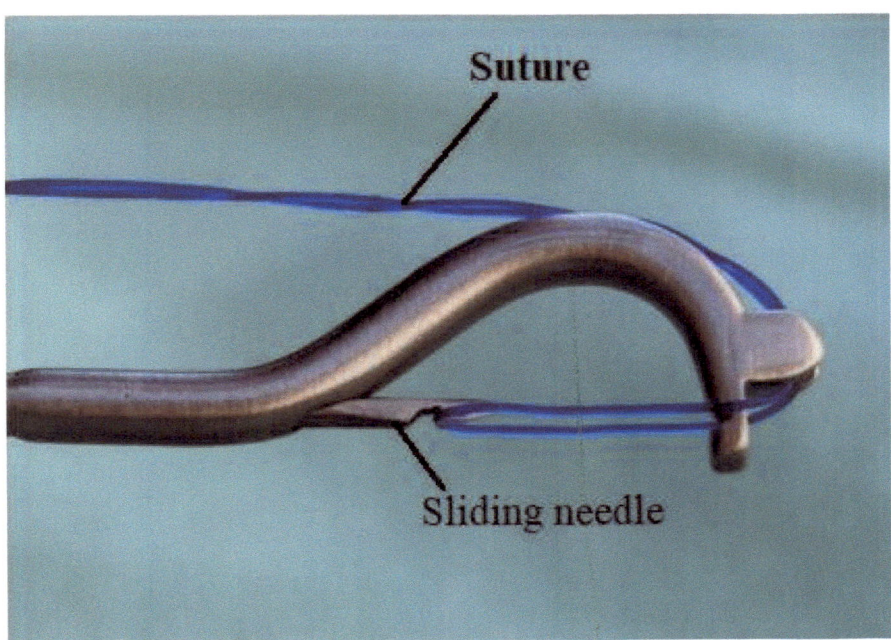

Fig. 7.104. Vaginal Viper, tip of the instrument. Example of the way the suture is grasped by the sliding needle

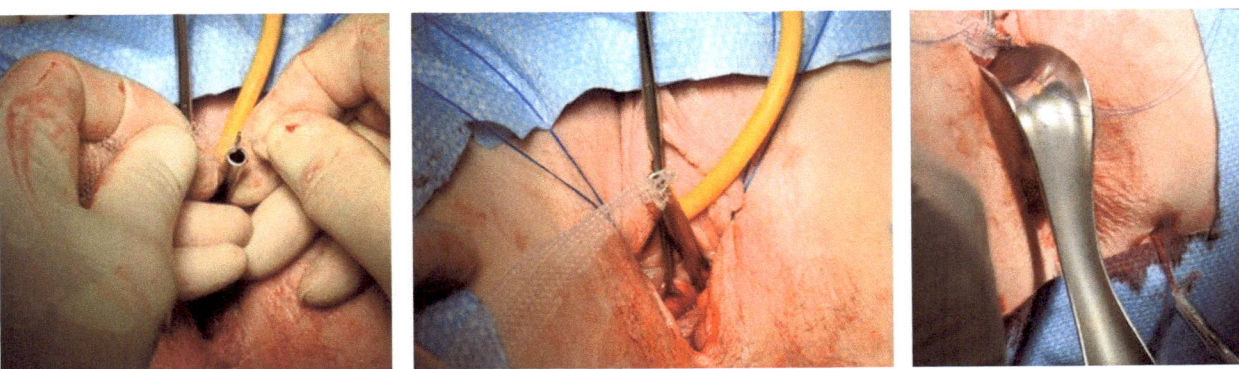

Fig. 7.105. Fixing the polypropylene mesh in the mandrel and its externalization
(from the archive of **Mueller-Funogea I-A**)

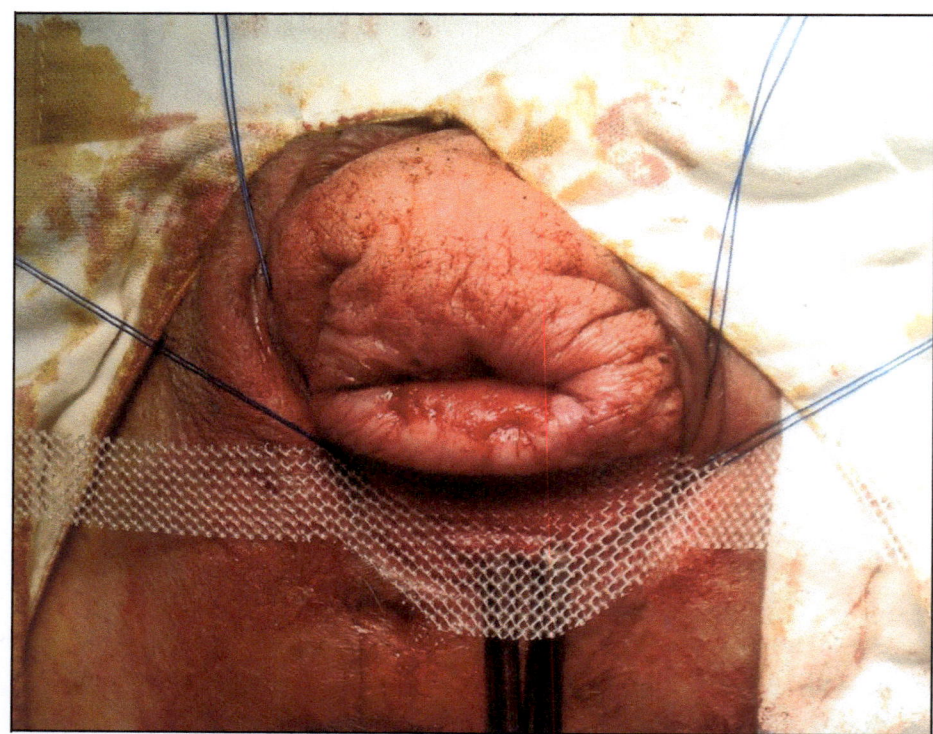

Fig. 7.106. Uterus prolapse and elitrocele corrected with a posterior intravaginal mesh with sacrospinous fixation
(from the archive of **Enache T.**)

9. After practicing the maneuver bilaterally, the mesh is anchored to the 2 sutures that were previously passed through the sacrospinous ligaments, Fig. 7.106.

10. Fixing the mesh at the level of cervix insertions of uterosacral ligaments.

11. Tying the ends of the sutures sacrospinous anchored with one another, with the reduction of uterus prolapse and elitrocele. The sutures are not tied until the sacrospinous ligaments are reached, but they are tied so that a part is left suspended.

12. After the surgical steps are achieved, suture of incisions at the level of vaginal mucosae is performed.

The patient is mesh-covered for 24 hours postoperatory, the discharge being made at the latest in 48 hours if no complications occur.

The final position of posterior intravaginal mesh, sacrospinous fixed, vectorally reproduces the biophysical structure physiologically met, Fig. 7.107. It is transversely disposed, parallel to the interspinous line, located at approximately 1 cm posterior. This disposition substitutes cardinal ligaments. Posterior anchoring to sutures passed sacrospinously restores the biomechanical role of uterosacral ligaments (**Aungst M.J.,** *et al.,* **2009**).

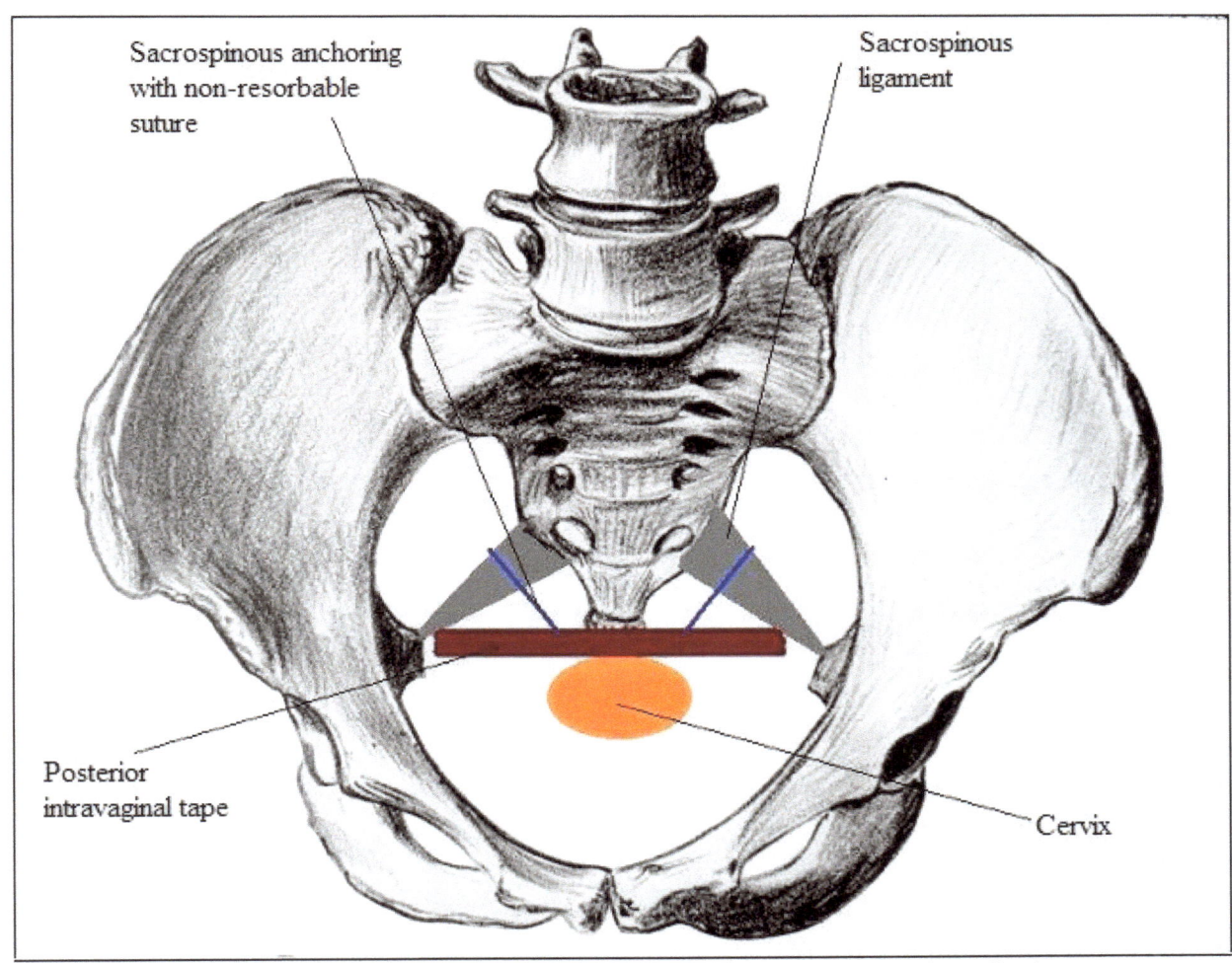

Fig. 7.107. Sketch of the postoperatory position of posterior mesh with sacrospinous fixation
(from the archive of **Enache T.**)

Although this technique conveniently restores anatomy at the cranial level of posterior compartment, DeLancey level I, many intraoperative accidents and incidents are reported, mainly due to the passage through the ischioanal fossa. The most important complications are perforation of the rectum and damage to a medium or large sized vessel followed by haemorrhage or hematoma of ischioanal fossa. Early complications such as postoperatory hematomas or infections may also occur, the most serious of which being the ischioanal postoperatory phlegmon with lethal potential. The vascular structures that can be injured during maneuvers are the artery and internal pudendal veins, the inferior rectal vascular-nervous structures, as well as numerous venous plexuses that pass through the fat of ischioanal fossa. Among the late complications, the following should be mentioned: rectovaginal fistulae, dyspareunia, and erosions.

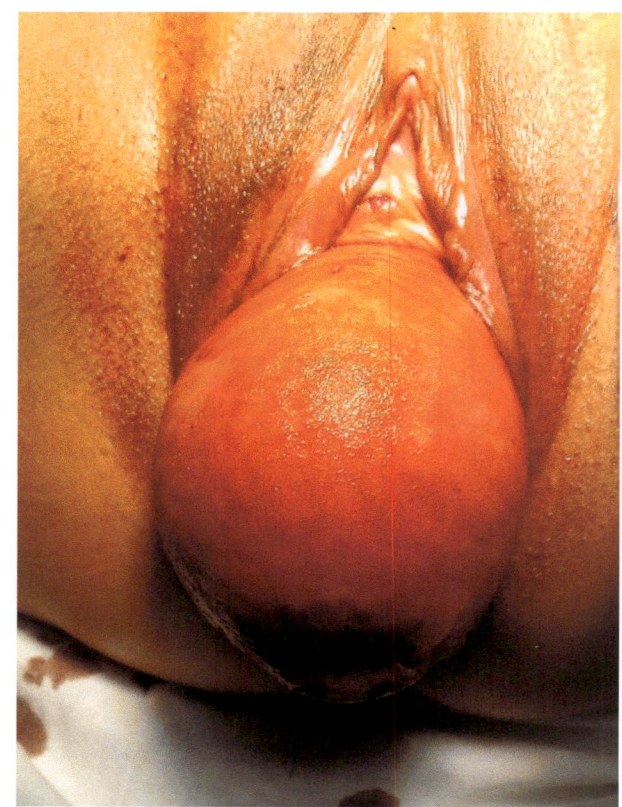

Fig. 7.108. Total uterine prolapse; preoperatory aspect
(from the archive of **Enache T.**)

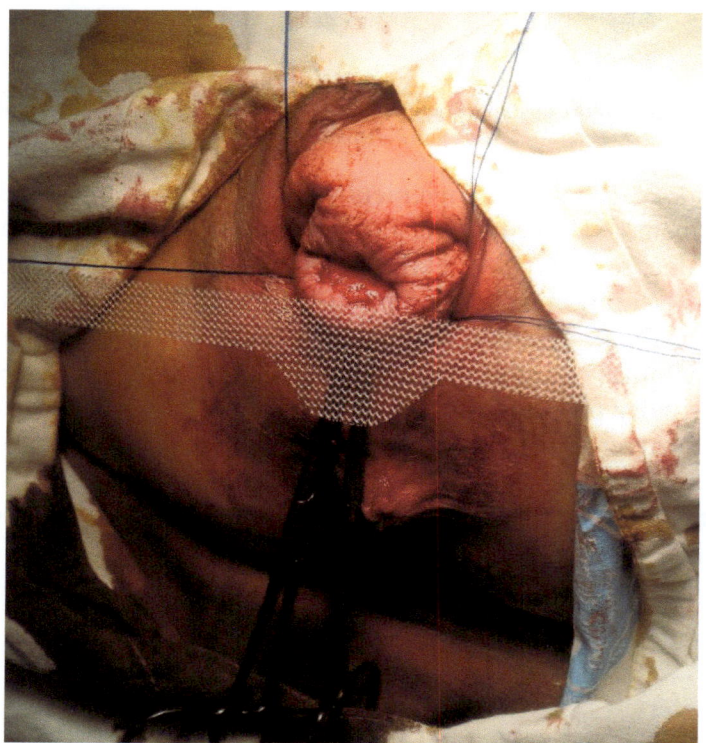

Fig. 7.109. Total uterine prolapse, mounting the posterior mesh; intraoperatory aspect
(from the archive of **Enache T.**)

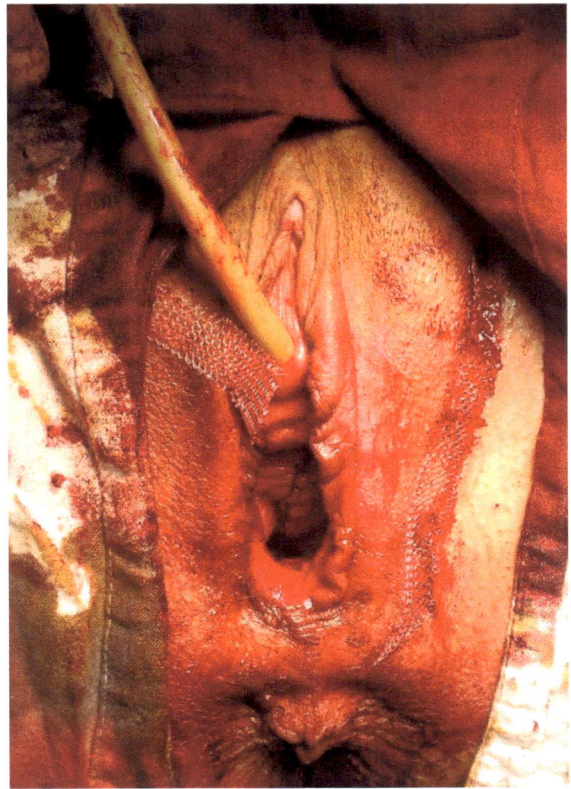

Fig. 7.110. Total uterine prolapse. Postoperatory aspect
(from the archive of **Enache T.**)

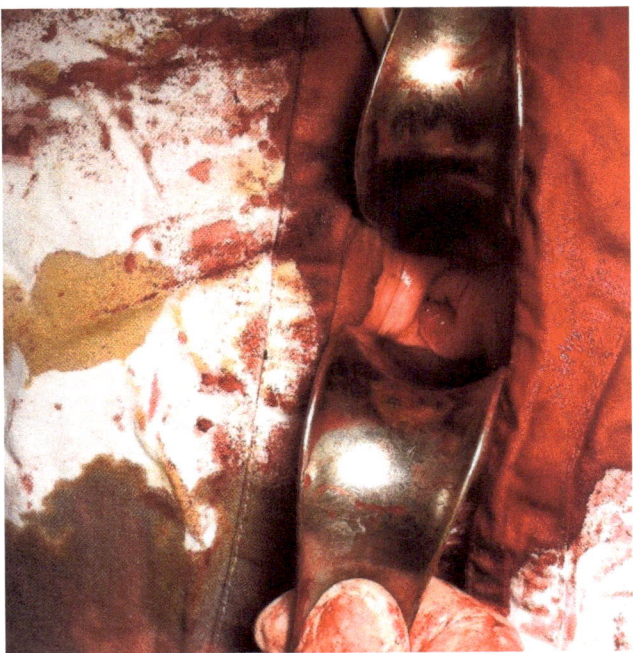

Fig. 7.111. Total uterine prolapse – postoperatory aspect: the high position of the cervix is observed
(from the archive of **Enache T.**)

Postoperatory results are favorable in the absence of complications. The most common complications at 5 years were dyspareunia and erosions.

However, anatomical results were satisfactory at five years, especially in cases with significant defects.

Below we present some cases with significant pelvic floor disorders, focusing on the apical correction with posterior mesh fixed sacrospinous.

Case 1

A 68-year-old patient with total uterine prolapse and defects affecting all three compartments. The posterior compartment was corrected with a posterior mesh fixed sacrospinous, to which a posterior "*bridge*" for the correction of rectocele and the restoration of perineal body was associated. The mesh was made so that it presented a posterior extension on the median line for the anchoring of the "*bridge*". The middle compartment was corrected with 4-arms anterior mesh – 2 passed transobturator and 2 laterocervical to strengthen the paracervix and fix to the sacrospinous wires. Six months later, the correction of anterior compartment with TOT suburethral mesh was associated, Fig. 7.108.–7.111.

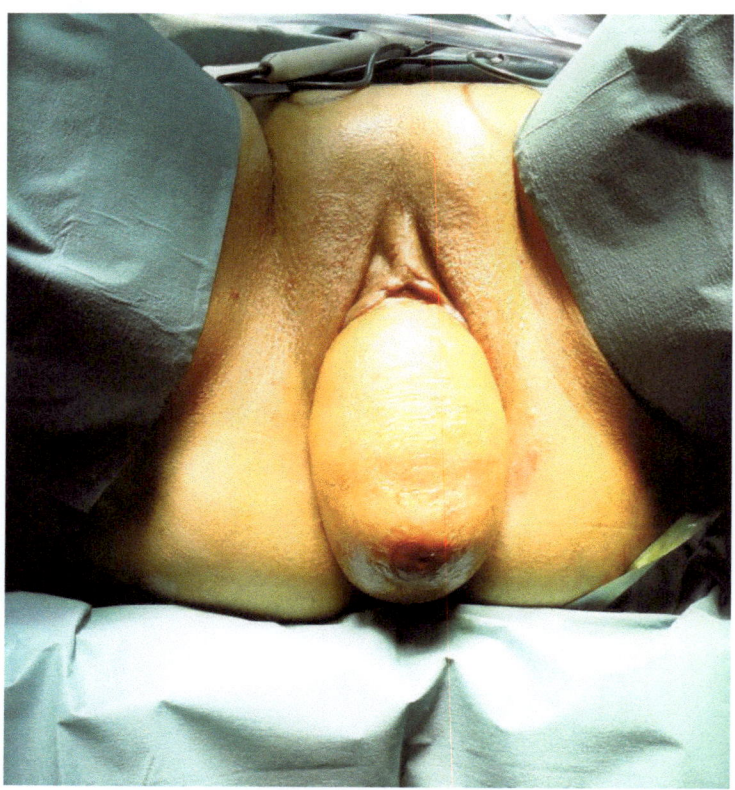

Fig. 7.112. Total uterine prolapse; preoperatory aspect
(from the archive of **Enache T.**)

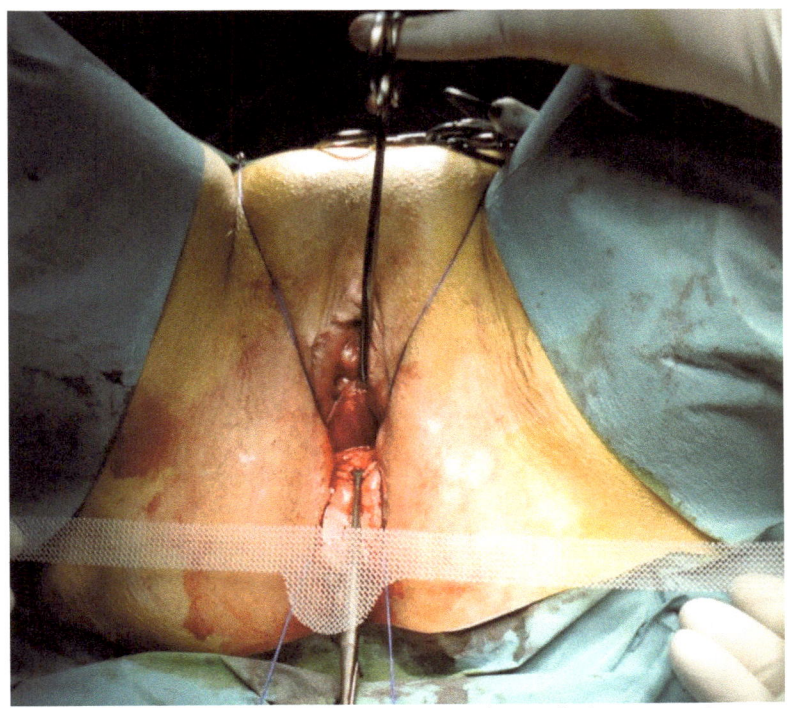

Fig 7.113. Total uterine prolapse – mounting the posterior mesh; intraoperative aspect
(from the archive of **Enache T.**)

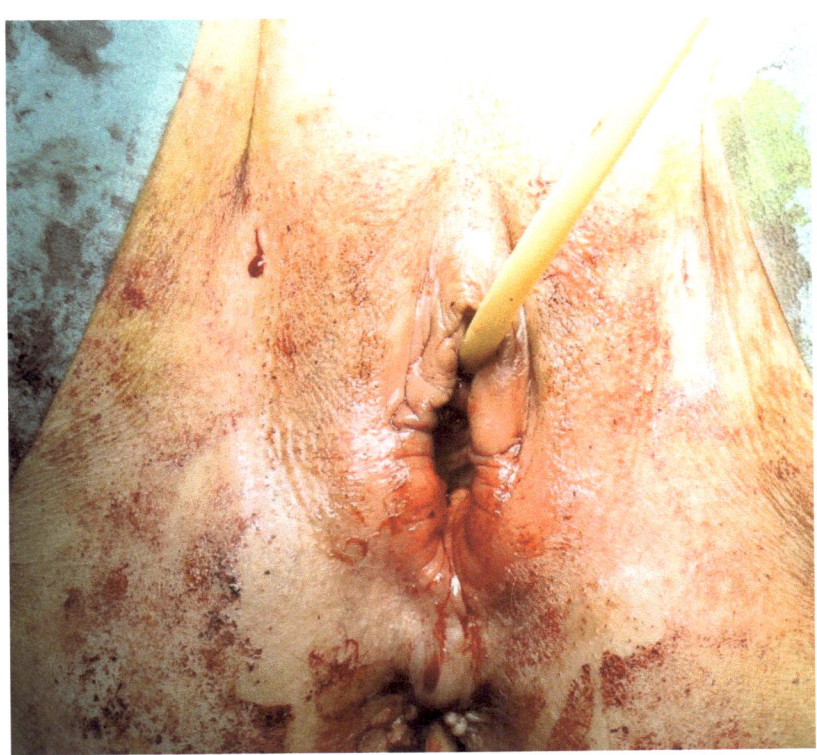

Fig. 7.114. Total uterine prolapse; postoperatory aspect
(from the archive of **Enache T.**)

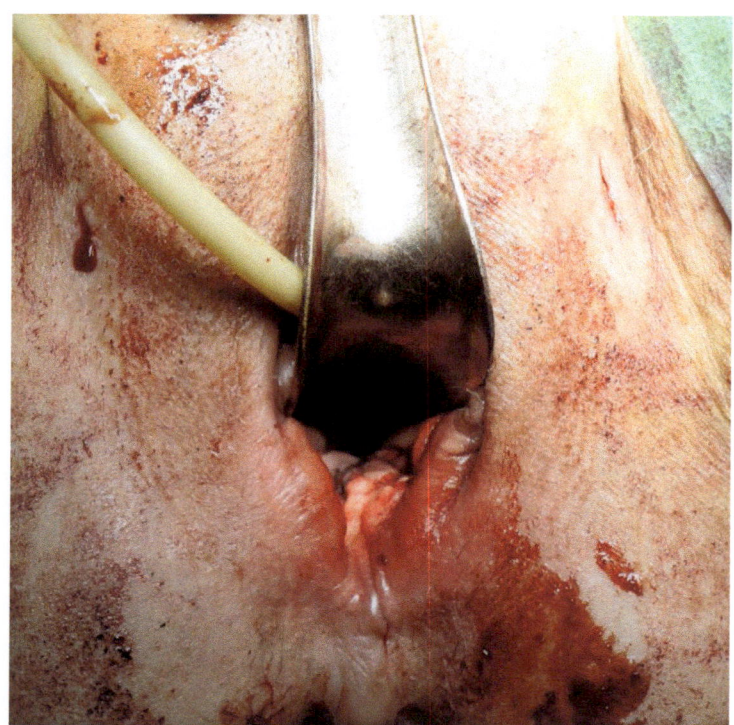

Fig. 7.115. Total uterine prolapse – correction of posterior compartment; postoperatory aspect
(from the archive of **Enache T.**)

Case 2

A 75-year-old patient with complex pelvic floor disorder, with all compartments affected: uterine prolapse 4th degree, elitrocele, rectocele, and cystocele. A posterior mesh was used with sacrospinous fixing, with posterior "*bridge*", the procedure being similar to the one presented before. The anterior and middle compartments were corrected the same way as in the previous case, Fig. 7.112.–7.115.

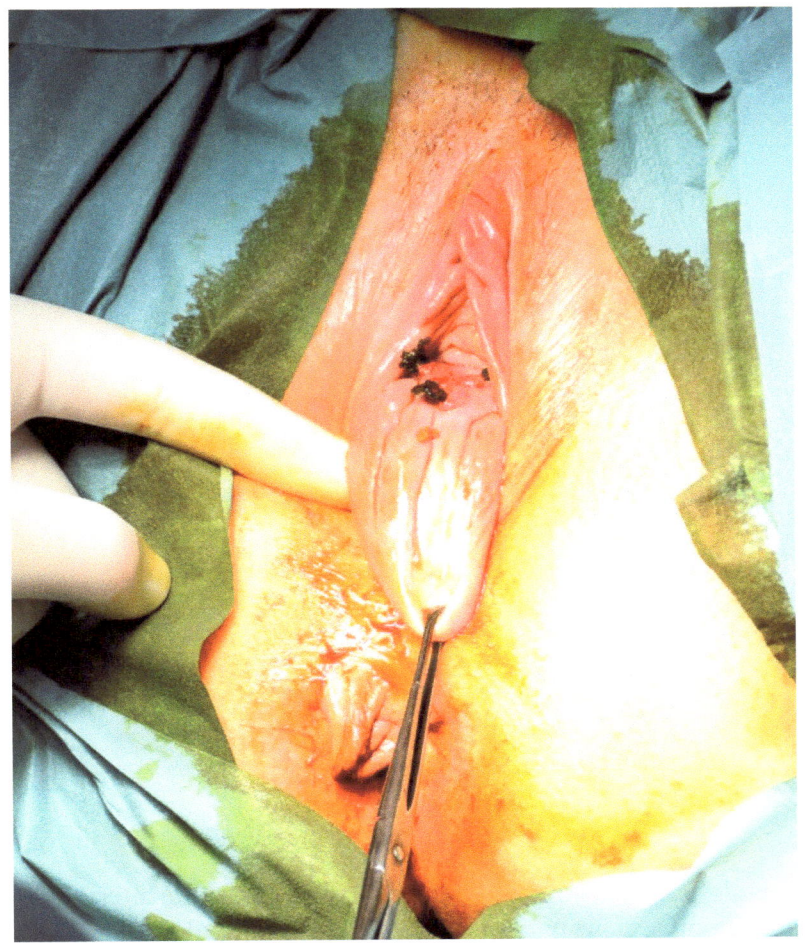

Fig. 7.116. Vaginal vault prolapse; preoperatory aspect
(from the archive of **Enache T.**)

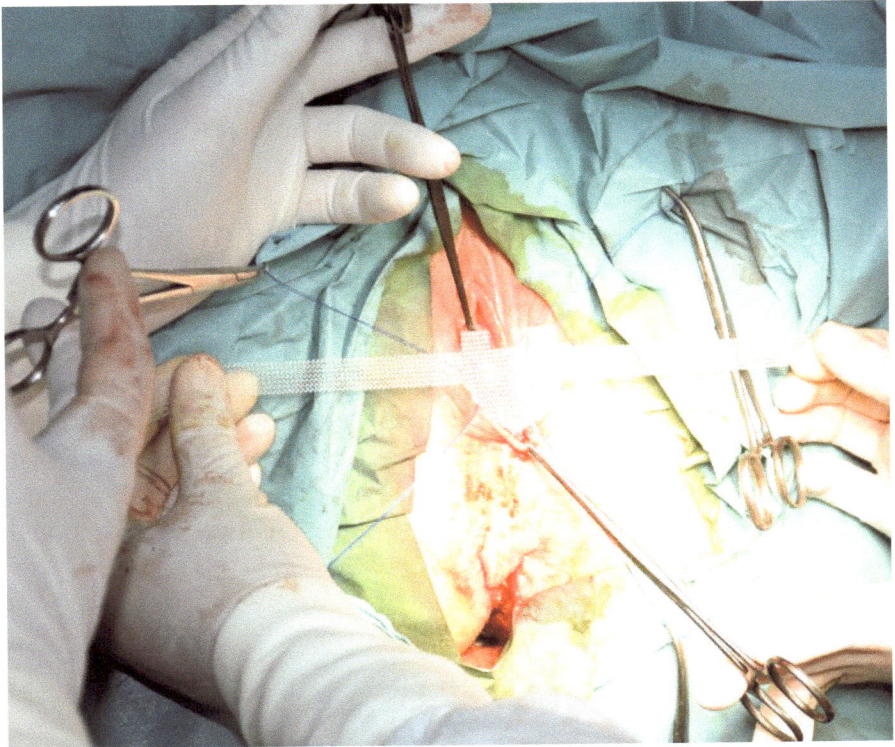

Fig. 7.117. Vaginal vault prolapse, mounting the posterior mesh; intraoperatory aspect
(from the archive of **Enache T.**)

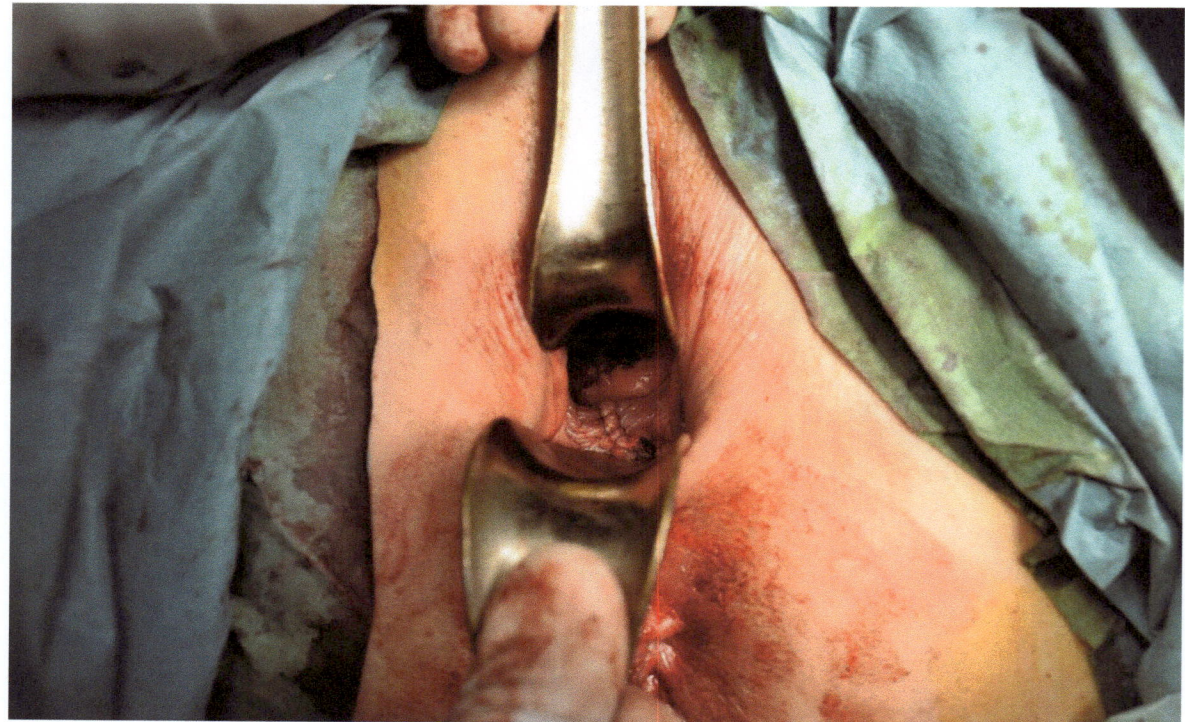

Fig. 7.118. Vaginal vault prolapse; postoperatory aspect
(from the archive of **Enache T.**)

Case 3

A 82-year-old patient with total vaginal hysterectomy for uterine prolapse, 4th degree, with relapse at 3 months. The patient presents with vaginal vault prolapse and rectocele, posterior compartment defect, however without associating disorders in the other compartments. In this case, a posterior mesh was mounted, fixed sacrospinous, to which a posterior "bridge" was associated like in the other cases. The mesh had two loops in the median area, 1 cm apart from one another. The sacrospinous wires were passed through the loops of the mesh at this level, Fig. 7.116.–7.118.

In all three cases presented, the evolution was favorable, without complications at the one-year check-up, but also at the 3 years one.

7.4.2.3. Posterior "patch" with sacrospinous fixation

Based on the analysis of the above-mentioned technique, we found that the part of the mesh located caudally from the plane of levator ani muscles is functionally inert, its presence at the level of ischioanal fossa being only the consequence of the insertion technique. Also, most associated complications are due to the mesh passage through the anatomical space mentioned above. Thus, we propose a new technique through which only the fragment of mesh between the two sacrospinous anchors is kept and the distal fragments of the mesh are abandoned. In addition, a "patch" that is inserted at the level of the transverse vaginal incision results, in the lateral sides the two sacrospinous wires being passed (**Enache T. *et al.*, 2016**).

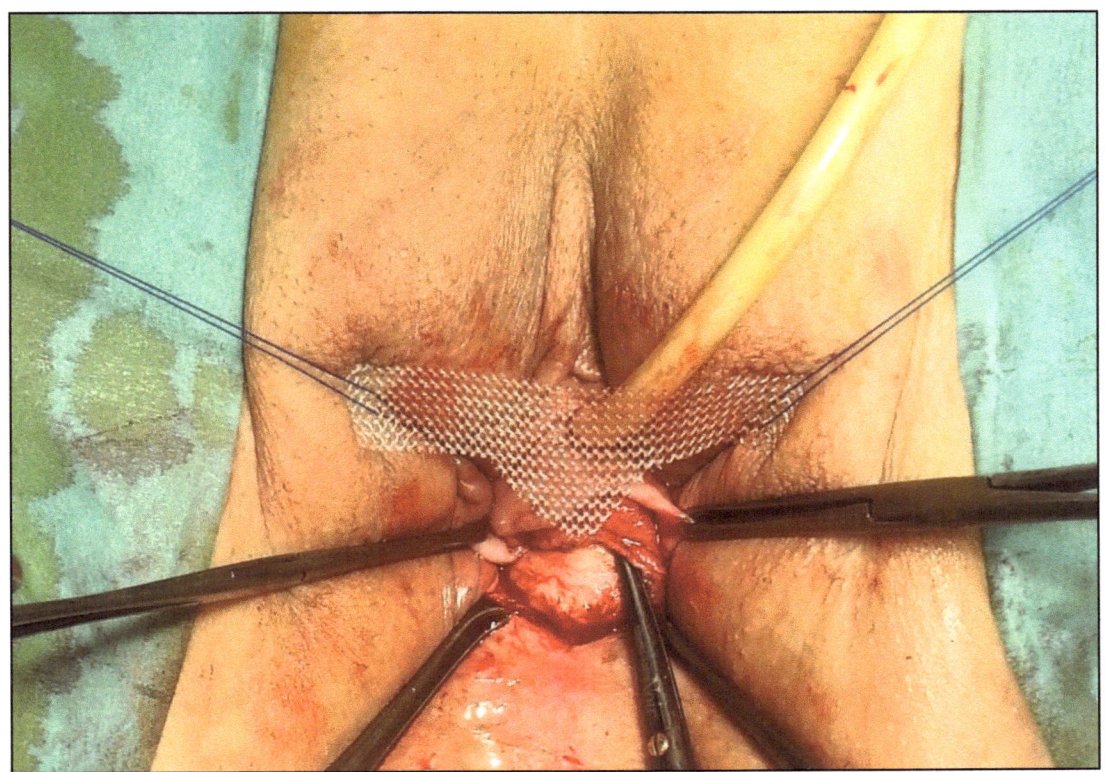

Fig. 7.119. Posterior "*patch*" with sacrospinous fixation in a patient in whom a posterior "*bridge*" is associated
(from the archive of **Enache T.**)

This polypropylene "patch" is made intraoperatively from a larger piece of mesh. Most often it has a rectangular shape with dimensions of 4/2 cm. Depending on the particularities of each case, its shape may undergo minor changes.

In cases of vaginal vault prolapse we left some extensions in the cranial parts, bilateral, where we anchored the sacrospinous wires to compensate for the lack of substance due to the absence of the cervix, Fig. 7.118. In patients who also associated rectocele and where it required its cure with posterior "bridge", we created a lower triangular or semicircular extension with a maximum size of 1.5 cm from the lower edge of the "*patch*", Fig. 7.119. Physiologically, the uterosacral ligaments provide the posterior vector component of the cervix and the cardinal ligaments provide the lateral component. Transposed in biomechanical language, we are talking about a "*tension in the wire*" that is opposed to the displacement of the cervix, one oriented posteriorly and the other one laterally.

The result of these forces is a vector with posterolateral orientation, Fig. 7.120.

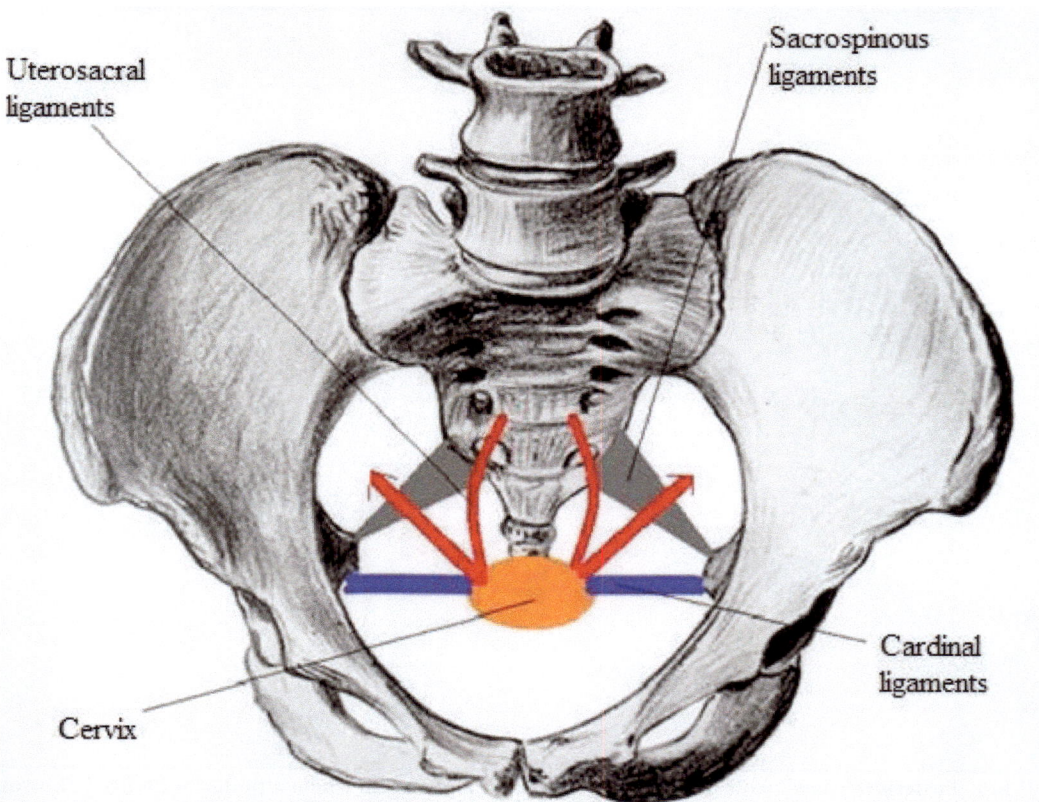

Fig. 7.120. Disposition of cardinal and uterosacral ligaments. Vector analysis.
The arrow is the vector result of the "tension in the wire" in the cardinal and uterosacral ligaments

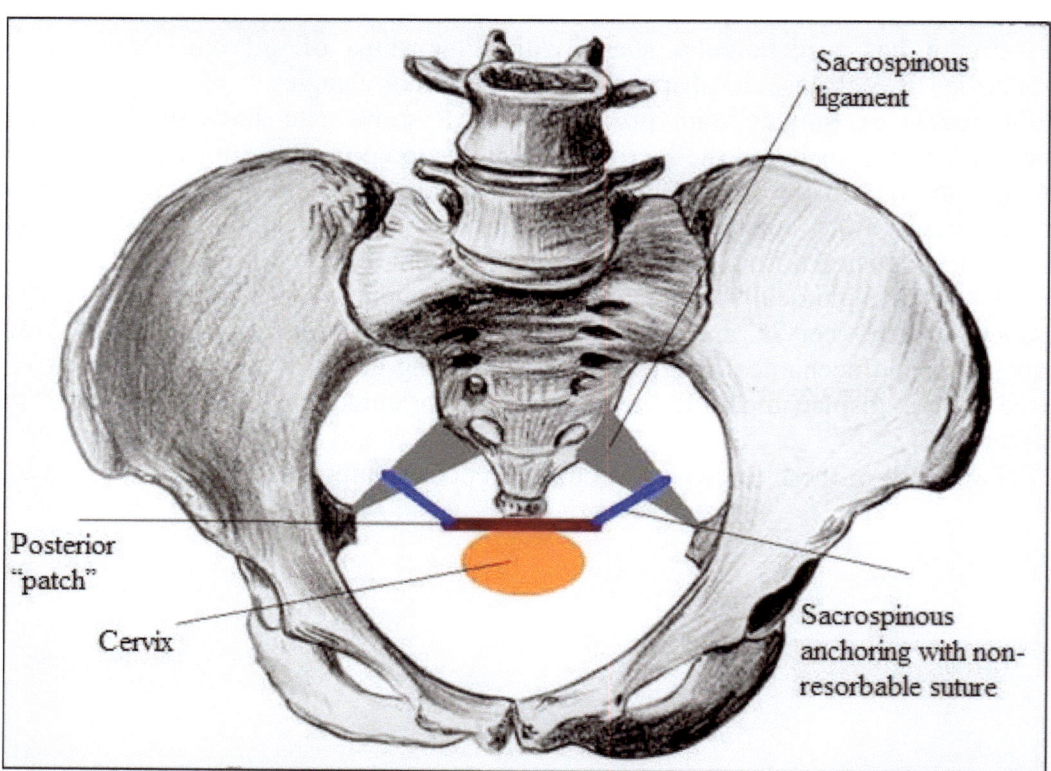

Fig. 7.121. Postoperatory position of the posterior "patch" with sacrospinous fixation

In the case of the posterior "*patch*", the sacrospinous anchoring wires also have a posterolateral direction, similar to that of the two ligament components, Fig. 7.121.

Thus, we can conclude that from a biophysical point of view, the posterior "*patch*" fixed sacrospinously has the prospect of a pathogenic correction of the defective anchoring of the cervix and the elitrocele. In the case of uterine prolaps, we preferred an additional technique depending on the possible pelvic floor disorders associated. For the cases in which an anterior vaginal prolapse coexisted, we preferred the 4-arms surgical cure, 2 passed transobturator and 2 laterocervical, subsequently fixed to the sacrospinous wires, thus also realizing the anchoring of the cervix. To the extent that there is no cystocele associated and there is only an apical defect, damage to uterosacral and cardinal ligaments, we practiced a pericervical cerclage with the anchoring of the edges of the mesh to the 2 sacrospinous wires. Vaginal vault prolapse benefits from the same surgical technique, the etiopathogeny being identical to that of uterine prolapse, as mentioned before.

Surgical steps

1. A transverse incision is made at the level of posterior vaginal mucosa, at 2 cm below its insertion on the cervix.

2. Digital dissection is performed with the index finger of the same hand posterolateral to the ischial spine and bilaterally.

3. The marking of sacrospinous ligaments with the index finger, bilateral, medial and in contact with the ischial spine.

4. Passing a 2/0 non-resorbable monofilament wire through each sacrospinous ligament using the "*Viper*" approximately halfway to the sacrospinous ligament, somehow more lateral than in the case of posterior mesh anchoring and marking the ends of the wires with an autostatic spreading-forceps. The maneuver is performed by positioning the instrument's handle in the hand opposite to the side of the patient operated on. Holding takes place so that the thumb is in contact with the plunger of the sliding needle (P), Fig. 7.103.

The instrument is inserted with the same hand corresponding to the side of the patient operated on, the index finger being in contact with the sacrospinous ligament at about 2 cm lateral to the ischial spine. The tip of the instrument is positioned so that in the concavity oriented inferiorly, to penetrate when in contact with the ligament. The tip of the "Viper" will be pressed on the ligament with the index finger, which it was marked with initially. At this point, with the thumb of the contralateral hand, the plunger is activated to the tip, with the movement of the sliding needle that will pierce the ligament and will meet the wire that is passed over the end of the instrument, Fig. 7.104.

The retraction of the plunger follows, also meaning the retraction of the needle that has the wire, thus realizing the anchoring of the wire to the sacrospinous ligaments. By retracting the instrument, both ends of the wire are at the level of the vaginal incision.

5. The insertion of the polypropylene "patch", passing the ends of the wires anchored sacrospinously through the loops of the mesh, in the lateral sides, bilaterally, Fig. 7.119.

6. Fixing the "*patch*" to the insertion on the cervix of sacrospinous ligaments, the wires will be located medial to the sacrospinous ones. In the case of patients with a history of total hysterectomy, the fixation of the "patch" is done at the posterior vaginal mucosa, 1 cm below the postoperatory scar.

7. Tying the ends of the wires anchored sacrospinous with one another, with consequent reduction of uterine prolapse and elitrocele. The sutures should not be strained excessively, thus avoiding overcorrection. A part of the wire will remain suspended, as mentioned above.

8. Suture of the vaginal cut. If there are additional steps, these will be made separately.

The technique described above has two advantages: avoiding most of the complications and it is simpler, four surgical steps disappearing. The "*in vivo*" provision of the "*patch*", with sacrospinous fixation, is schematically represented in Fig 7.121., and represents a technical solution that respects the vector distribution, thus providing the premises for the restoration of pelvic organs physiology. The patient is mesh-covered for 24 hours postoperatory, the discharge being made at 48 hours at the latest if no complications occur.

The results at three years are favorable, with a relapse rate of less than 1% in a group of 150 patients, but is also requires a statistical confirmation at five years. However, prospects are encouraging. The method was registered at the State Office for Inventions and Trademarks (OSIM) in Romania with the title "*Surgical kit and method for elitrocele correction vaginally*" and the Patent No. 130607/29.11.2016 was obtained.

In the following, we will offer examples of the application of the method in some cases that associated the apical defect and its correction by the above-mentioned method.

Case 1

A 57-year-old patient, presented with posterior vaginal fornix symptomatology, nocturia, urge incontinence, dyspareunia and medium pelvic pains. The clinical examination revealed a posterior compartment defect at all three levels: elitrocele with minimal uterine prolapse, rectocele, and perineal body defect. The surgical correction was performed with a "*patch*" posteriorly fixed to the sacrospinous ligaments, and, additionally, the cure of rectocele with posterior "*bridge*", Fig. 7.122. – 7.124.

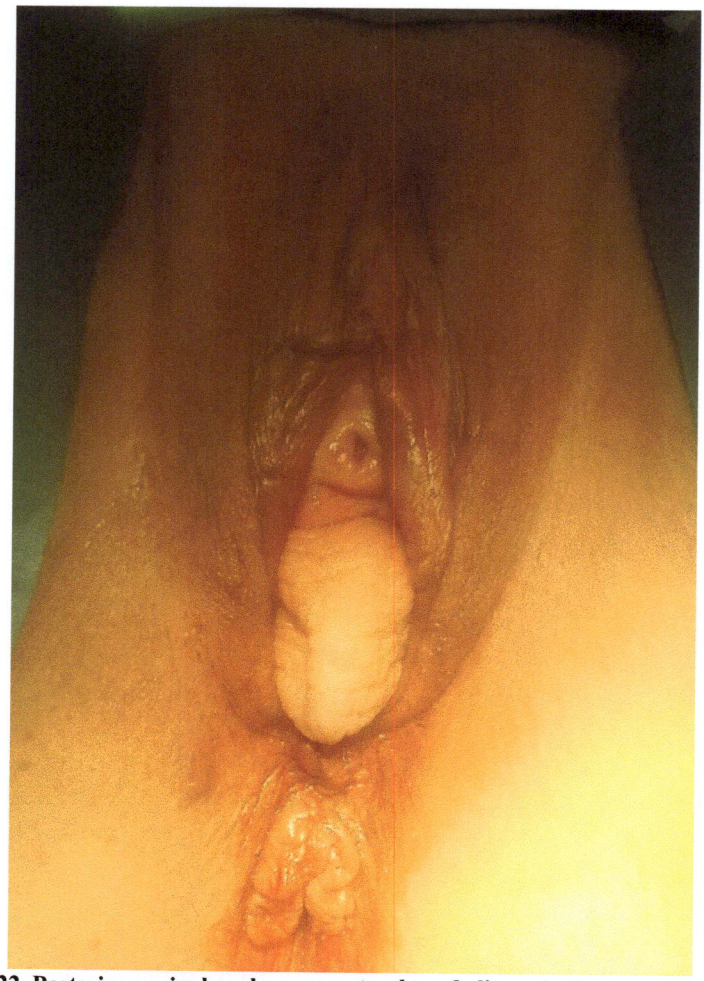

Fig. 7.122. Posterior vaginal prolapse – rectocele and elitrocele. Preoperatory aspect
(from the archive of **Enache T.**)

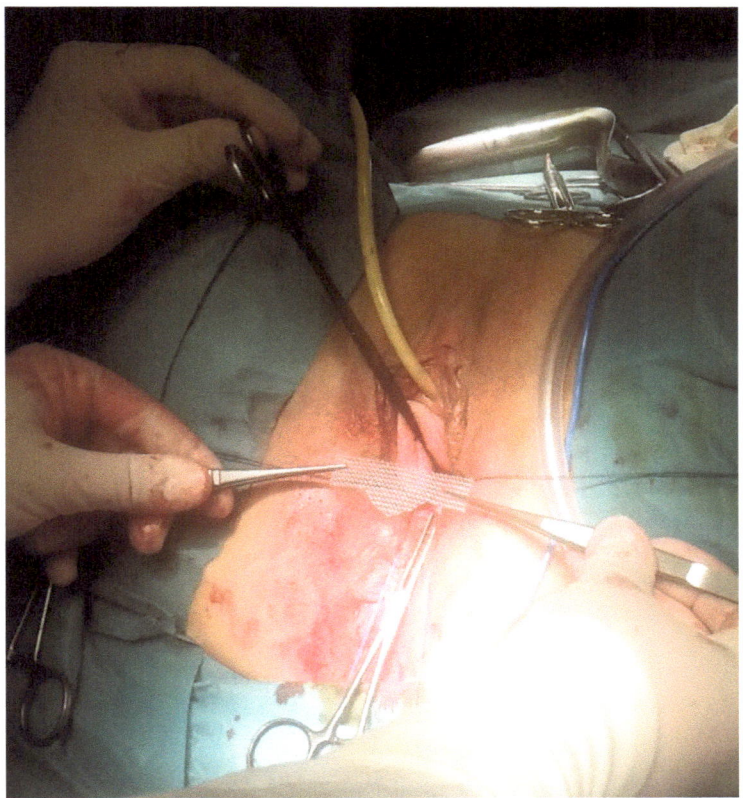

Fig. 7.123. Posterior vaginal prolapse. Intraoperatory aspect
(from the archive of **Enache T**.)

At six months, the patient returned with a satisfactory anatomical result and a significant clinical improvement, however, nocturia was still persistent, but with a lower frequency from 6 to 3 episodes per night. Moreover, a significant reduction of hemorrhoidal disease was observed, which the patient also noticed.

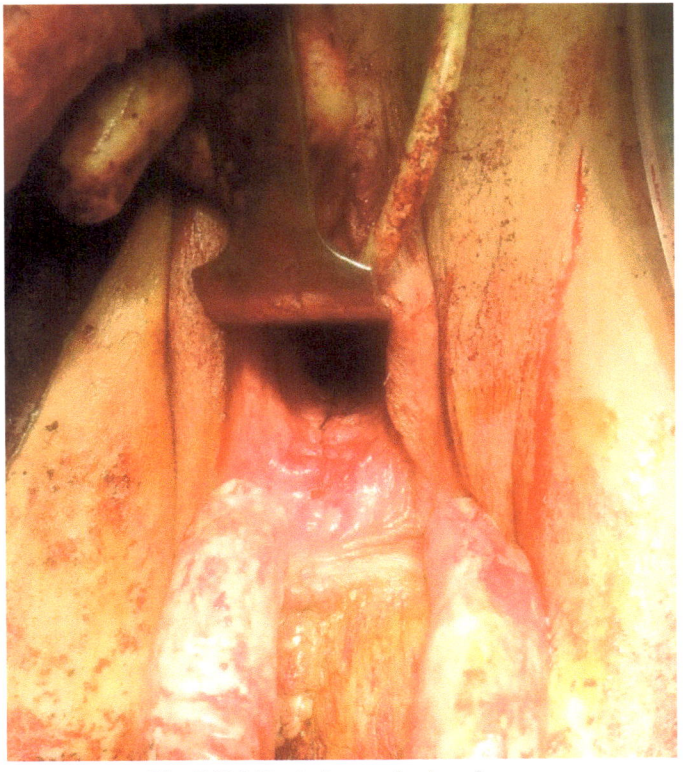

Fig. 7.124. Posterior vaginal prolapse.
Postoperatory aspect (from the archive of **Enache T**)

Case 2

A 54-year-old patient presented for a formation that came out from the vaginal introit, nocturia, and urge incontinence, that she declared it was however variable. The objective examination revealed a 2nd degree uterine prolapse, elitrocele and 3rd degree rectocele, Fig. 7.125 and 7.126.

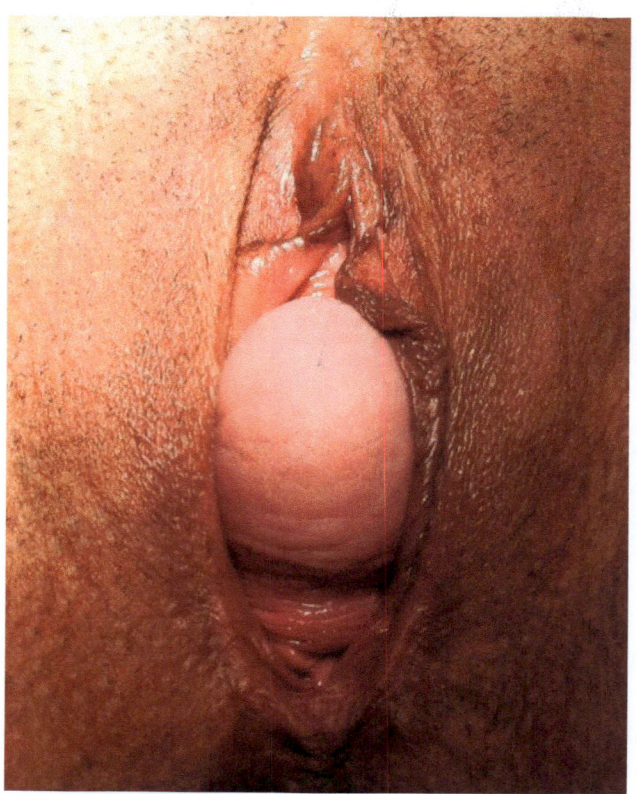

Fig. 7.125. Posterior uterine and vaginal prolapse
Preoperatory aspect (from the archive of **Enache T.**)

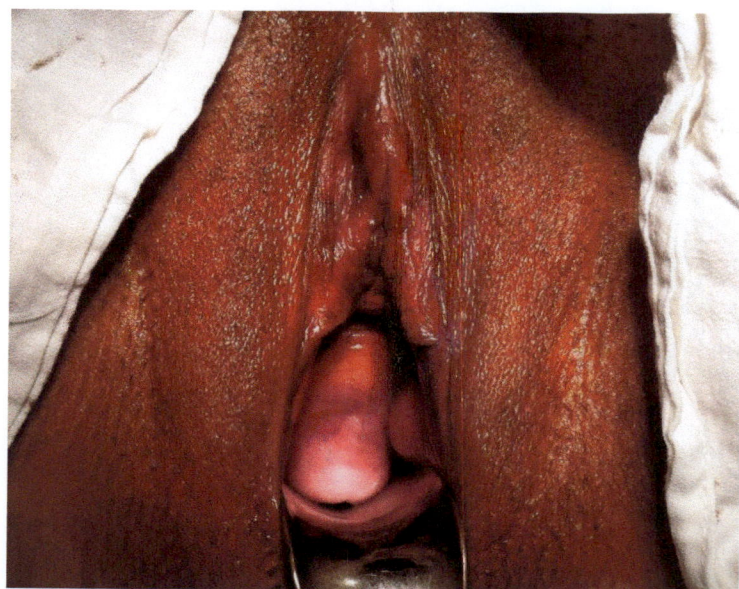

Fig. 7.126. Posterior uterine and vaginal prolapse. Presentation of the unharmed anterior wall.
Preoperatory aspect (from the archive of **Enache T.**)

Surprisingly, the anterior wall did not present any pelvic floor disorder. Surgical treatment consisted in mounting a posterior "patch" with sacrospinous fixation, which reconstructed the cardinal and uterosacral ligaments vectorally. A more difficult moment was the dissection of the hernial sac and the reduction of elitrocele, Fig. 7.127. In this case, a patch with a particular shape was made, Fig. 7.128., with two extensions anteriorly and laterally, and through their loops, the sacrospinous wires were passed, and, with an inferior and median extension, the posterior "bridge" was attached for the correction of rectocele, Fig. 7.129. Postoperatory progression was favorable at six months, with the disappearance of symptoms and the restoration of the anatomy.

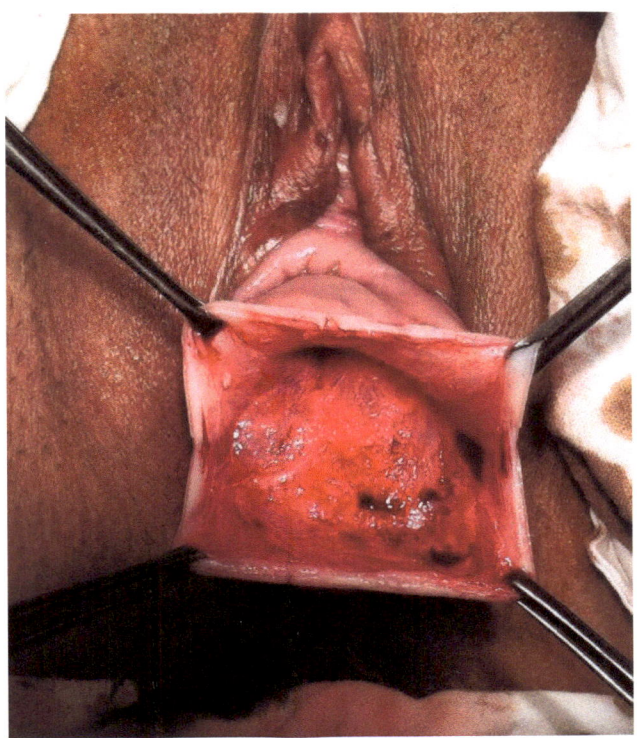

Fig. 7.127. Posterior uterine and vaginal prolapse, dissection of hernial sac.
Intraoperatory aspect (from the archive of **Enache T.**)

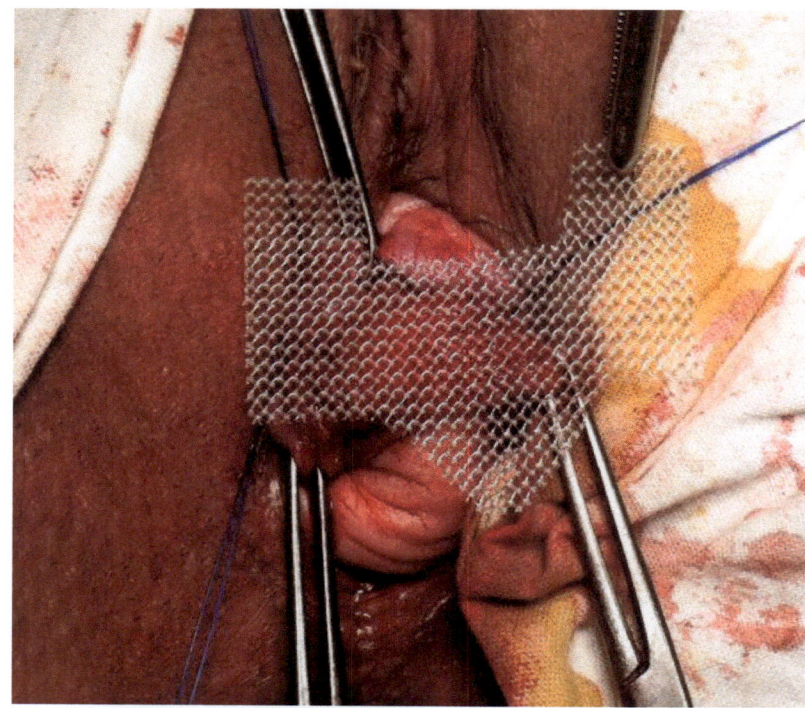

Fig. 7.128. Posterior uterine and vaginal prolapse: posterior "*patch*".
Intraoperatory aspect (from the archive of **Enache T.**)

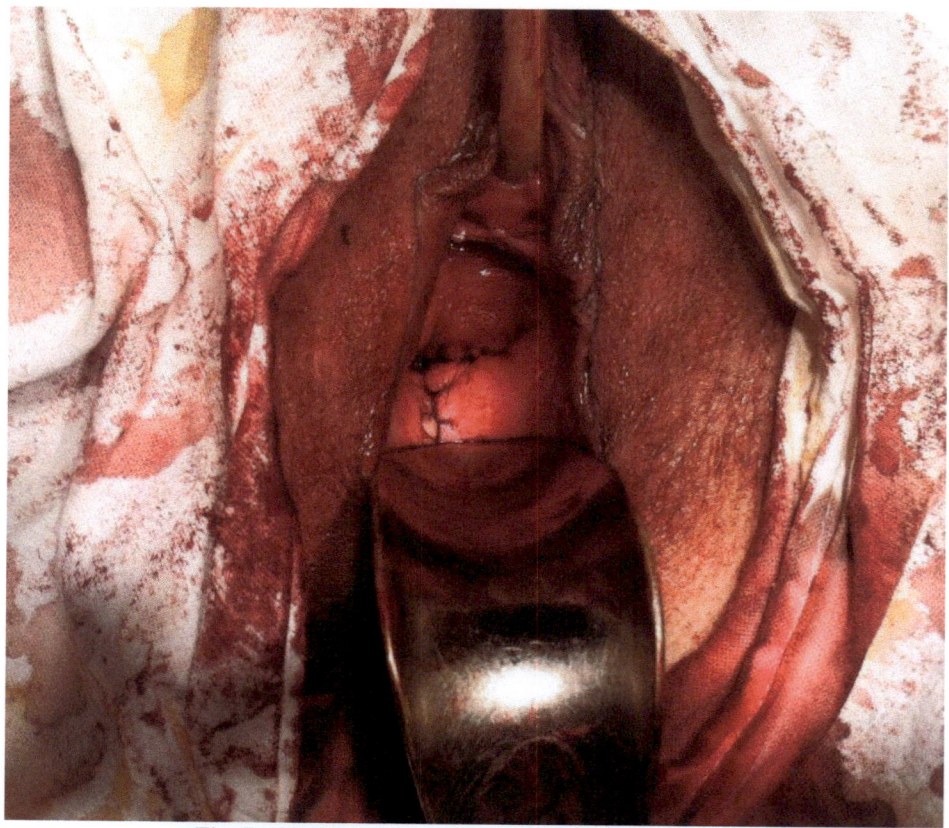

Fig. 7. 129. Posterior uterine and vaginal prolapse.
Postoperatory aspect (from the archive of **Enache T.**)

7.4.2.4. Posterior patch, homograft with sacrospinous fixation

We present a surgical technique that has been successfully applied in some cases and which has prospects of imposing as an alternative to surgical treatment with alloplastic materials. Patients who have benefited from this method were generally elderly with significant atrophy, multiple relapses, some with erosions registered in the medical history. The surgical indication was determined by a noisy symptomatology: bladder globe with significant prolapse, low intestinal occlusion, and decubitus superinfected lesions. In these cases, it was preferred to give up the polypropylene patch, attempting to change it so that the pelvic floor disorder is efficiently neutralized.

We replaced the polypropylene "*patch*" with a homograft made up of desepithelised vaginal mucosa, with the same shape and same anchoring style, Fig. 7.130.

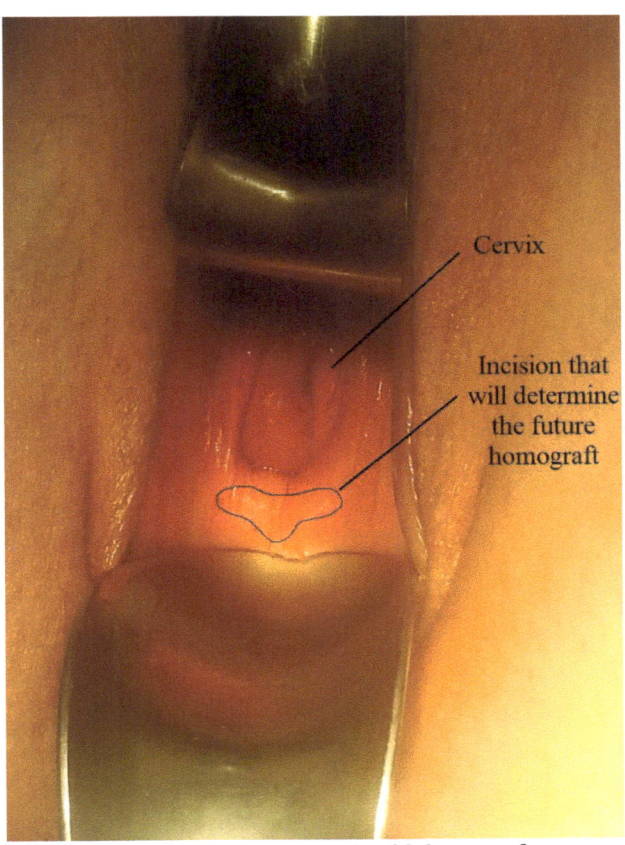

Fig. 7.130. Posterior patch with homograft
(from the archive of **Enache T.**)

Surgical steps is identical to the one of sacrospinous fixation of posterior "*patch*", except for 1 and 5.

1. An elliptical incision is made in the posterior vaginal mucosa, at 2 cm below its insertion into the cervix, with the delimitation of a mucosa fragment of the approximate dimensions of a "*patch*" that would have been made for that case.

2. Digital dissection with the index finger of the same hand in the posterolateral direction towards the ischial spine bilaterally.

3. Marking the sacrospinous ligaments bilaterally with the index finger, medial, and in contact with the ischial spine.

Passing a 2/0 non-resorbable monofilament suture through each sacrospinous ligament by using the "*Viper*", approximately halfway the sacrospinous ligament, somewhat more lateral than in the case of anchoring the posterior mesh and marking the ends of the wires with an autostatic spreading-forceps. The maneuver is done by positioning the instrument handle in the opposite hand to the side of the patient being operated on. The holding is done so that the thumb is in contact with the plunger of the sliding needle (P), Fig. 7.103. The instrument is inserted with the same hand corresponding to the side of the patient operated on, the index finger being in contact with the sacrospinous ligament at about 2 cm lateral to the ischial spine. The tip of the instrument is positioned so that in the concavity oriented inferiorly, to penetrate when in contact with the ligament. The tip of the "Viper" will be pressed on the ligament with the index finger, which it was marked with initially. At this point, with the thumb of the contralateral hand, the plunger is activated to the tip, with the movement of the sliding needle that will pierce the ligament and will meet the wire that is passed over the end of the instrument, Fig. 7.104.

4. The retraction of the plunger follows, also meaning the retraction of the needle that has the wire, thus realizing the anchoring of the wire to the sacrospinous ligaments. By retracting the instrument, both ends of the wire are at the level of the vaginal incision.

5. Desepithelation of the vaginal mucosa patch with the electrocautery to destroy any glands at this level and to provide increased resistance. The ends of the sutures anchored sacrospinous through the lateral sides of the mucosa patch are passed through a needle bilaterally.

6. Fixing the mucosa patch to the cervix insertion of sacrospinous ligaments, the sutures will be located medial to the sacrospinous ones.

7. Tying the ends of the wires anchored sacrospinously with one another, with consequent reduction of uterine prolapse and elitrocele. The sutures should not be strained excessively, thus avoiding overcorrection. A part of the wire will remain suspended, as mentioned above.

8. Suture of the vaginal cut. If there are additional steps, these will be made separately.

The patient is mesh-covered for 24 hours postoperatory, the discharge being made at 48 hours at the latest if no complications occur.

7.4.2.5. Pericervical cerclage with sacrospinous fixed mesh

It is a method of restoring uterosacral and cardinal ligaments, similar to the method of posterior "patch", but which stabilizes the paracolpos, a structure that interconnects all connective tissue with a role in pelvic floor anatomy.

It is preferred especially in patients with apical defect, which mainly manifests by uterine prolapse and secondly by elitrocele, but does not associate anterior vaginal prolapse. Pericervical cerclage is performed with polypropylene sling, whose posterior ends are anchored to the sacrospinous ligaments. Also, this technique implies the use of a posterior intravaginal sling or a posterior "*patch*" with sacrospinous fixation. The sling used to perform the cerclage is generally anchored to the same sutures to which the posterior sling or "*patch*" is suspended. This way, the posterior vector component is reconstructed, with the corresponding support of vaginal fornix and cervix (**Bradley C.S. & Nygaard I.E., 2005**), Fig. 7.131.

The surgical steps for the insertion of pericervical cerclage were systematized as it follows:

1. A transverse incision is made at the level of posterior vaginal mucosa, at 2 cm below its insertion on the cervix.

2. Digital dissection is performed with the index finger of the same hand posterolateral to the ischial spine and bilaterally.

3. The marking of sacrospinous ligaments with the index finger, bilateral, medial and in contact with the ischial spine.

4. Passing a 2/0 non-resorbable monofilament wire through each sacrospinous ligament using the "*Viper*" approximately halfway to the sacrospinous ligament, somehow more lateral than in the case of posterior mesh anchoring and marking the ends of the wires with an autostatic spreading-forceps. The maneuver is performed by positioning the

instrument's handle in the hand opposite to the side of the patient operated on. Holding is done so that the thumb is in contact with the plunger of the sliding needle (P), Fig. 7.103.

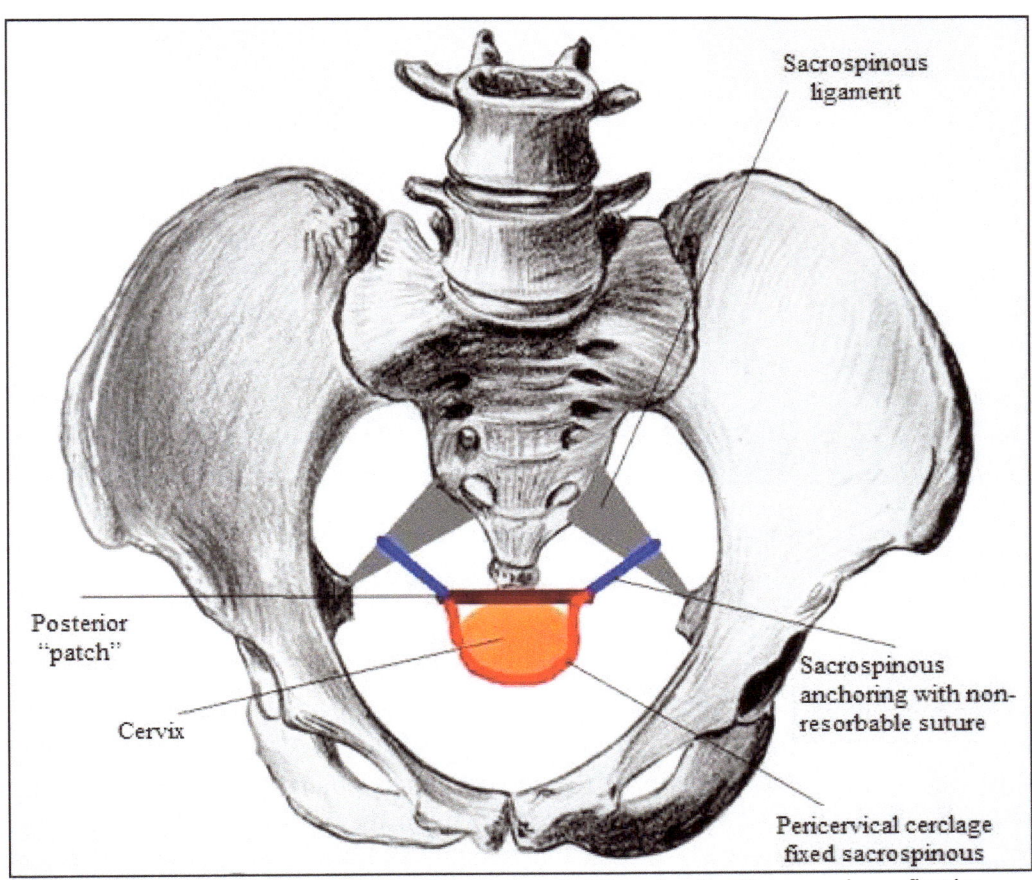

Fig. 7.131. Postoperatory position of the pericervical "cerclage" with sacrospinous fixation
A posterior "*patch*" is also used

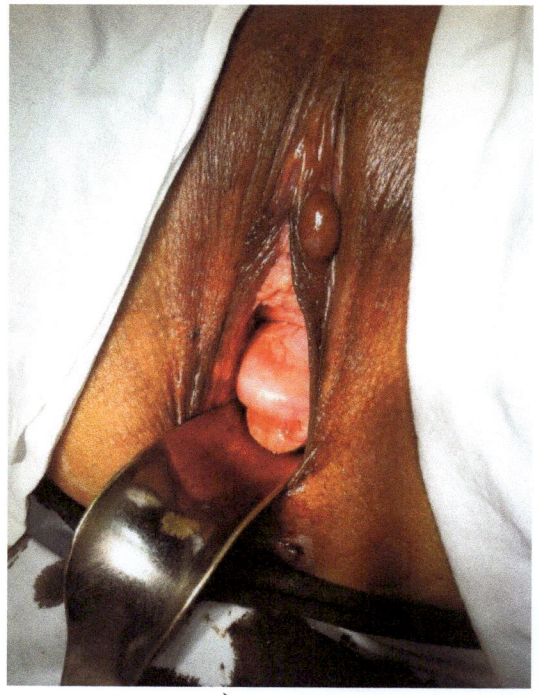 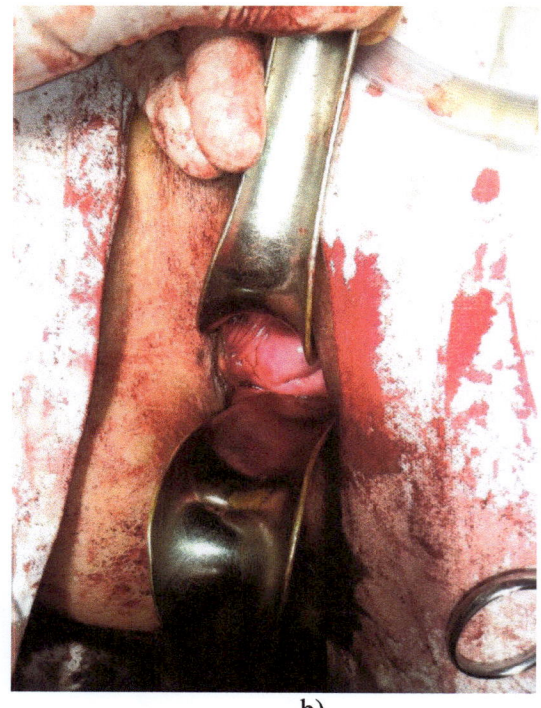

a)   b)

Fig. 7.132. Uterine prolapse in a 28 year-old-patient
Clinical aspect.
a) preoperatory b) postoperatory

The instrument is inserted with the same hand corresponding to the side of the patient operated on, the index finger being in contact with the sacrospinous ligament at about 2 cm lateral to the ischial spine. The tip of the instrument is positioned so that in the concavity oriented inferiorly, to penetrate when in contact with the ligament. The tip of the "Viper" will be pressed on the ligament with the index finger, which it was marked with initially. At this point, with the thumb of the contralateral hand, the plunger is activated to the tip, with the movement of the sliding needle that will pierce the ligament and will meet the wire that is passed over the end of the instrument, Fig. 7.104. The retraction of the plunger follows, also meaning the retraction of the needle that has the wire, thus realizing the anchoring of the wire to the sacrospinous ligaments. By retracting the instrument, both ends of the wire are at the level of the vaginal incision.

5. An approximately 2 cm longitudinal incision is performed on the anterior side of the cervix, on its cranial side.

6. The submucosa space located juxta vesical is tunneled with the surgical scissors.

7. The laterocervical tunneling is completed by penetrating from posterior side, from the level of posterior vaginal incision to the anterior side, towards the anterior longitudinal incision, with an Overholt forceps.

8. Insertion of each end of the sling with the Overholt forceps and its retraction from the laterocervical tunnel.

9. Passing the sacrospinous sutures through the ends of the sling, which are located on the posterior side of the cervix and tying the ends of the sutures until the cervix is set in the physiological position. A part of these sacrospinous sutures remain suspended, the ends of the sling not reaching the ligaments.

10. After the associated time has passed, the suture of incisions at the level of vaginal mucosae is performed.

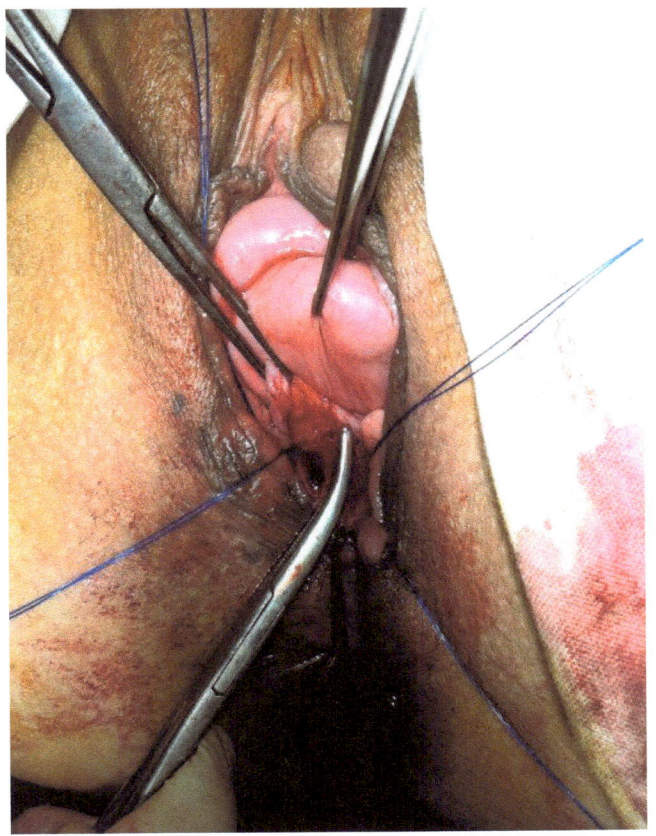

Fig. 7.133. Pericervical cerclage and posterior patch, intraoperatory aspect
(from the archive of **Enache T**.)

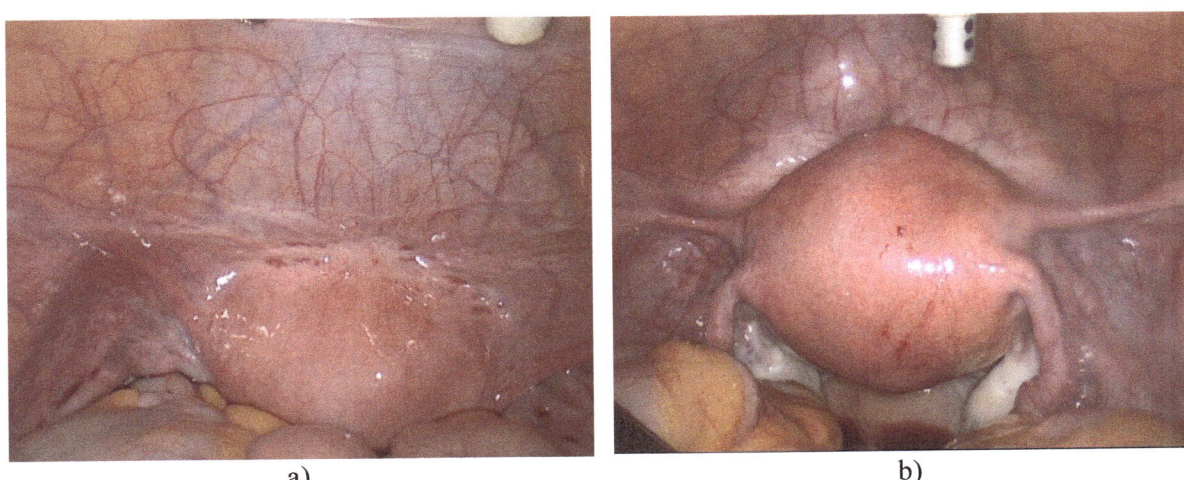

a)   b)

Fig. 7.134. Uterine prolapse in a 28-year-old patient. Laparoscopic aspect.
a) preoperatory b) postoperatory

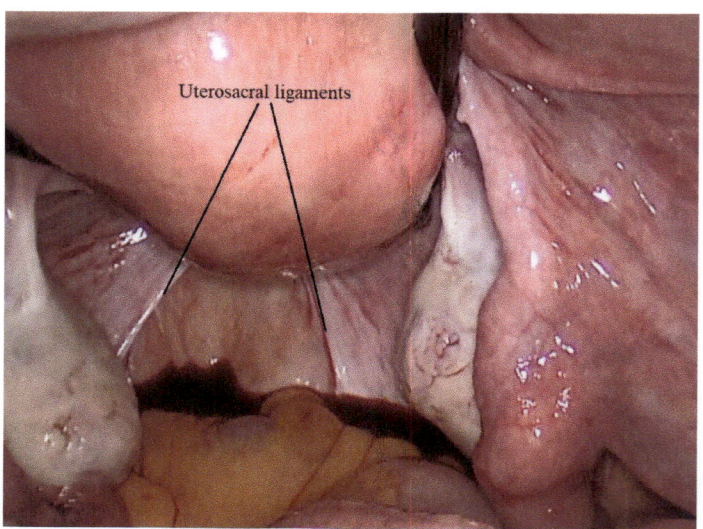

Fig. 7.135. Uterine prolapse
Preoperatory laparoscopic aspect. Analysis of support means (from the archive of **Enache T.**)

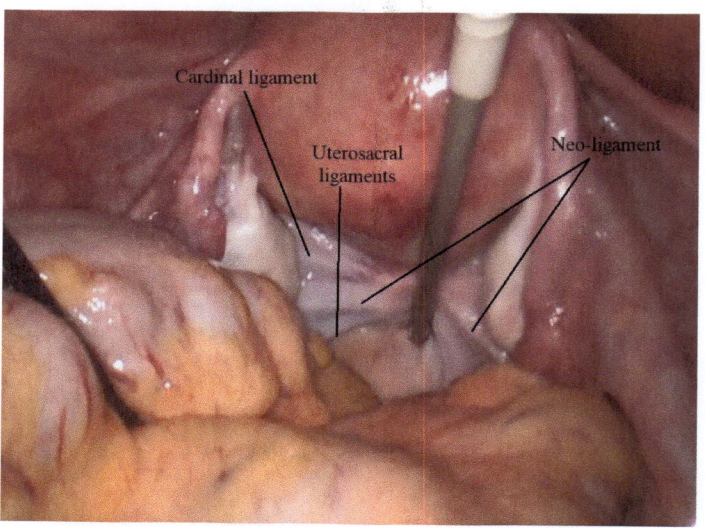

Fig.7.136. Uterine prolapse
Postoperatory laparoscopic aspect. Analysis of support means (from the archive of **Enache T.**)

The result is a uterus support device made up "*de novo*" of alloplastic material.

To offer an example, we present the case of a 28-year-old patient with two births, who presented with a 2nd-3rd degree prolapse and who presented as a primary symptom dyspareunia along with pelvic pains. Its intensity severely affected the quality of life, the patient mentioning the lack of sexual activity for about two years.

Surgical reconstruction consisted in mounting a pericervical cerclage fixed to sacrospinous ligaments and a posterior "*patch*", also with sacrospinous fixation, Fig 7.133. Considering the intensity of the pains, it was decided to perform a diagnostic laparoscopy at the same surgical time to exclude concomitant intraperitoneal lesions. This way, we were able to evaluate the preoperatory and postoperatory aspect both clinically and laparoscopically, Fig. 7.132.–7.134.

The laparoscopic evaluation gave us the possibility of analyzing the anatomical modifications postoperatory, as well as the position of the sacrospinous wires, which are actually neoligaments.

Preoperatively, an enlarged pouch of Douglas with concomitant elongation of uterosacral ligaments was observed, Fig. 7.135. After surgery, the laparoscopic aspect changed essentially. All anatomical elements are normally represented by the tensioning and highlighting of the round ligaments, but also by the appearance of the support means. In Fig. 7.136., the normal compliable pouch of Douglas can be observed, along with a physiological position of uterosacral ligaments. We can also analyze the disposition of cardinal ligaments and the intermediate position of neoligaments.

Laparoscopic control after pelvic floor disorders correction surgeries performed vaginally, provides a new perspective on results. Intraperitoneal, a *"restitutio ad integrum"* of pelvic anatomy can be observed. The analysis of the structures thus assessed highlights the physiological aspect of pouch of Douglas, with the prominence of uterosacral and cardinal ligaments, but also with the appearance of a new plication, which is the *"neoligament"*, the new means of posterior anchoring of the cervix. Its direction is posterolateral, between the directions of the two ligaments, lateral and posterior.

In the case presented, the evolution was very good, with the disappearance of symptoms at five years and a satisfactory sexual life.

7.4.2.6. Tissue fixation system for the posterior compartment

The surgical procedure involves the anchoring system described in tissue fixation system (TFS) for SUI treatment. Correction of the posterior compartment requires the restoration of the vector role of uterosacral ligaments (USL) and the cardinal ligaments, the two being functionally interconnected. The cardinal ligaments repair has been described in a tissue fixation system for the middle compartment. Recovery of USL by TFS is accomplished by their reinforcing, this method being preferred to a suspension to sacrospinous ligaments due to the position of approximately 3 cm below the USL in orthostatism. However, the vector direction remains the same, Fig. 7.137.

Surgical steps

1. Surgery begins with a 5 cm incision on posterior vaginal mucosa, approximately 3-4 cm below its insertion on the cervix or under the posthysterectomy scar. As far as there is a 3rd or 4th degree prolapse, an incision of 1-2 cm below the mentioned markers is performed because the sling should shorten the length of the USL. A longitudinal incision can also be made.

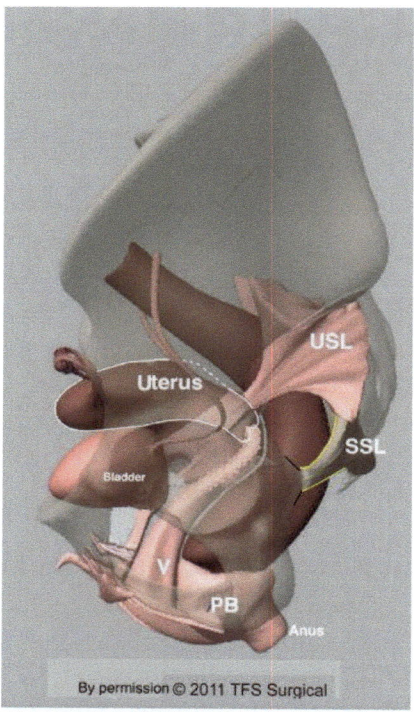

Fig. 7.137. **The ratio of uterosacral ligaments compared to sacrospinous ligaments**
(with approval of **TFS Surgical**)

2. Dissection of elitrocele so that we have access to the USL. These are located at 2 and 10 o'clock and are highlighted by the anterior movement of the cervix and their tension. They are spotted with Chaput forceps. The direction of the ligaments is established, being important to make the tunnel and for the insertion of the sling. Xyline is injected in the thickness of the ligaments so that their dilation occurs. At this point, a vertical incision is made at the upper edge of the ligaments. While tense, a tunnel is created with a thin Metzenbaum scissors inserted in the USL, which reaches 1 cm towards the sacrum. Rectal control is very important.

3. By tensioning the vaginal mucosa, the preformed canal is penetrated with the TFS applicator up to 1 cm towards the sacrum and the anchor is fixed in the tissue. The maneuver is also repeated contralateral, where the sling is tensioned until it becomes fixed.

4. A second vertical incision of about 5 cm length, starting at about 1 cm distal to the vesical trigone area, is performed.

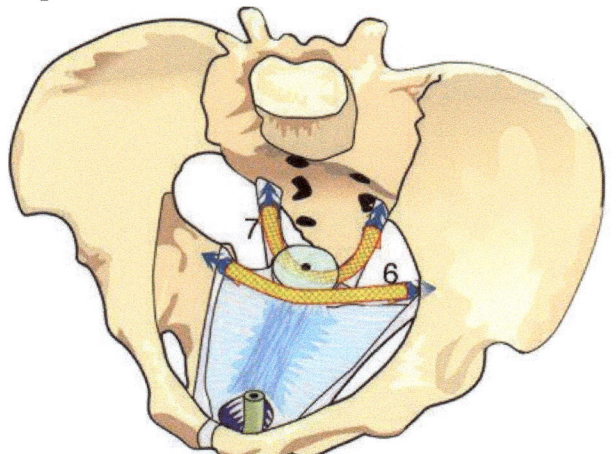

Fig. 7.138. **TFS correction of posterior apical compartment**
(according to **Petros P., 2010**)
6– reconstruction of cardinal ligaments; 7 – uterosacral ligaments reconstruction

5. The bladder is dissected from the vaginal mucosa to create a channel wide enough to be able to insert the sling. The tunnel is made with the dissection scissors, and its orientation is from the inner side of the ischiopubic ramus towards the ATFP insertion on the pubis.

6. Through this channel, the TFS applicator is introduced until resistance is encountered. At that level, the fascia is perforated with the tip of the anchor, and then the applicator is removed. The process is also repeated contralateral. The sling is tensed until resistance is encountered, then the applicator is extracted, the sling remaining fixed.

7. Vaginal layers are sutured with separate wires.

The patient can be discharged at maximum 24 hours after surgery, in case no complications have occurred.

The postoperatory aspect is schematically represented in Fig. 7.138. Apical anchoring is observed by restoring the lateral and posterior fixation means.

7.4.2.7. Surgical treatment with posterior vaginal wall prolapse (rectocele) *"bridge"*

The reconstruction of the rectovaginal fascia is difficult to do due to its being close to the rectum. Even if it does not imply the use of alloplastic material, it requires a homograft. The „bridge" is made of a desepithelised mucosa fragment that is clogged, thus reducing the posterior vaginal wall prolapse.

The technique was described by Petros and later modified by Goeschen, Fig. 7.139. (**Petros P., 2010**). From a pathogenic point of view, the DeLancey level 2 correction is performed.

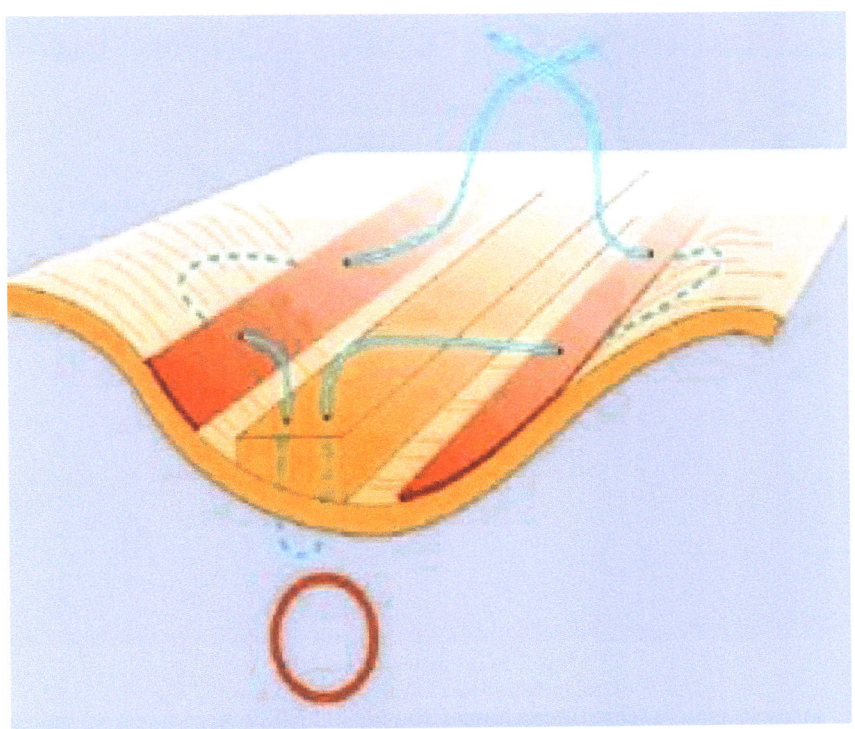

Fig. 7.139. Posterior *"bridge"*
(according to **Petros P., 2010**)

Surgical steps

1. Initially, an elliptical incision is made in the posterior vaginal wall to create a membrane of about 4 cm in length and 1 cm in width. It remains adherent to the submucosa

layer of the anterior wall of the rectum, Fig 7.140.

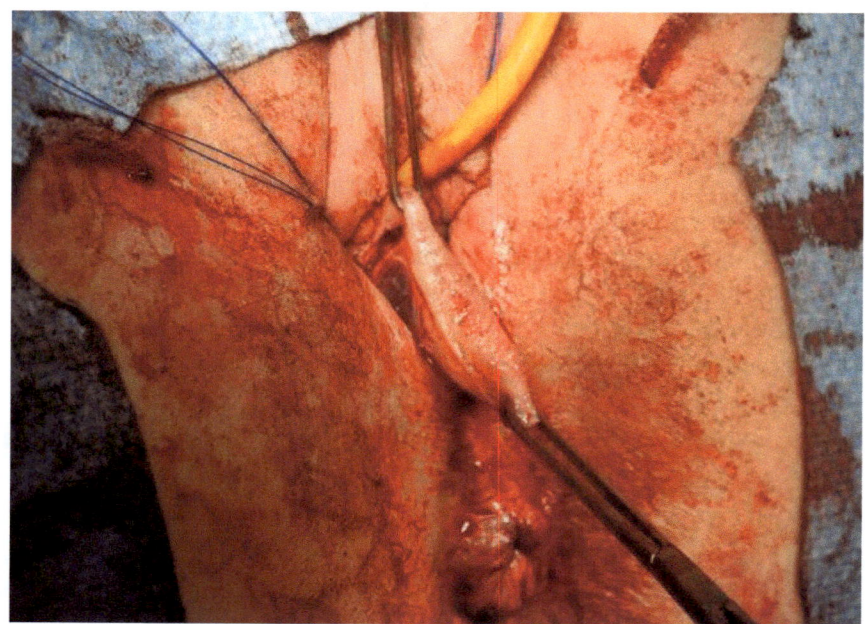

Fig. 7.140. Posterior "*bridge*".
The aspect of vaginal mucosa membrane after the incision
(from the archive of **Mueller-Funogea I-A**)

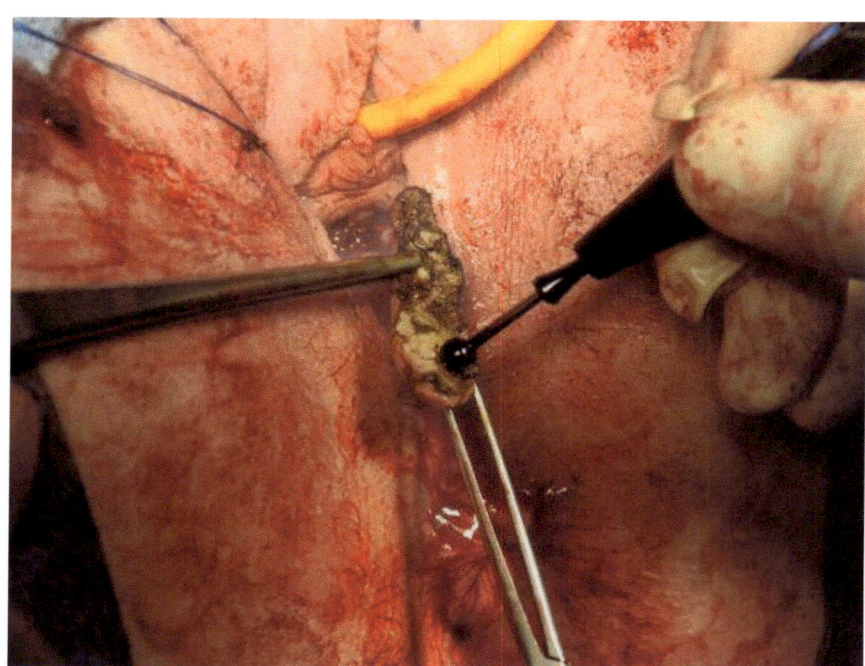

Fig. 7.141. Posterior "*bridge*".
Desepitheliation of mucosa membrane
(from the archive of **Mueller-Funogea I-A**)

2. The membrane is desepithelised with the monopolar electrocautery. This step is necessary to destroy the secretory glands of the mucosa that could give rise to retention cysts after positioning the membrane under the vaginal mucosa, Fig. 7.141.

3. The lateral edges of the membrane are joined by some resorbable sutures, polyglycolic acid, giving rise to a double plate, which is fixed in its cranial part with a

resorbable suture in the middle of the posterior sling or the polypropylene "*patch*" and to the vaginal submucosa or to the posterior cervical wall, when the uterus is present, Fig. 7.142.

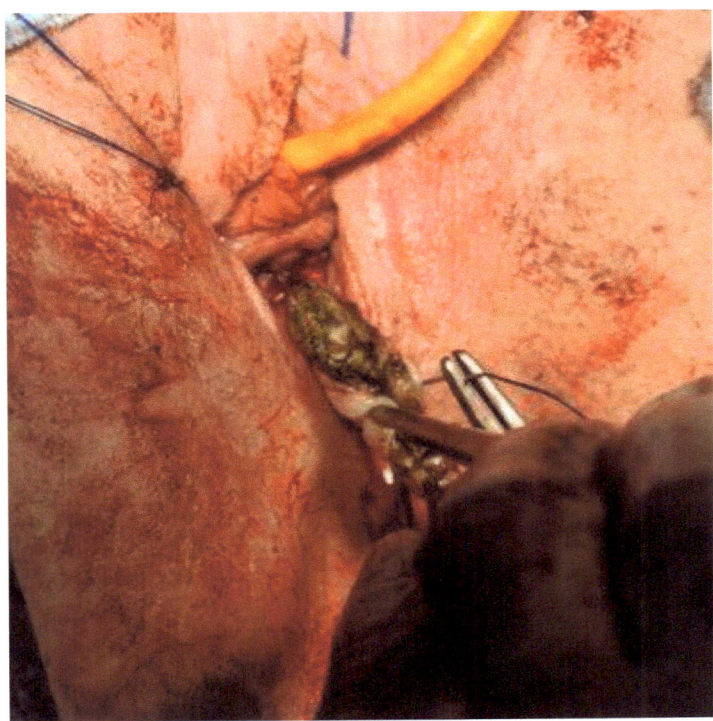

**Fig. 7.142. Posterior "*bridge*".
Creating the double plate**
(from the archive of **Mueller-Funogea I-A**)

4. Lateral endopelvic fascia and levator plate will be connected to the contralateral side with 2-3 monofilament slowly resorbable sutures (2/0), integrating in the middle by suture, the previously prepared flap. These steps need increased attention due to the high risk of rectum injury. Thus, a careful dissection is performed up to the ischioanal fossa, lateral to the rectum, until the levator plate is felt. At this level, the sutures are passed so that they are perpendicular on the direction of muscle fibers to offer resistance.

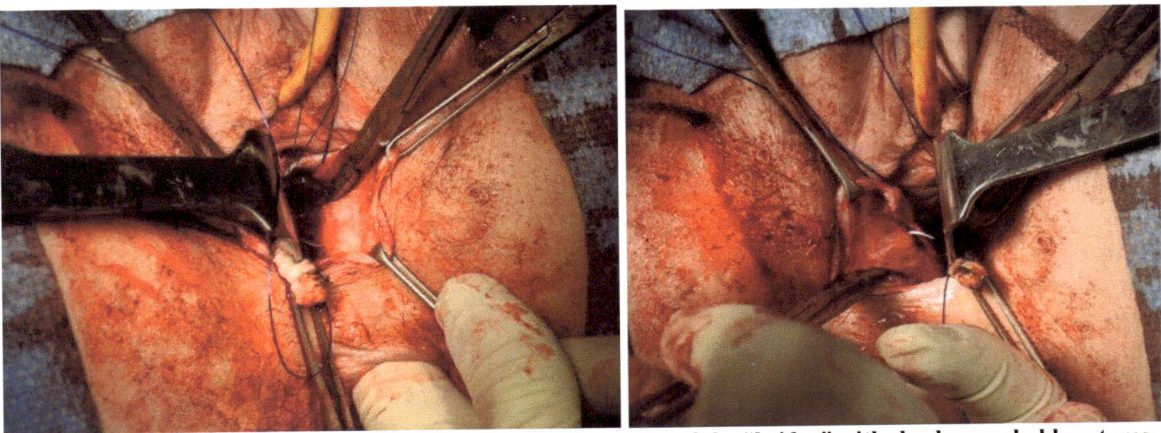

Fig. 7.143. Posterior "*bridge*": rectocele reduction by the suture of the "bridge" with slowly resorbable sutures to the levator plate
(from the archive of **Mueller-Funogea I-A**)

When these sutures are tied, the posterior vaginal wall becomes soft and is lifted and angulated in its anatomical direction (horizontal) towards the sacral concavity, Fig 7.143.

5. Suture of vaginal mucosa with the restoration of posterior vaginal wall continuity. Postoperatory, the suture trance will be disposed longitudinally, Fig. 7.144.

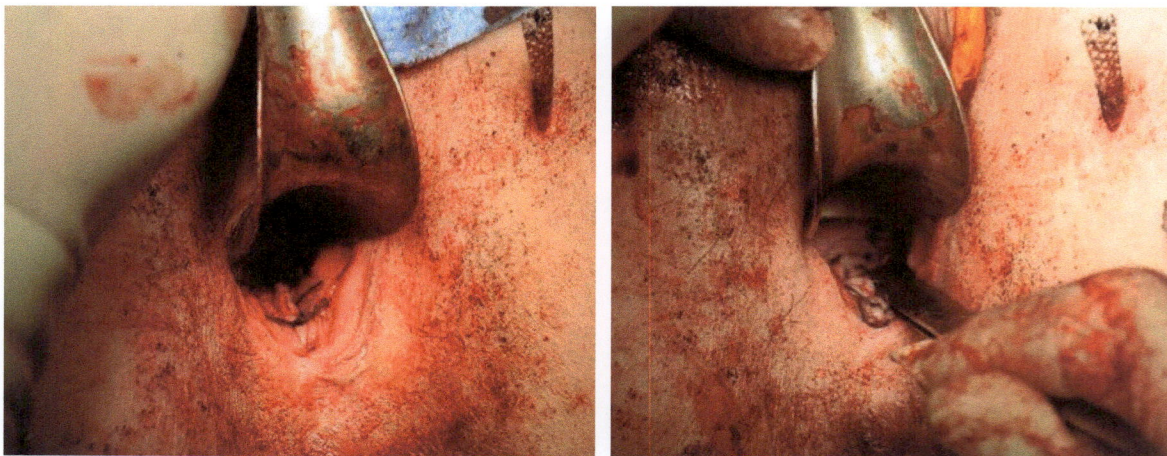

Fig. 7.144. Posterior "*bridge*": final aspect of posterior vaginal wall
(from the archive of Mueller-**Funogea I-A**)

The patient is mesh covered for 24 hours postoperatory, being discharged from hospital not later than 48 hours if no complications occur.

7.4.2.8. Perineal body restoration

In case of perineal body dilation or widening of genital hiatus by lateralizing the muscles inserted at the level of perineal body, the so-called plasty is performed, according to the technique developed by Professor Klaus Goeschen. Correction of perineal body corresponds to the level 3 restoration, according to DeLancey classification. Even though methods that use alloplastic materials have been described, such as TFS for example, the easiest restoration is achived by placing "*U*" shaped sutures at its level.

Surgical steps:
1. The technique starts when, during lateral pararectal preparation, both the muscles and the lateral recto-anal endopelvic fascia have already been highlighted. A suture with a 2.0 resorbable suture loads "*en-bloc*" the musculo-fascial side of the left perineal on the needle, being united with the lower side of the flap with the desepithelised vaginal mucosa, the posterior "*patch*", previously created.

2. The next step implies the loading of the contralateral side of lateral perineal body. By tying the suture, the perineal body is repositioned centrally, being united with the lower side of the "*bridge*" and providing a strong static structure that allows the correct transmission of the muscular force vectors of this region to the recto-anal structure.

The technique most often complements the complex surgery of the posterior compartment and is therefore not performed as a stand-alone surgical procedure (**Petros P. & Inoue H., 2013**).

An alternative way for performing this plasty using alloplastic material is the *tissue fixation system* (TFS), proposed by Peter Petros.

Surgical steps
1. A transverse incision of 5 cm is performed right next to the hymen.
2. The dissection of the vagina from the rectum is performed and the separate fragments of the perineal body are identified laterally. These are whitish. Due to the fact that deep perineal transverse muscles are inserted on it and on the ischiopubic ramus, the medial

pulling of the tendinous fragments must tension this muscle.

3. Using a curved needle with a multifilament resorbable suture, the two tendinous fragments are highlighted, each end being kept with a forceps. Using a Metzenbaum scissors, a small tunnel is created on each side, passing through the tendinous side and medial side of the deep perineal transverse muscle. The tip of the scissors should be oriented horizontally, any lower angulation risking injuring the pudendal nerve at the exit from the Alcock's canal (pudendal canal).

4. The TFS applicator is inserted through the canal thus formed and the anchor is fixed in the muscle fat, Fig 7.145. The maneuver is also repeated contralateral, being tensioned until a tension is recorded, at which point the applicator is extracted, the sling remaining fixed. By tensioning the sling, the two dislocated fragments of the perineal body will come into contact one with the other, Fig. 7.146.

The patient is mesh covered for 24 hours postoperatory, being discharged from hospital not later than 48 hours if no complications occur.

Thirty patients with third degree rectocele, low obstructive constipation symptoms, or who required compression maneuvers of the posterior vaginal wall to defecate, were operated by restoring the perineal body with TFS. Additionally, the recovery of uterosacral ligaments was also performed with TFS. At 12 months, the healing rate was 90% (27 patients).

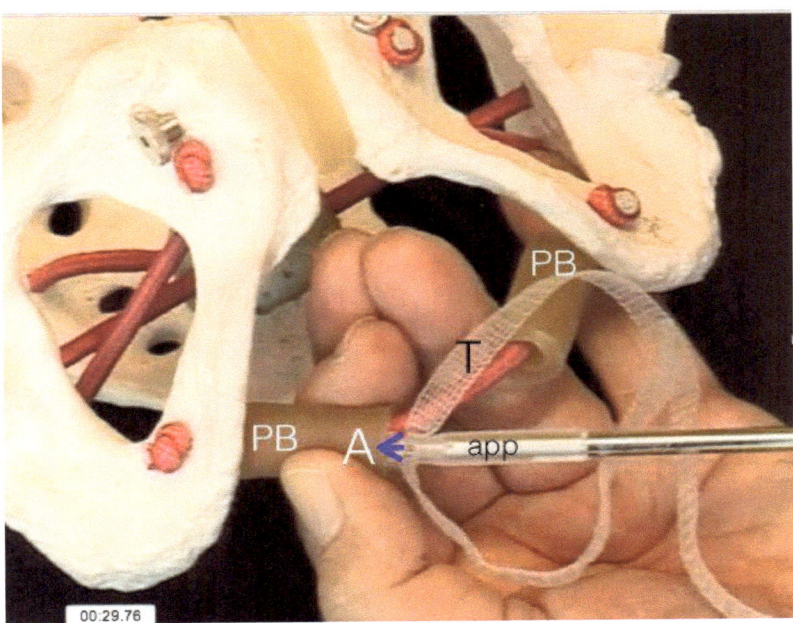

Fig. 7.145. Surgery of restoration of perineal body with TFS
(according to **Petros P., 2010**) PB – perineal body

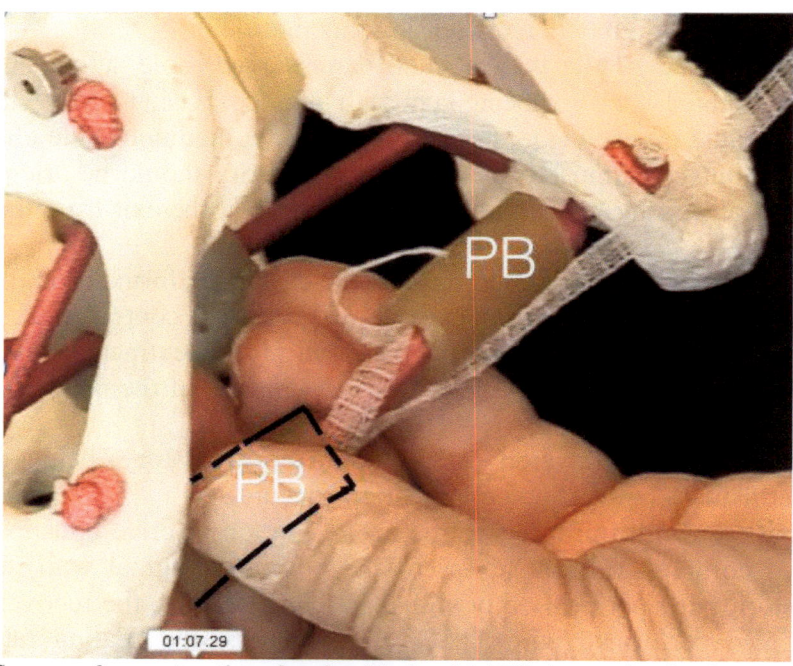

Fig. 7.146. Surgery of reconstruction of perineal body with TFS. Aspect simulated at the end of surgery
(according to **Petros P., 2010**) PB – perineal body

7.4.2.9. Uterosacral ligaments restoration

In order to restore the uterosacral ligaments, we proposed a new technique, *"VALASURE"*, which uses a combined approach, both vaginal and laparoscopic. The method is similar to the TFS technique, but is currently the only strictly anatomical correction solution by inserting two slings that are fixed at the level of sacral insertion of the uterosacral ligaments: S3-S4 sacral bone periosteum, Fig. 7.147.

The TFS system uses some anchors that are fixed in ligament and connective structures and not in the periosteum and thus do not have an adequate resistance. For the *"VALASURE"* technique, the topographic anatomy of the plexus sacralis and the presacral trajectory of the sympathetic nerve chain should be considered. The roots of the somatic nerves have a medial-to-lateral trajectory, and the slings are anchored to the lateral edge of the sacral bone, Fig. 7.148.

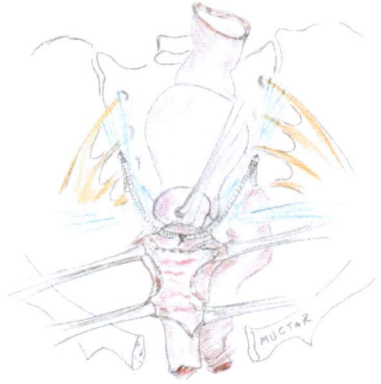

Fig. 7.147. Reconstruction of uterosacral ligaments
(drawing by **Muctar S.**)

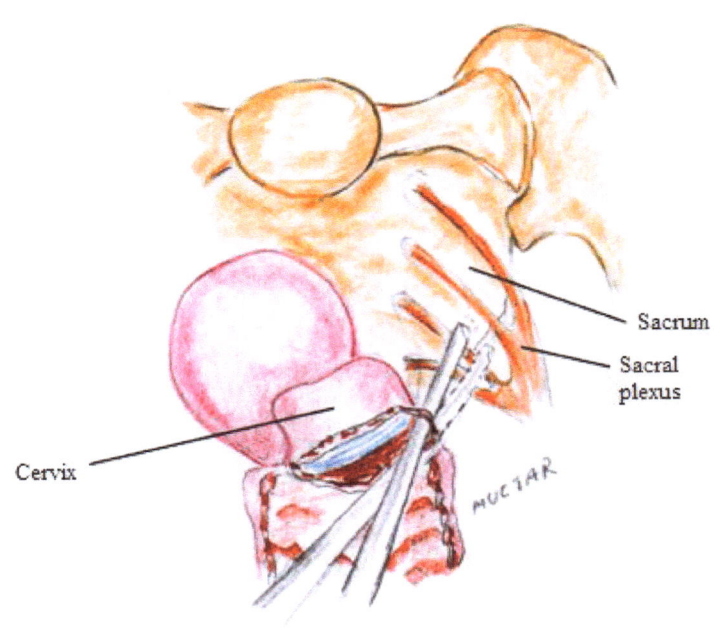

Fig. 7.148. Anchoring of the sling to the lateral edge of the sacral bone
(drawing by **Muctar S.**)

Surgical steps

1. The cervix is tensioned anterior and caudally with a Tierball forceps to highlight the posterior pouch of Douglas. After infiltration with physiological serum for hydrodissection, a transverse incision of approximately 2 cm below the cervix, at the level of the posterior vaginal wall, is performed, Fig. 7.149.

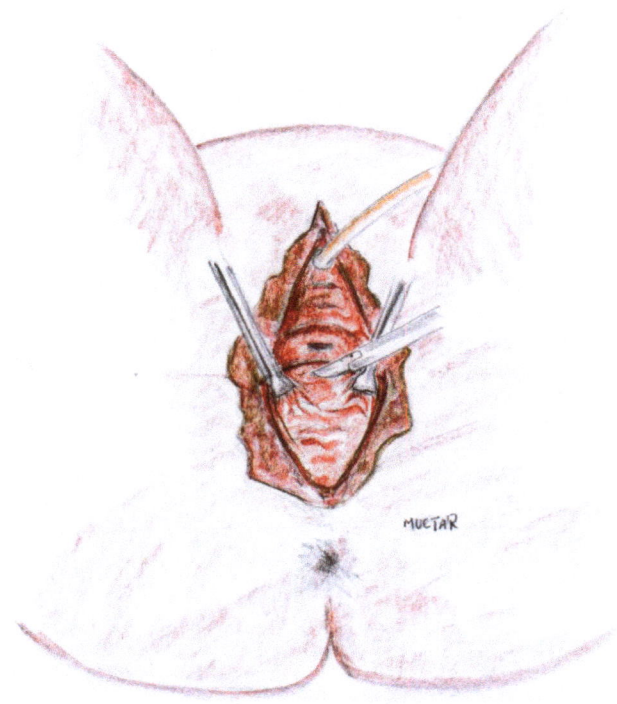

Fig. 7.149. Incision of posterior pouch of Douglas
(drawing by **Muctar S.**)

2. The distal part of the uterosacral ligaments is digitally dissected. Below the uterosacral ligaments, cardinal ligaments are inserted into the cervix, Fig. 7.150. The preparation of the ligaments is done laterally, in order not to accidentally pierce the pouch of Douglas. An atraumatic tunnel of approximately 3 cm length is created, Fig. 7.151.

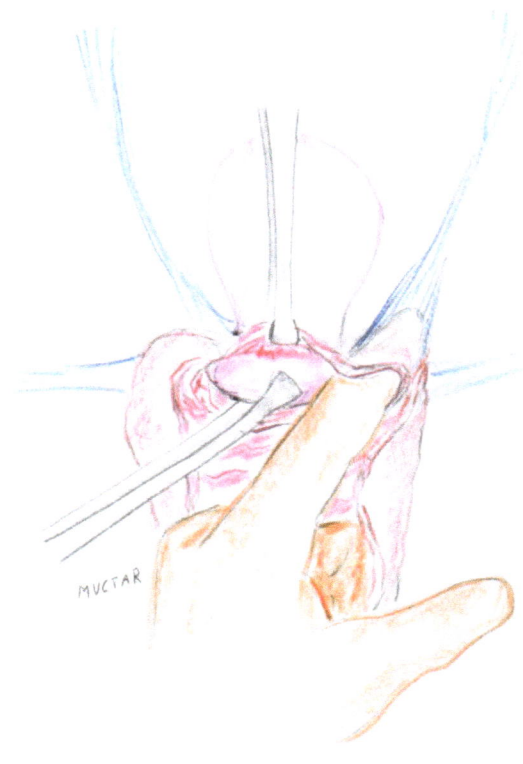

Fig. 7.150. Tactile detection of uterosacral ligaments
(drawing by **Muctar S.**)

3. The distal part of uterosacral ligaments is highlighted with a Kocher clamp and is tensioned caudally. This maneuver facilitates the blunt preparation of ligaments and the subsequent blind dissection along the ligaments, Fig. 7.152.

4. After tunneling, a non-resorbable suture is passed at the level of the cervix bilaterally, each of which will anchor the slings to the cervix, Fig. 7.153.

5. From this moment on, the laparoscopic approach is applied. The lower limbs of the patient are placed in extension and the surgical trocars are inserted. The aim of laparoscopy in this technique is to track the slings along the ligaments and to avoid the perforation of neighboring organs such as the uterus, sigmoid colon, etc., but also to exclude other comorbidities that induce a similar symptomatology, such as the pelvic congestion syndrome of endometriosis.

6. After the laparoscopic inspection of the abdomen, a 24-charrier cystoscope is inserted lateral to the uterosacral ligament. Its insertion through the medial side can lead to the perforation of the pouch of Douglas and gas losses that lead to the loss of pneumoperitoneum and impossibility of continuing the laparoscopy operation, Fig. 7.154.

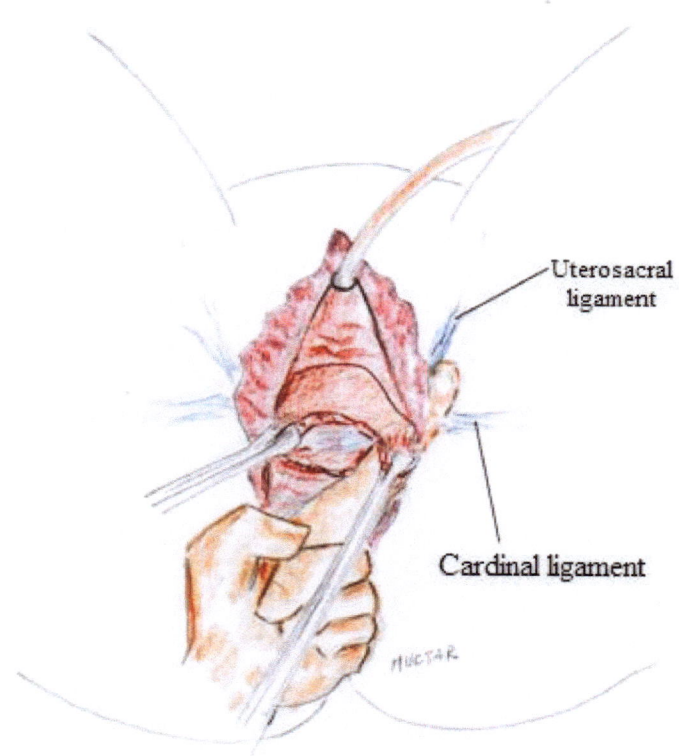

Fig. 7.151. Making a tunnel lateral to the uterosacral ligaments
(drawing by **Muctar S.**)

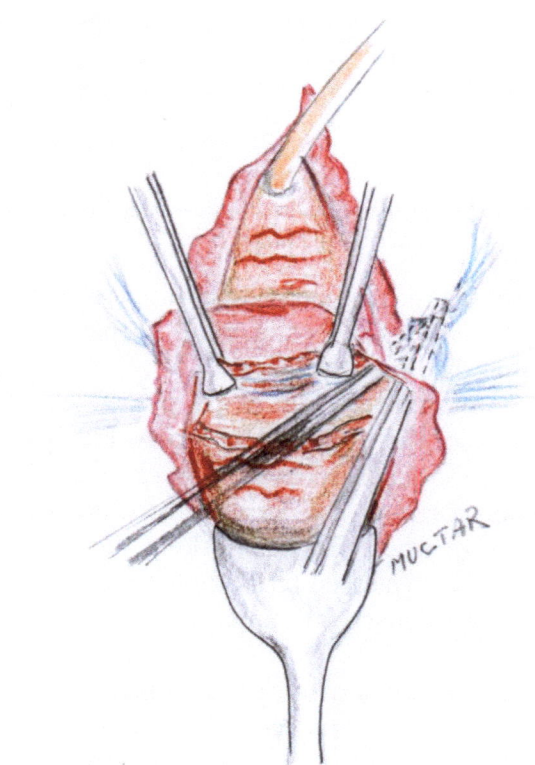

Fig. 7.152. Pulling the uterosacral ligament with a Kocher forceps
(drawing by **Muctar S.**)

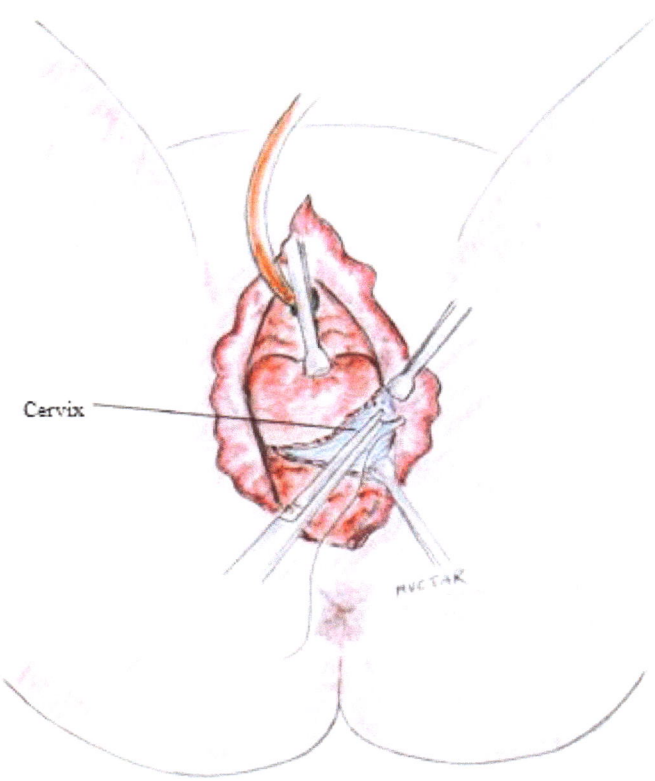

Fig. 7.153. Passing the non-resorbable sutures at the level of the cervix
(drawing by **Muctar S.**)

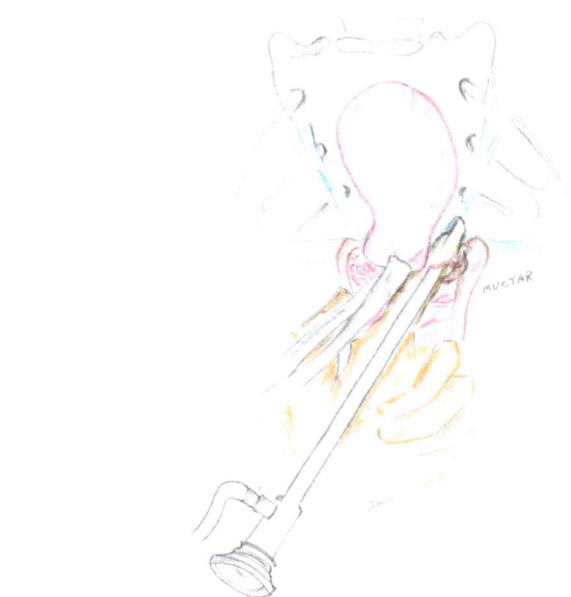

Fig. 7.154. Insertion of cystoscope lateral to the uterosacral ligaments
(drawing by **Muctar S.**)

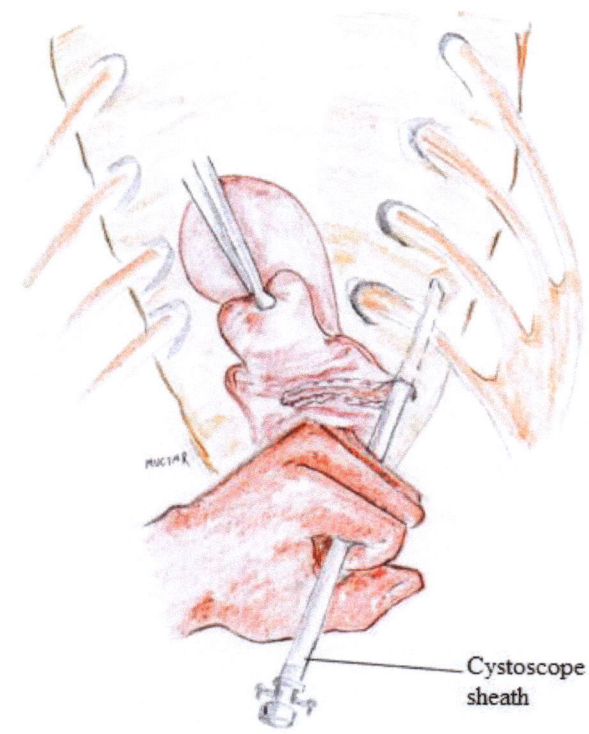

Fig. 7.155. Retraction of the optic device and preservation of the cystoscope sheath
(drawing by **Muctar S.**)

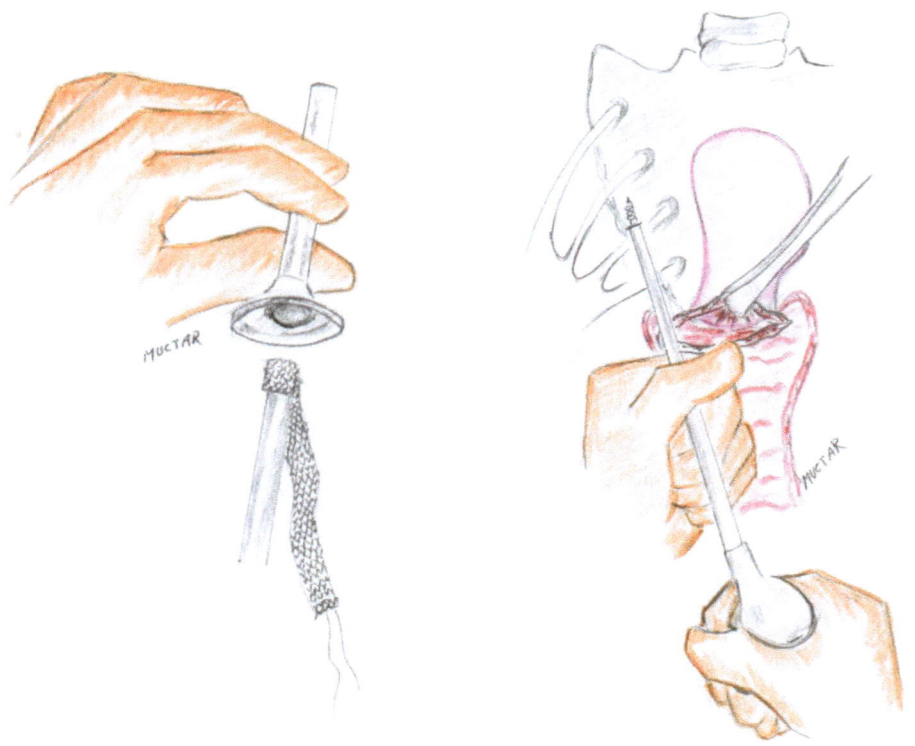

A)   B)

Fig. 7.156. Insertion of the sling through the cystoscopic tube and its fixation with clips
(drawing by **Muctar S.**)

246

7. The cystoscope sheath is positioned so that it is laparoscopically visible at the edge of the sacrum. It is possible to visualize the periosteum and the possible nerve branches. In order to avoid nerve damage, the cystoscope is rotated 90 degrees, thus the tip of the cystoscope comes in direct contact with the periosteum. Keeping the contact with the periosteum, the cystoscope is rotated counterclockwise and the telescope is retracted, thus leaving only the external sheath. The sling is inserted through the sheath and will be attached to the periosteum, thus excluding the nerve tract lesions, Fig. 7.155.

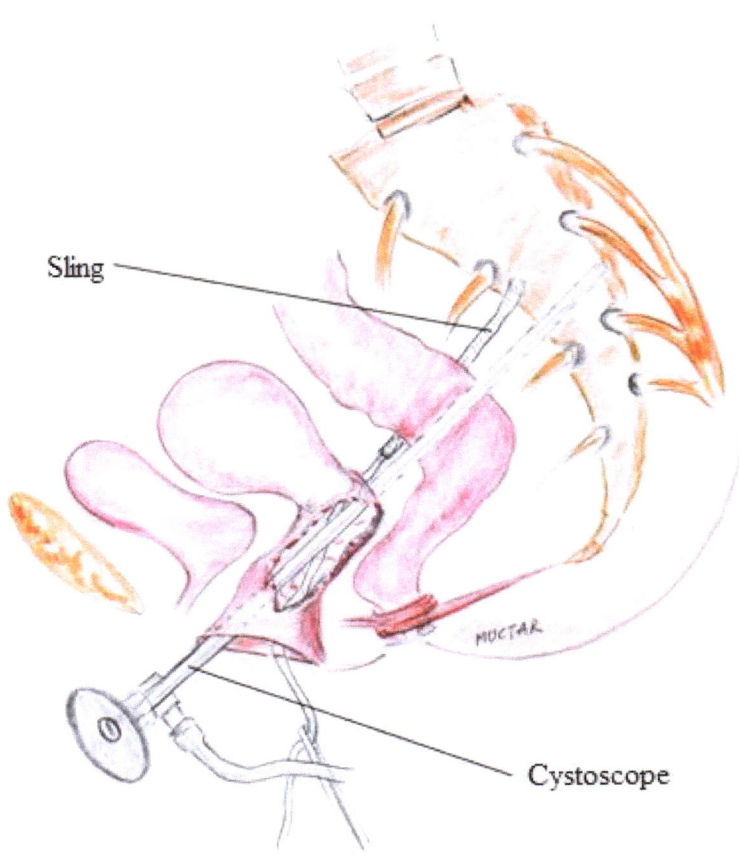

Fig. 7.157.A Anchoring of the sling bilaterally
(drawing by **Muctar S.**)

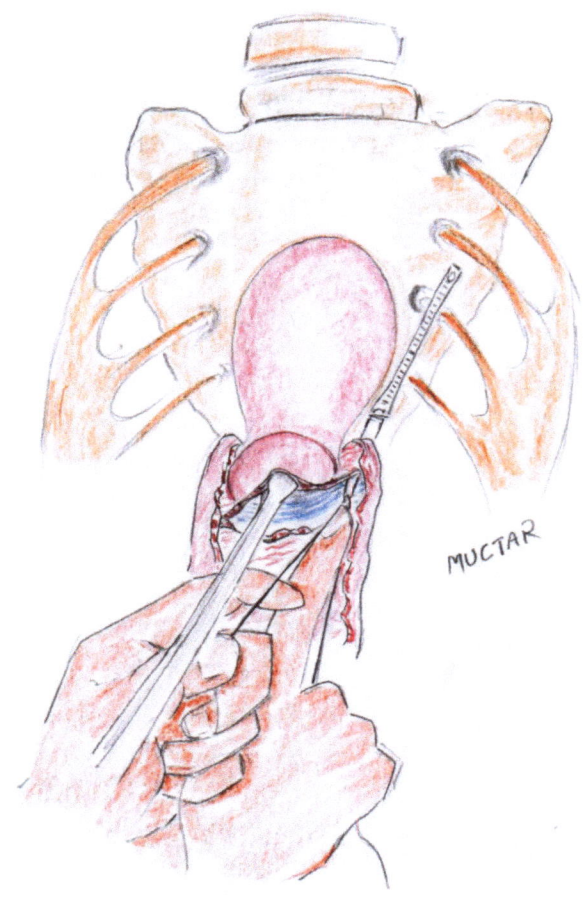

Fig. 7.157 B. Tying the sutures and reduction of prolapse
(drawing by **Muctar S.**)

8. The operator can make the polypropylene sling. It is 1 cm wide and has a "*pocket*" at its cranial end, where the instrument is fixed with clips.
Together with the sling, it is inserted through the cystoscope sheath and fixes the clips to the periosteum by triggering an insertion mechanism. Only one clip is often enough, Fig. 7.156.A and B. The technique is performed bilaterally, Fig. 7.157.A. The caudal end is anchored to the waiting sutures passed at the level of the cervix at moment 4. By tying and pulling the sutures, the uterus is pushed in the cranial direction with the consequent reduction of the prolapse, Fig. 7.157.B.

9. The suture of vaginal incision is done with separate resorbable sutures. It is recommended that a marginal mesh is left for 2 days.

The postoperative evolution is favorable, no significant pains associated to the procedure being described up until this moment, Fig. 7.158.

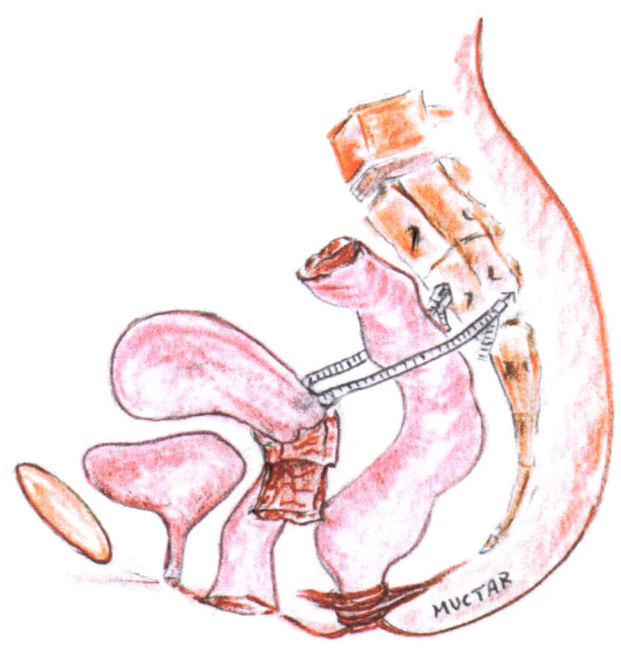

Fig. 7.158. Final aspect after the reconstruction with a sling
(drawing by **Muctar S.**)

7.5 Laparoscopic surgery in pelvic floor disorders

Although it is not a disease that may endanger the lives of the patients, pelvic prolapse induced by pelvic floor disorders is one of the most common disorders among women over 50 years old and leads to a significant decrease in their quality of life (**Hoshino K.,** *et al., 2016*). In addition, Women's Health Organization reported that the incidence of cystocele is of 34% in women between 50 and 79 years old, the one of rectocele can reach 19%, while the incidence of uterine prolapse is around 14% (**Hendrix S.L.,** *et al., 2002*).

Moreover, studies conducted by Olsen (**Olsen A.L.,** *et al., 1997*) and Wu (**Wu J.M.,** *et al., 2014*) estimated that the incidence of incontinence and pelvic floor prolapse can reach 11% and 20% respectively, at 80 years old. Also, with the global increase in life expectancy, it is estimated that the prevalence of pelvic floor disorders will increase significantly (**Gadonneix P.,** *et al., 2004*). Regarding the need for surgical treatment of these conditions, it is estimated that 58% of these surgeries are practiced in women under 60 years old, with 29.2% of them developing at some time the recurrence of prolapse, which will require another surgery (**Gadonneix P.,** *et al., 2004*).

7.5.1 Laparoscopic treatment of uterine and vaginal vault prolapse - sacrocolpopexy

In the case of uterine prolapse and vaginal vault prolapse, the surgical approach can be vaginal or abdominal; the abdominal approaches can be practiced as open surgery or laparoscopic surgery. The main surgical interventions that can be used in the treatment of uterine prolapse and vaginal vault prolapse include the sacrospinous fixation, iliococcygeus fixation, uterosacral suspension or colpocleisis, via a vaginal approach and sacrocolpopexy or hysteropexy, via an abdominal approach (classical or laparoscopic).

Laparoscopic sacrocolpopexy

Laparoscopic sacrocolpopexy is one of the most effective methods that address both uterine and vaginal vault prolapse, as well as pelvic multi-compartment defects (**Brown J.S., et al., 2002**). The success rate of this procedure is 74-98%, the recurrence rate being significantly lower compared to the other procedures, while the long-term adverse effects rate is significantly reduced compared to the sacrospinous fixation (**Maher C.M., et al., 2012**). The purpose of surgery is to fix the vaginal vault to the anterior longitudinal ligament from the anterior side of the promontory with polypropylene textile prosthesis (**O Sullivan O.O. & Reilly B., 2016**).

To achieve laparoscopic sacrocolpopexy, the patient will be placed in a Trendenlenburg position (30° C), with both upper and lower limbs in abduction position. Preparation will continue by mounting a Foley catheter.

After the induction of pneumoperitoneum, with a Veress needle inserted at the level of left side, the optic port will be placed at the umbilical level, while the 5 mm trocars will be placed paraumbilical bilaterally and, respectively, a 12 mm trocar in the right iliac fossa or suprapubic. Then, the uterine manipulator will be inserted under visual control.

The exposure of the pelvic working area will be ensured by the cranial mobilization of the *intestinal loops*, a systematic maneuver, starting with the greater omentum that will be positioned subfrenically on the left, the transverse colon, the jejunal loops, and then the ileal ones. The orientation of the operating table in *Trendelenburg position* favors, by gravitational force, the cranial movement, and the maintenance of the small intestine outside the pelvic excavation. Also, surgical access to pelvic structures may be facilitated by the *suspension of the sigmoid colon* with a suture passed through the mesocolon or omentum tassel and fixed transabdominal and externalized in the left side.

Mounting the uterine manipulator will help in the mobilization, exposure and anterior dissection, respectively posterior dissection of the vaginal walls.

Anteriorly, the dissection starts by sectioning the vesical-uterine peritoneal plication with an electrode hook, and, in case of uterine prolapse, the limited bladder dissection, while, in the case of vaginal vault prolapse, the mobilization of the anterior vaginal wall is also necessary. The main intraoperatory incident that can occur at this moment is bladder damage.

The dissection continues *posteriorly* by accessing the *rectovaginal space*. At this point of surgery, dissection can be facilitated by mounting a *rectal manipulator* to better expose the inter-rectovaginal space better. The dissection of the posterior space starts by sectioning the peritoneal reflexion at the level of the pouch of Douglas, which is afterwards continued with the dissection of the posterior vaginal wall on the anterior side of the rectum. Thus, the dissection continues downwards up to the level of levator ani muscles, while at the upper level, the peritoneum sectioning continues at the presacral level up to the identification of anterior longitudinal ligament. During this surgery time, the main intraoperative incidents may be the lesion of the rectum, the hypogastric plexus, and the presacral vessels that can induce hemorrhages that are hard to control. In terms of vaginal walls damage, this incident can occur at any moment of electrical or sharp dissection, and may predispose to late complications that include vaginal prosthesis erosion that will be placed at the moment of the reconstruction phase.

The *reconstructive* phase begins with the insertion of the T-shaped polypropylene prosthesis, which will be fixed posteriorly at the level of levator ani muscles and respectively at the level of posterior vaginal wall, and anteriorly, at the level of the anterior vaginal wall, adjacent to the internal urethral meatus. The cranial extremity of the prosthesis will be fixed, at relative tension to the anterior longitudinal ligament of the promontory, using titanium metal clips (Protack, Medtronic), or preferably sutures, passed by a crimped needle, of non-resorbable material, polypropylene monofilament 1. In this maneuver, increased attention should be paid to the risk of damage to the hypogastric nerve plexus or iliac vessels.

The last surgical moment consists of covering the polypropylene prosthesis by closing the posterior peritoneal loop originally created. In this regard, we recommend the use of a resorbable monofilament suture (PDO 2.0) or a self-locking suture (V-Lock, Medtronic or Stratafix PDS, Ethicon).

Verification of the suspension by vaginal examination, careful control of hemostasis, placement of the pouch of Douglas drainage and exudation of pneumoperitoneum end the surgical intervention.

Laparoscopic hysteropexy

Transvaginal hysterectomy has long been the treatment of choice in patients diagnosed with uterine prolapse, but this procedure has been questioned in recent decades because it does not treat the cause that led to the prolapse, and because it involves the ablation of a healthy organ (**Price N. & Jackson S., 2016**). As a result, various other techniques have been imagined, based on suspension uterine ligaments plication or the placement of textile prostheses that lead to uterine suspension, known as *hysteropexy*. These procedures can be performed both as open surgery and laparoscopic surgery and include *sacrospinous hysteropexy, hysteropexy by uterosacral ligaments plication, sacral hysteropexy, Manchester procedure and, more recently, Oxford procedure*.

Manchester procedure was first described in 1888 and consists of cervical amputation transvaginally, colporrhaphy, and fixation of the cervical blunt to the uterine cardinal ligaments. The procedure is for patients with cervical elongation and intact cardinal ligaments (**Krause H.G., et al., 2006**).

The purpose of *laparoscopic hysteropexy by Oxford procedure* is to restore the normal position of the uterus in the pelvic cavity, strengthen its suspension, restore the normal length and anatomy of the vagina, and treat the possible concurrent prolapses – cystocele and rectocele, provided that their degree is low (**Price N. & Jackson S., 2016**). The intervention consists in placing a polypropylene prosthesis that has an anterior bifurcation around the cervix and its fixation to the promontorium.

The patient will be placed in Trendelenburg position, with her hips in adduction; then a Foley catheter will be mounted. The optical trocar will be inserted at the umbilical level while the working trocars will be inserted on the sides, a trocar of 5 mm on each side and a 12 mm trocar suprapubian. Subsequently, under visual control, the uterine manipulator will be mounted.

Exposure of the working area by mobilization of the intestinal mass and parietal suspension of sigmoid colon will be performed as in the case of laparoscopic approach of uterine prolapse.

The dissection begins at the level of the paucivascular area of large ligaments, near the cervico-isthmic junction and continues anteriorly by sectioning the peritoneum of vesical-uterine plication. Subsequently, the dissection of pelvic parietal peritoneum is continued at posterior level, from the pouch of Douglas to the promontorium, with its exposure, Fig. 7.159., 7.160. and 7.161. The two bifurcations of the polypropylene textile prosthesis are inserted through the two braches created at the level of large ligaments and are fixed anterior to the cervix with non-resorbable sutures. The prosthesis thus positioned is oriented and then fixed with titanium sutures or clips to the anterior longitudinal ligament of the sacral promontorium so that to create a lifting of the uterus.

In other variants of this technique, the dissection of the pouch of Douglas is continued until the identification of uterosacral ligaments that can be used as caudal fixation points of the prosthesis, Fig. 7.162. and 7.163.

Subsequently, the peritoneum is sutured over the entire dissection surface with slowly resorbable sutures (PDO, 2.0), thus ensuring that the prosthesis is fully covered. This way, the procedure ensures the correction of the pelvic anatomy by using the cervix and the anterior longitudinal ligament as fixation points for the polypropylene prosthesis (**Rahmanou P.,** *et al.,* **2014**), Fig. 7.152.*a,* and 7.152.*b,* Fig. 7. 7.153.

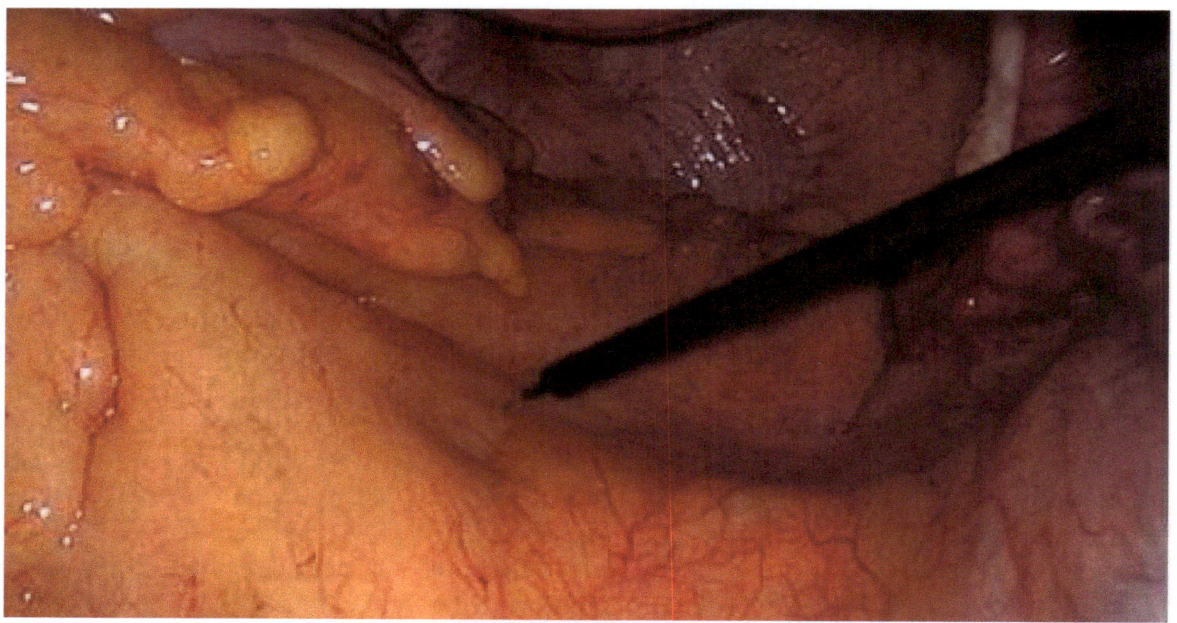

Fig. 7.159. Identification of promontorium

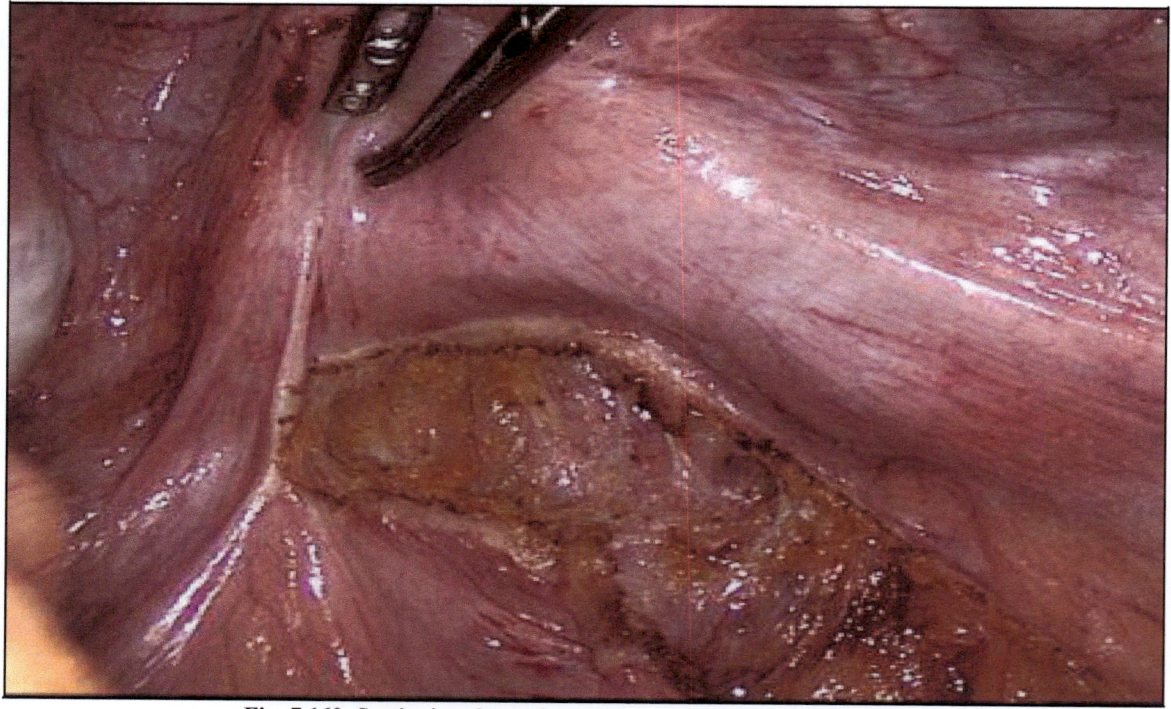

Fig. 7.160. Sectioning the peritoneum at the pouch of Douglas level

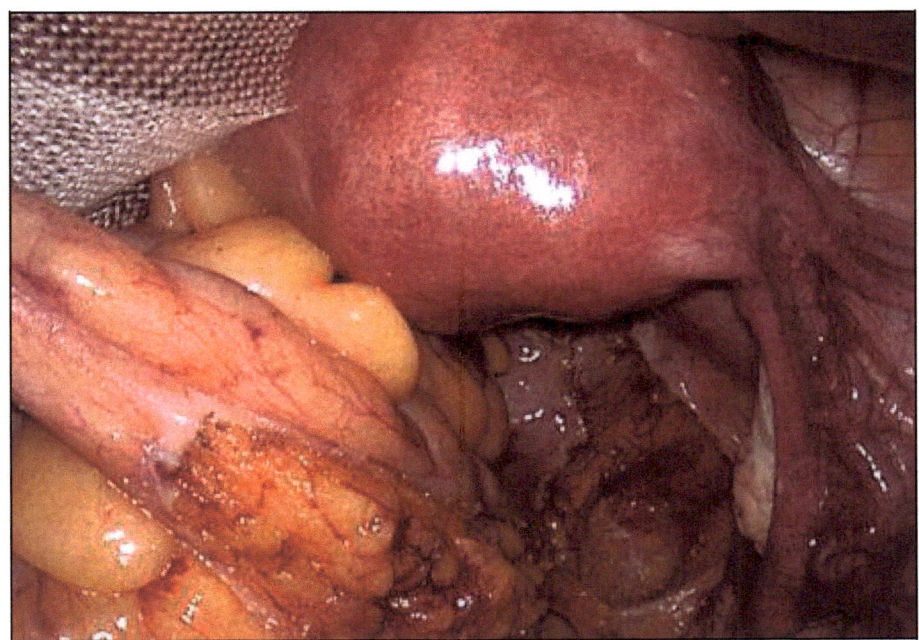
Fig. 7.161. Final aspect of peritoneal breach in which the polypropylene textile prosthesis will be inserted

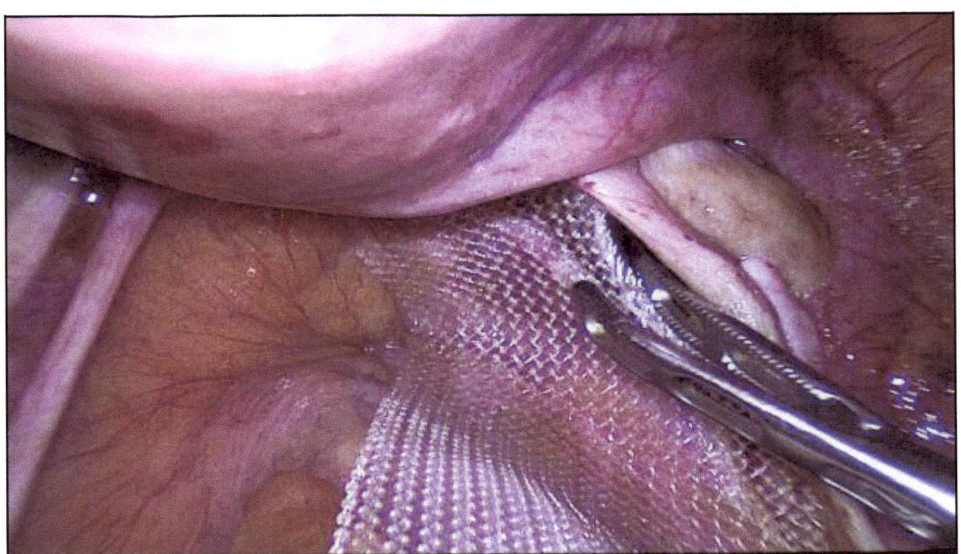
Fig. 7.162. Placing the textile prosthesis in the inter-recto-uterine lifting area

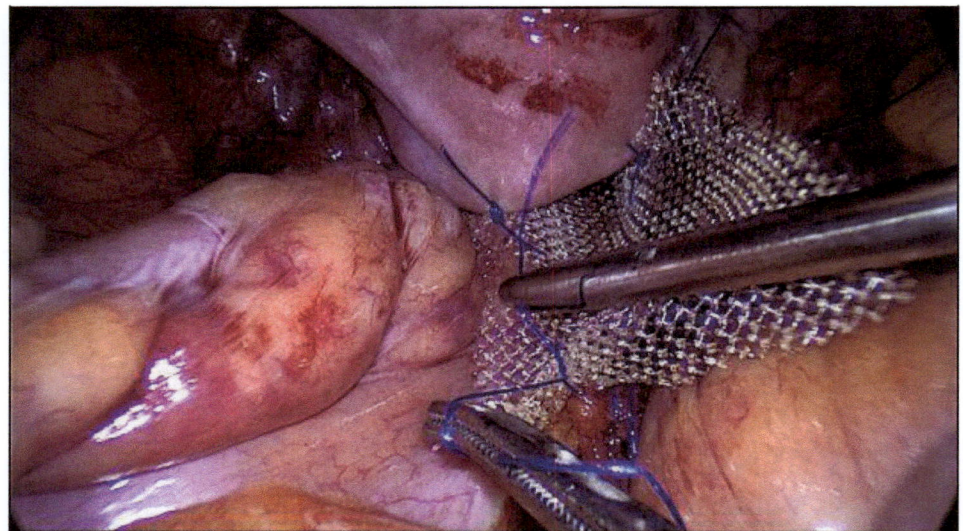

Fig. 7.163. Fixing the prosthesis at the level of uterosacral ligaments, subsequently at the level of anterior longitudinal level

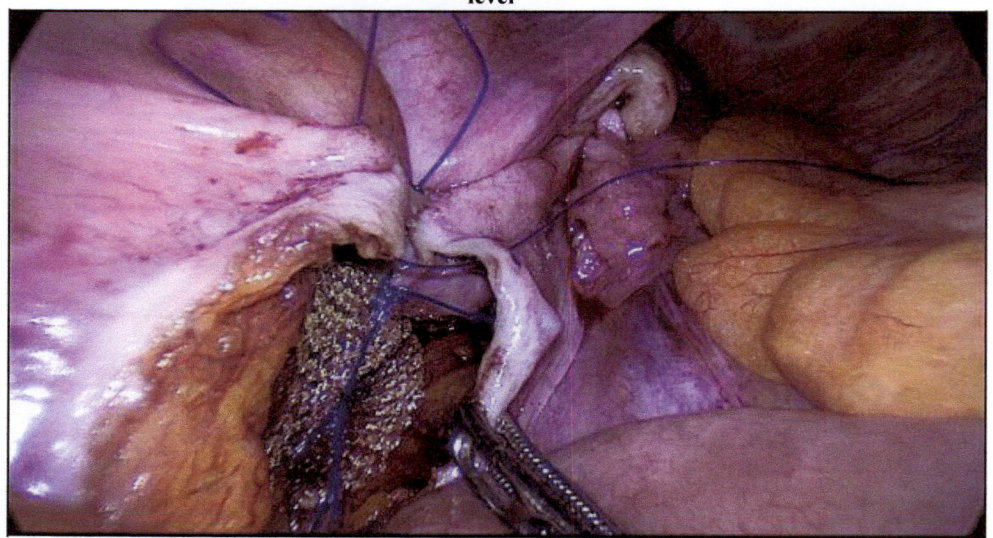

Fig. 7.164.*a* Closing the breach of pelvic peritoneum while covering the textile prosthesis

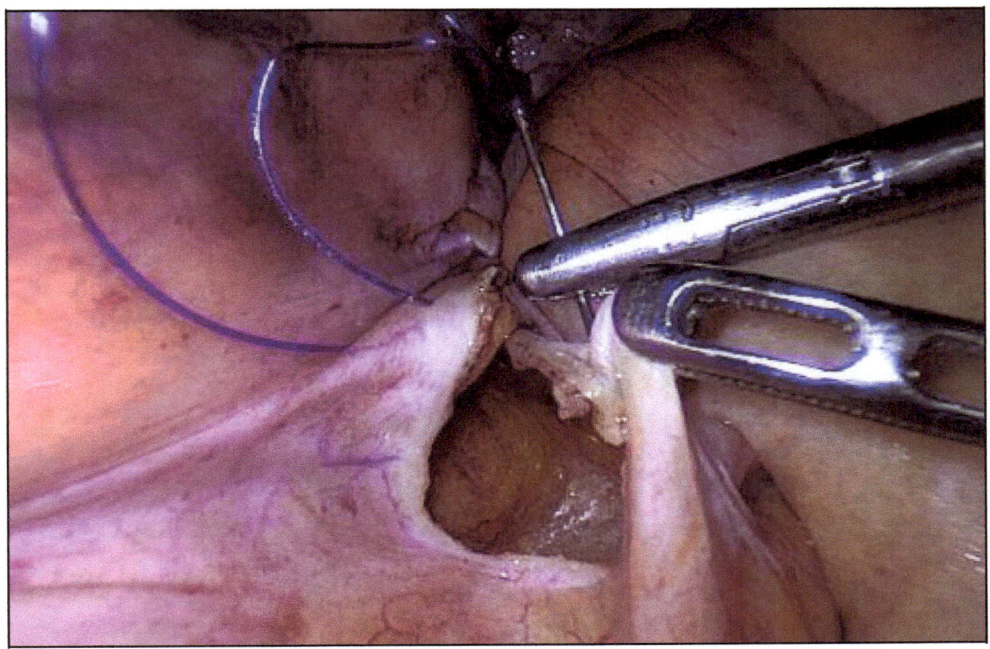
Fig. 7.164.*b*. Closing the breach of pelvic peritoneum while covering the textile prosthesis

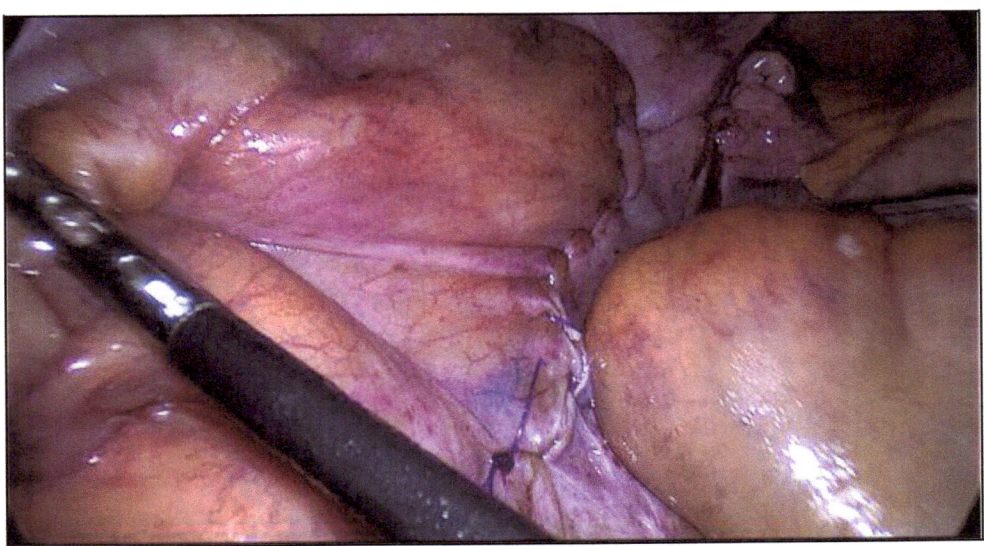
Fig. 7.165. Final aspect of hysteropexy – initial peritoneal breach is sutured on its entire length, thus isolating completely the pelvic prosthesis

7.5.2. Laparoscopic rectopexy

Rectopexy aims at eliminating rectal prolapse and correcting the continence and defecation disorders that are most common in patients who are diagnosed with rectocele and can be performed both abdominally and perineal (**Kellokumpu I.H.**, *et al.*, **2000**; **Bruch H.P.**, *et al.*, **1999**).

Abdominal rectopexy is considered the first-line treatment for complete rectal prolapse, together with an up to 75% improvement of fecal continence, while the recurrence rate is between 0 and 12%. Abdominal rectopexy, which has long been practiced by open surgery, has been replaced more and more frequently in the last few decades by laparoscopic surgery (**Nunoo-Mensah J.W.**, *et al.*, **2007**).

Laparoscopic rectopexy retains all the benefits of the classical procedure, but has the benefit of avoiding a median laparotomy that may predispose to a more difficult recovery, especially in elderly patients (**Kwok S.P.**, *et al.*, **1994**). Once the rectum is fully mobilized, it will be suspended with a polypropylene prosthesis interlocked to the rectal wall and fixed at the sacral level with titanium clips (Protack) (**Duthie G.S. & Bartolo D.C., 1992; Berman I.R., 1992**) or with non-resorbable sutures.

Laparoscopic rectopexy is initiated by induction of pneumoperitoneum by a Veress needle or by Hasson technique, followed by placing the optical trocar at the umbilical level. The working trocars, two of 5 mm and the third of 12 mm, are placed on the two sides, respectively suprapubian. Once the working trocars are mounted, the uterine manipulator will be inserted under visual control.

The exposure of the pelvic field will be ensured by the *cranial mobilization of intestinal loops*, a systematic maneuver, starting with the greater omentum that will be positioned subfrenically left, the transverse colon, the jejunal loops, and then the ileal loops. The orientation of the operating table in *Trendelenburg position* favors, by gravitational force, the cranial movement, and the maintenance of the small intestine outside the pelvic excavation. Also, surgical access to pelvic structures can be facilitated by the *suspension of sigmoid colon* by a suture through the mesocolon or an epiploic tassel and fixed transabdominal and externalized to the left side.

The dissection begins with the mobilization of the sigmoid colon from the lateral to the medial side by sectioning the peritoneum at this level, Fig. 7.166. and 7.167., followed by the identification of the left ureter and the left iliac vessels. The sectioning of the peritoneum will be extended distally from the promontorium to the left prerenal level. This dissection will then allow the identification of the avascular area and the proper mobilization of the mesorectum, Fig. 7.168. The dissection will then continue medially, to the right of the rectosigmoid junction, with the peritoneum sectioning at this level. Opening the retroperitoneal space will lead to the identification of the right uterus. The dissection at this level will continue in the posterior side until it joins with the dissection area that was made on the left side. Subsequently, the intervention continues by sectioning the peritoneal layer from the pouch of Douglas, between the rectum and the vagina, progressing up to the level of the anal canal. At this point, dissection maneuvers could cause injuries to the posterior wall of the vagina and the anterior rectal wall respectively. In this sense, the anterosuperior mobilization of the uterus by the uterus manipulator will facilitate the identification of anatomical features and the reduction of the risk of mechanical or electrical lesions of the rectum or vagina, Fig. 7.169. and Fig 7.170.*a,b*.

Once the rectum is fully mobilized and physiologically restored, it will be fixed directly by non-resorbable sutures, *tackers*, that will regard the pararectal tissues and the presacral area, (**Nunoo-Mensah J.W., et al., 2007**) or by polypropylene prostheses, Fig. 7.171. (**Kaiwa Y., et al., 2004**). If the choice is made to place a polypropylene textile prosthesis, a technique that we recommend, it will be fixed to the posterior side of the rectum with non-resorbable sutures and by *tackers* or polypropylene sutures to the promontorium and the presacral fascia, Fig. 7.172. and Fig. 7.173. The half or third of the rectum will remain free by using this technique (**Kaiwa Y., et al., 2004**). At the end of the intervention, the peritoneal breach will be closed with a non-resorbable suture, thus preventing contact of the prosthesis with the pelvic viscera, Fig. 7.174. and Fig. 7.175.

If the rectocele has a considerable size and after its full intraabdominal mobilization, a significant excess of the left colon results, it will be decided to resect the redundant sigmoid loop (**Kaiwa Y., et al., 2004**). We recommend that, if sigmoid resection is required, to be performed laparoscopically at a later stage after a detailed functional evaluation and after certification of correct prosthetic material integration.

The last surgical time is to cover the polypropylene prosthesis by closing the peritoneal breach created initially. In this regard, we recommend the use of an resorbable monofilament suture (PDO 2.0) or a self-locking suture (V-Lock, Medtronic or Stratafix

PDS, Ethicon).

Careful check of hemostasis, placement of a proximal drainage and exudation of pneumoperitoneum end the laparoscopic rectopexy surgery.

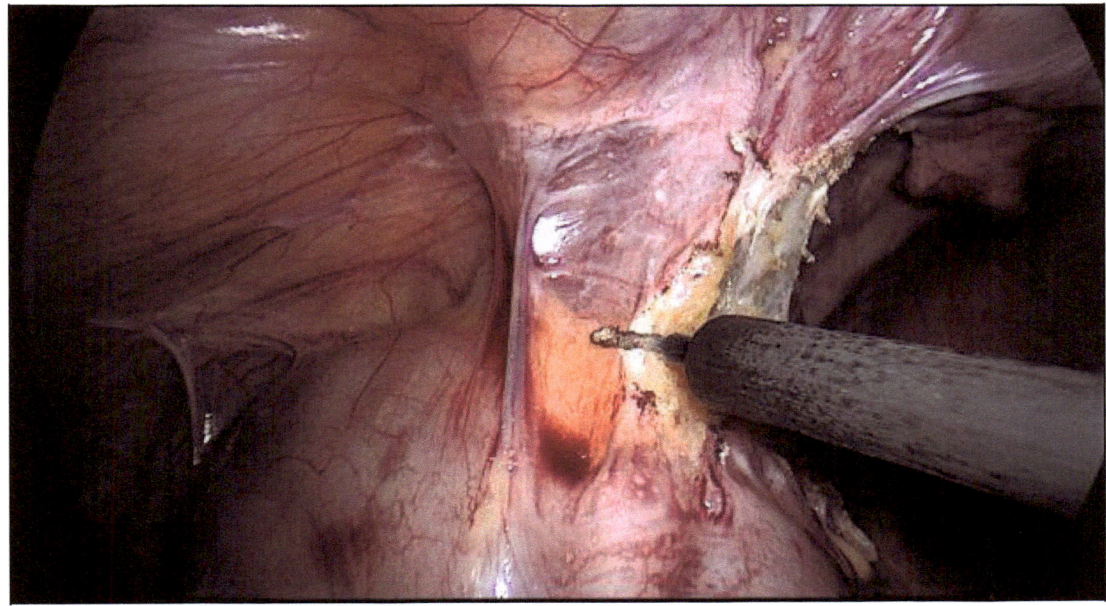

Fig. 7.166. Dissection of sigmoid loop – sectioning of parietal pelvic peritoneum

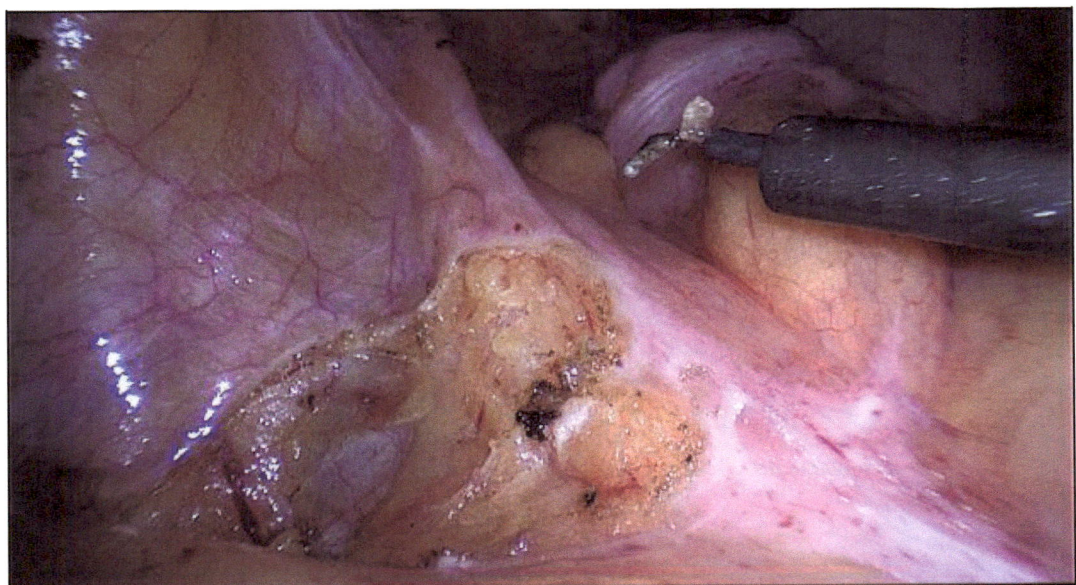

Fig. 7.167. Dissection of sigmoid loop - sectioning the parietal pelvic peritoneum progressing towards the pelvis

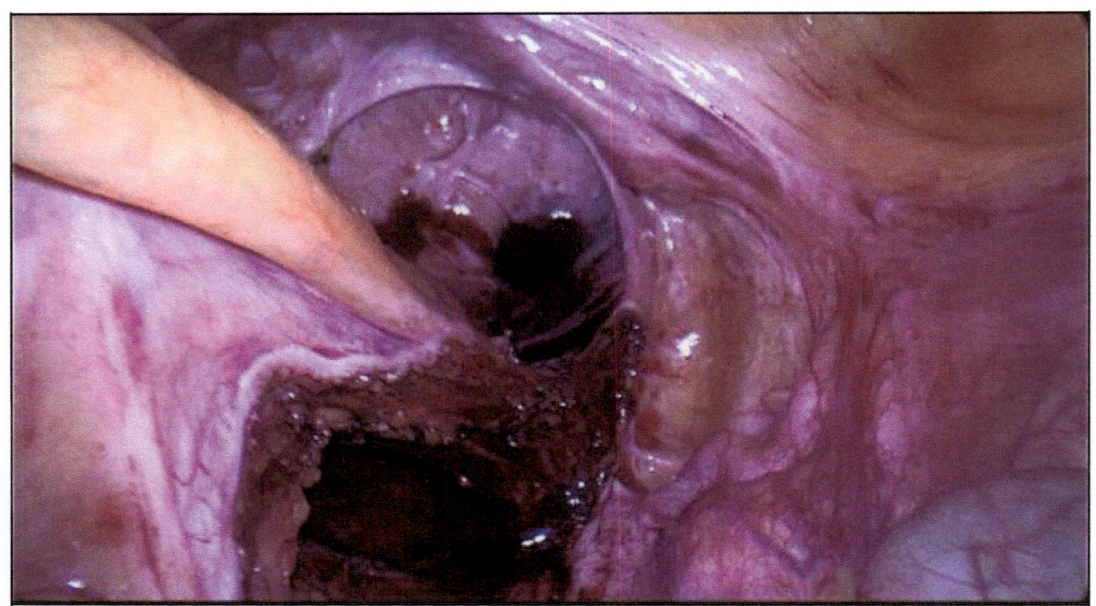
Fig. 7.168. Rectum dissection – mobilized en bloc with the mesorectum in the avascular area

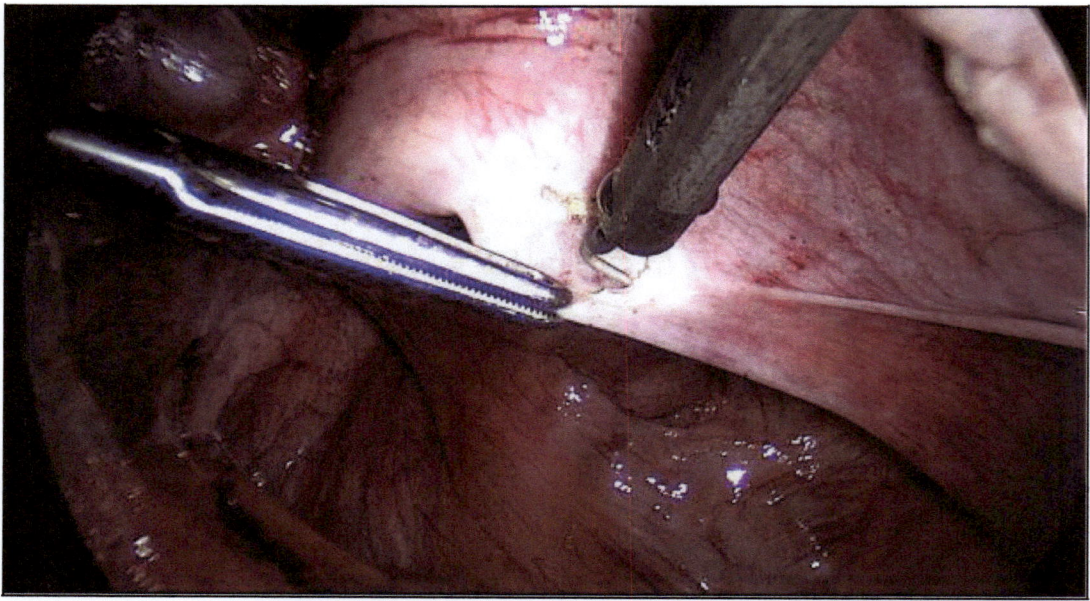
Fig. 7.169. Inter-recto-vaginal sectioning of the peritoneum with rectal prolapse in a hysterectomised patient

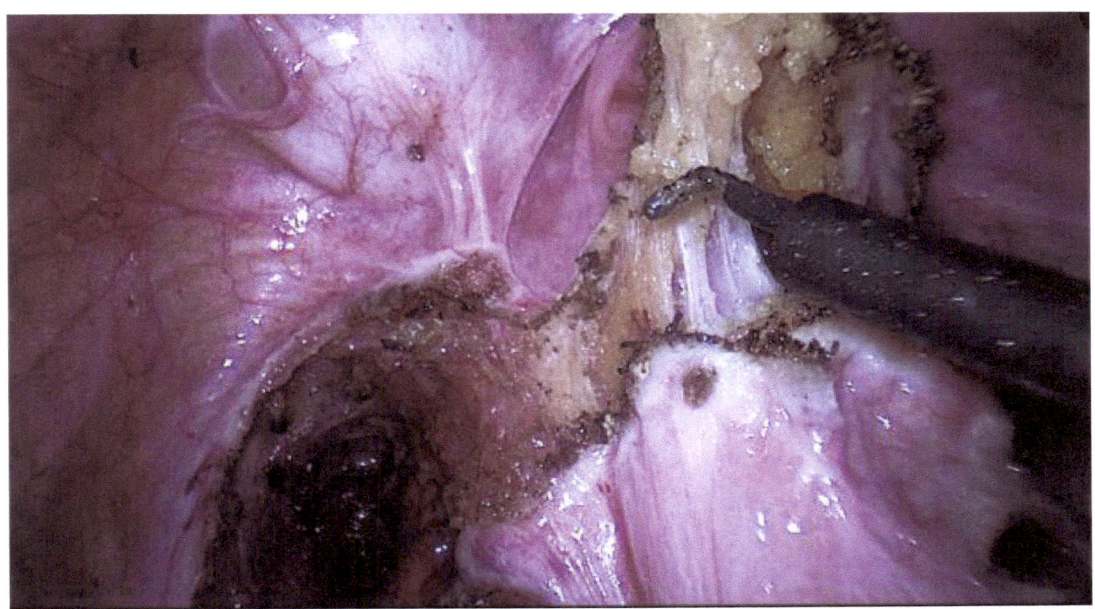
Fig. 7.170.*a* Inter-recto-vaginal dissection with rectal prolapse in a hysterectomised patient

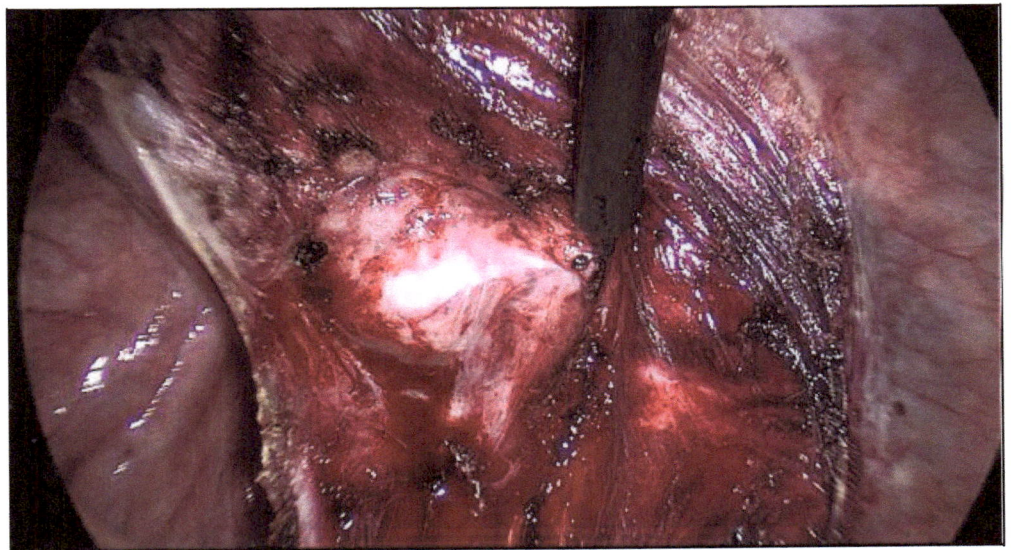
Fig. 7.170.*b* Inter-recto-vaginal dissection with rectal prolapse in a hysterectomised patient

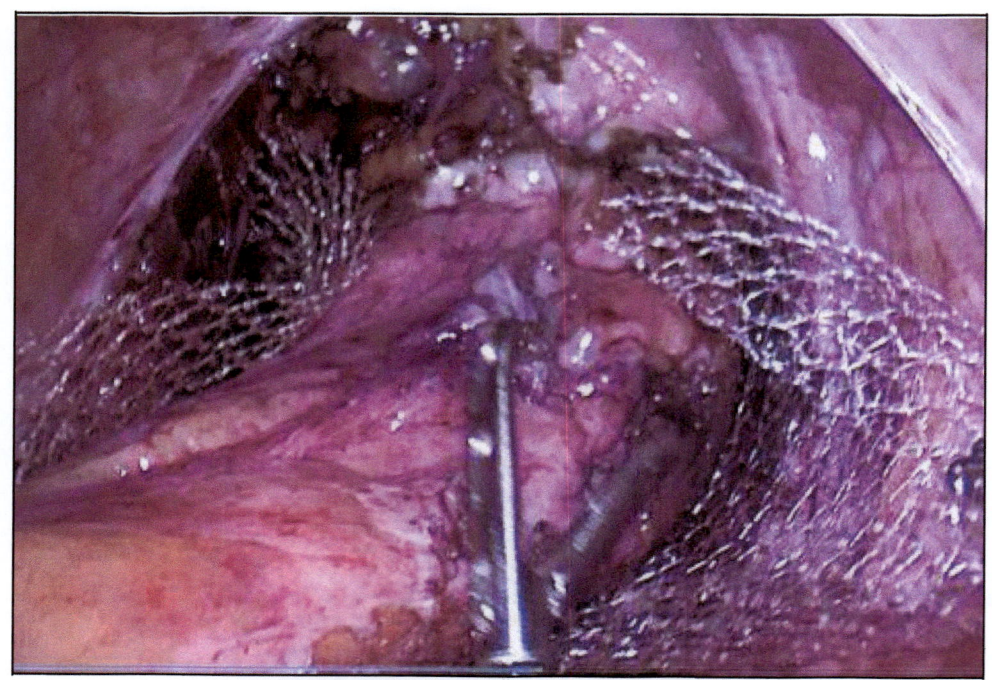
Fig. 7.171. Placing the textile prosthesis posterior to the rectum

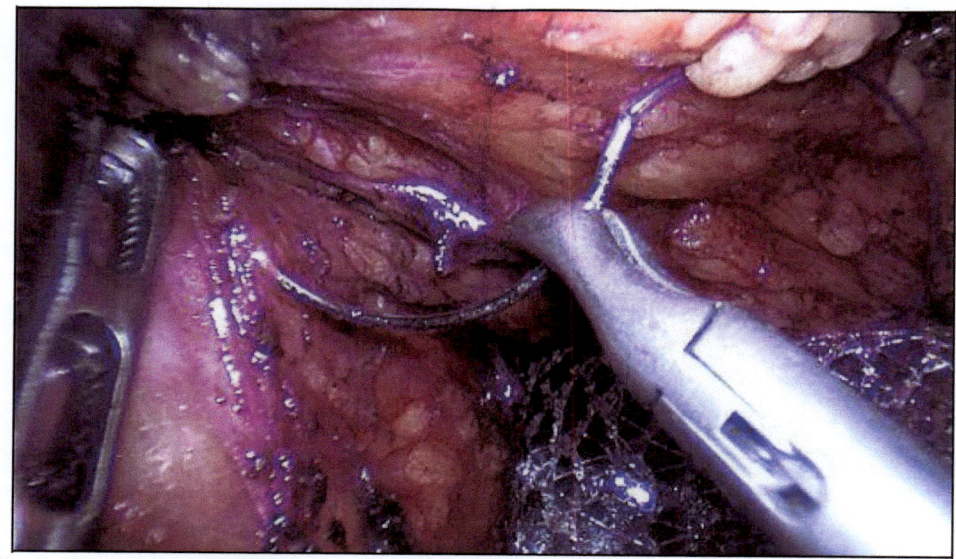
Fig. 7.172. Fixing the textile prosthesis on the posterior side of the rectum, at the mesorectum level

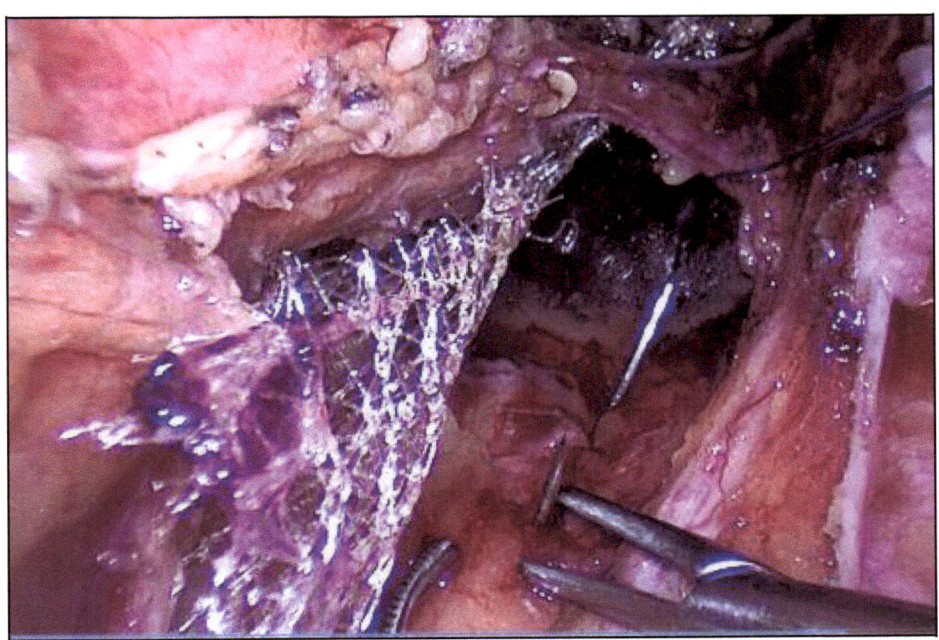
Fig. 7.173. Fixing the textile prosthesis at the promontorium level

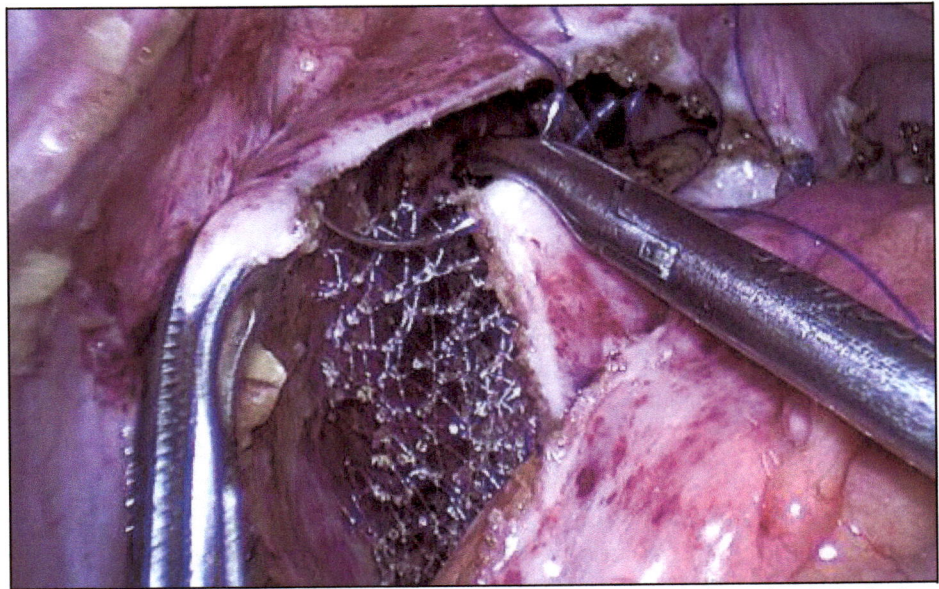
Fig. 7.174. Closing the peritoneal breach to isolate the textile prosthesis from the abdominal cavity

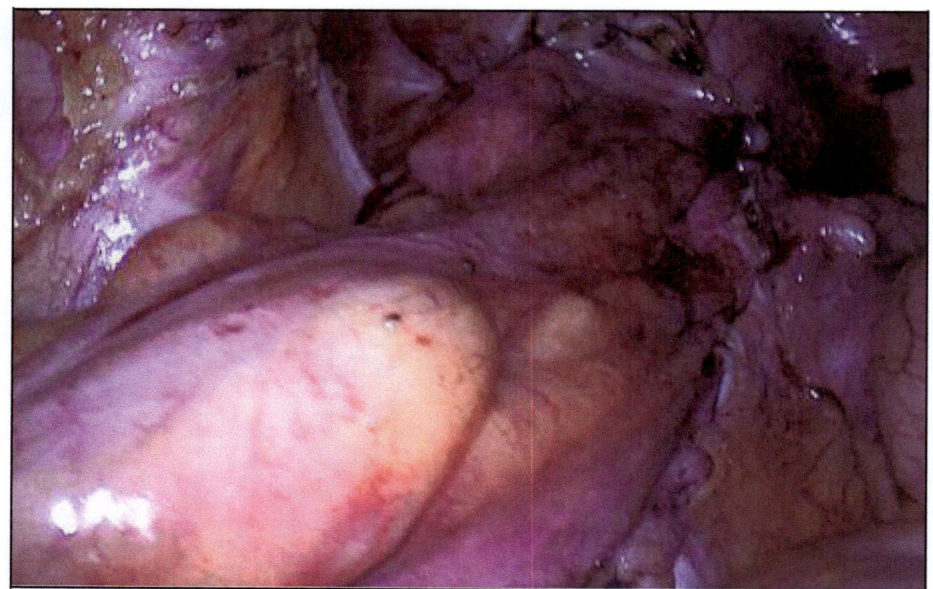
Fig. 7.175. Final aspect after closing the peritoneal breaches and full covering of the prosthesis

7.5.3. Laparoscopic Burch surgery

With the introduction of Kelly Plication as a surgical procedure for the treatment of urinary incontinence, over 100 surgical techniques that address this pathology have been reported, the choice of surgical procedure to be practiced being significantly influenced by the surgical and gynecological medical history of the patient (**Kelly H.A., 1913**; **Park G.S. & Miller E.J. Jr., 1988**). However, over the past decades, *Burch surgery* has become the *gold standard* in the treatment of stress urinary incontinence. Initially, the procedure was conducted by open surgery, being associated with the need for prolonged antialgic administration, with a longer hospital stay and, at the same time, with a more difficult recovery of the patient, which is why some surgeons abandoned it in favor of vaginal approach procedures (**Ross J.W., 1995**). However, with the development of laparoscopic surgery, Burch surgery has become increasingly used, making it the most recommended method in the treatment of urinary incontinence treatment (**Liu C.Y. & Paek W., 1993**). Regardless of the approach, Burch surgery consists of suspending the pouch of Douglas, paracolpos, and automatically the paravesical tissue to Cooper ligament, thus achieving *colposuspension* (**Burch J.C., 1961**).

The intervention can be done both transperitoneal and extraperitoneal, with a success rate of over 80% (**Saidi M.H.**, *et al.*, **1998**), although the technique originally described by Burch was preperitoneal, there are currently no studies to conform the superiority of one of the two approaches, transperitoneal, or preperitoneal (**Burch J.C., 1961**). As for the suspension modalities, different methods have been proposed, from colposuspension with sutures to tackers, clips, textile materials or even fibrin based products (**Ou & Rowbotham R., 1999; Lyons T.L., 1994; Hannah S.L. & Chin A., 1996; Kiilholma P.**, *et al.*, **1995**).

Transperitoneal technique

After the induction of pneumoperitoneum, the optical trocar will be inserted at umbilical level and three 5 mm working trocars in the right side, two trocars and on the left side one trocar. Subsequently, the patient will be placed in Trendelenburg position and, after cranial mobilization of the intestines, pelvic inspection will be carried out, correct positioning of the Foley catheter and the mounting of the uterine manipulator will be undergone. The intervention starts with the identification of the umbilical ligament and the dissection of the peritoneum in a transversal approach. Dissection continues inferiorly until the identification of Cooper ligaments. Subsequently, the dissection continues bilaterally paravesical to the identification of paravaginal fascia. Once the dissection is completed, the intervention continues by fixing the vaginal fornix and the paracolpos to Cooper ligaments, but without the passing of these sutures transfixed via the vagina. This surgical time is performed with vaginal control, one of the helps being asked to perform a vaginal touch, thereby lifting and maintaining the vagina in the position in which it will be fixed (**Bulent T.M.,** *et al.,* **2004**). Regarding the exact placement of the sutures at the paraurethral level, this should be 2 cm lateral to the urethra and the bladder neck (**Tanagho E.A., 1976**).

Retroperitoneal technique

The intervention starts with a 1.5 cm horizontal incision to 1.5 cm subumbilical incision up to the level of anterior sheath of the right abdominal muscles. This is then sectioned vertically and the right abdominal muscle is leaned laterally, thus making it possible to identify the posterior sheath of muscle aponeurosis of the right abdominal muscles. A workspace is created by inserting a 12 or 15 mm trocar without a nail, which will make the blunt dissection of the preperitoneal space to the level of the pubic symphysis. Once this space is created, the island hose will connect to the trocar, thus creating the preperitoneal space distension. Subsequently, the working trocars will be inserted at the suprapubic level and the lateral sides of the right abdominal muscles. The blunt dissection at the level of the preperitoneal space will continue until the same key elements as in transperitoneal technique are identified periurethral tissue, paracolpos, and Cooper ligaments, Fig. 7.176. and Fig. 7.177. The intervention then continues with the Foley catheter balloon observation and the identification, under transvaginal digital control, of the lateral vaginal fornix, which are suspended to Cooper ligaments with some non-resorbable sutures on each side, Fig. 7.178., 7.179., 7.180., 7.181. and 7.182. What should be mentioned is that the sutures will not be fully tightened, thus preventing excessive urethral angulation. The intervention ends with the vaginal exploration, whose purpose is to confirm the suspension of the anterior vaginal wall, without the sutures being transfixed (**Bulent T.M.,** *et al., 2004*).

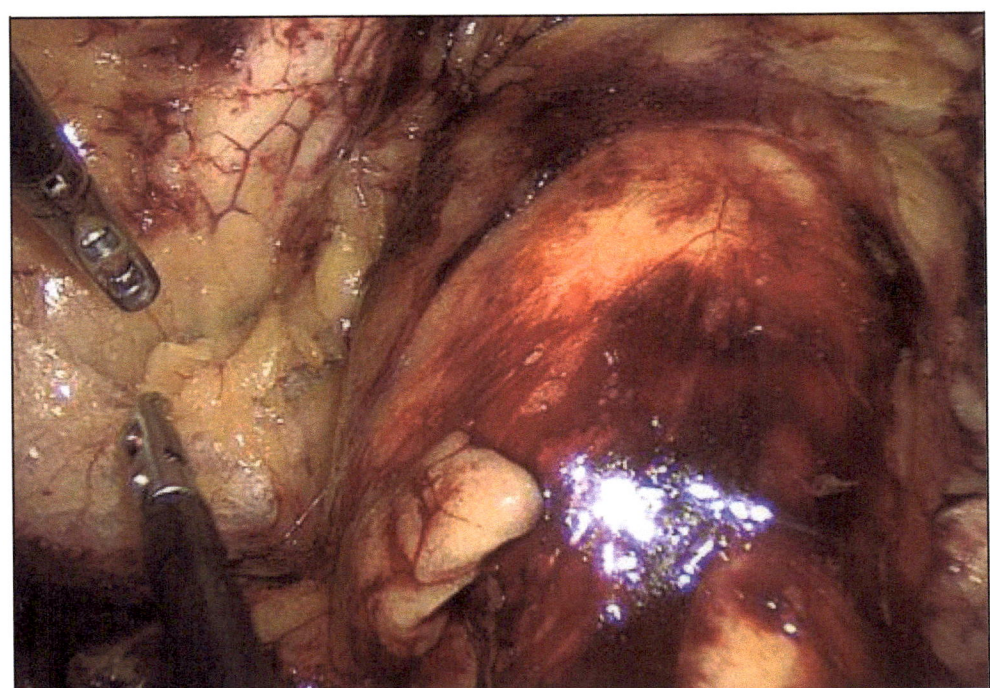

Fig. 7.176. Dissection in the preperitoneal space with the identification of Cooper ligament on the left side

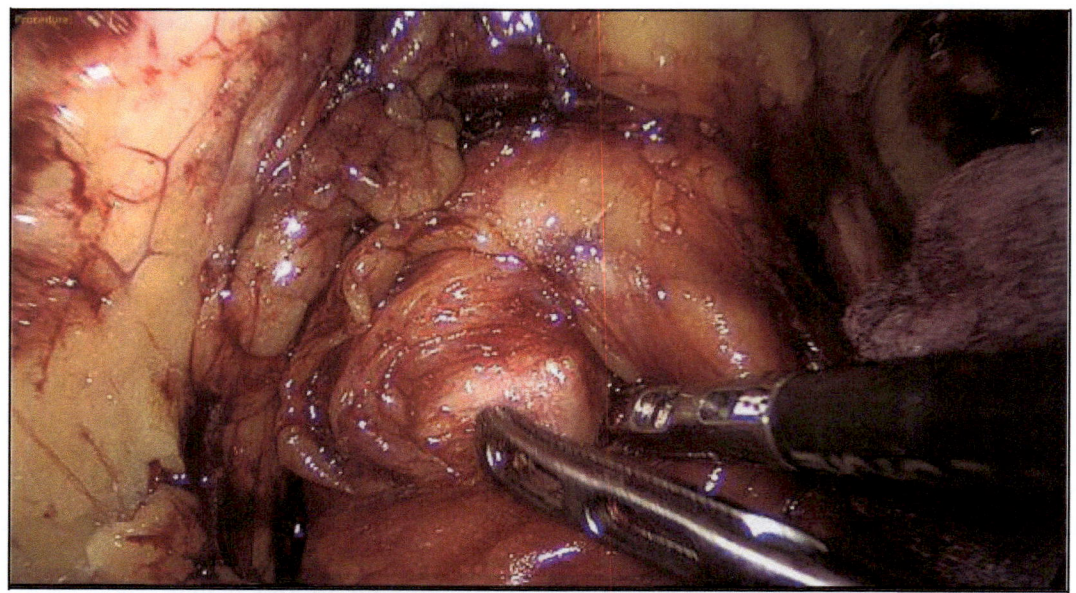

Fig. 7.177. Dissection in the preperitoneal space with the identification of vaginal fornix on the left side

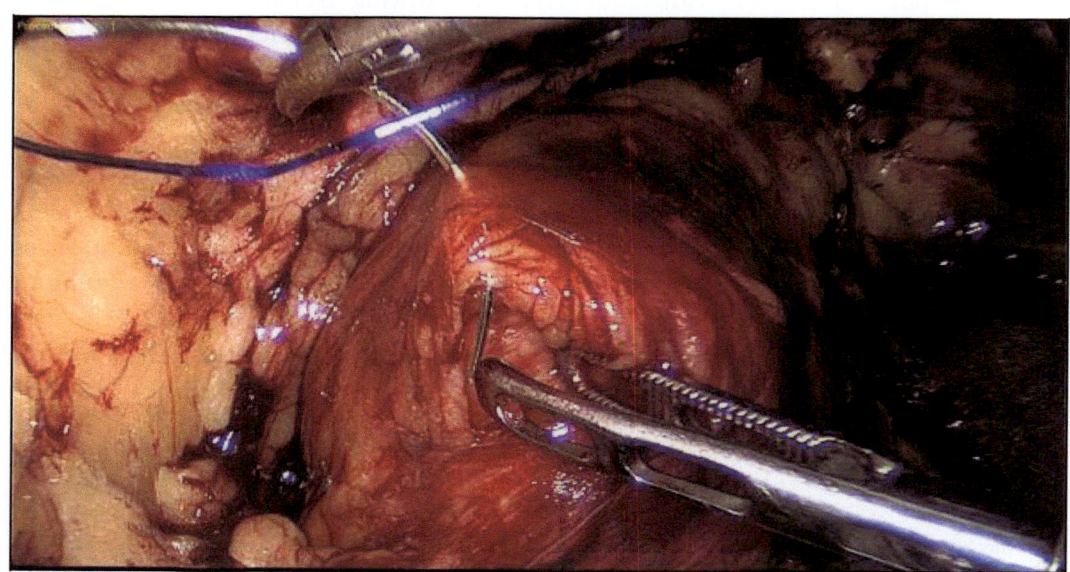

Fig. 7.178. Passing the sutures at the level of the left vaginal fornix

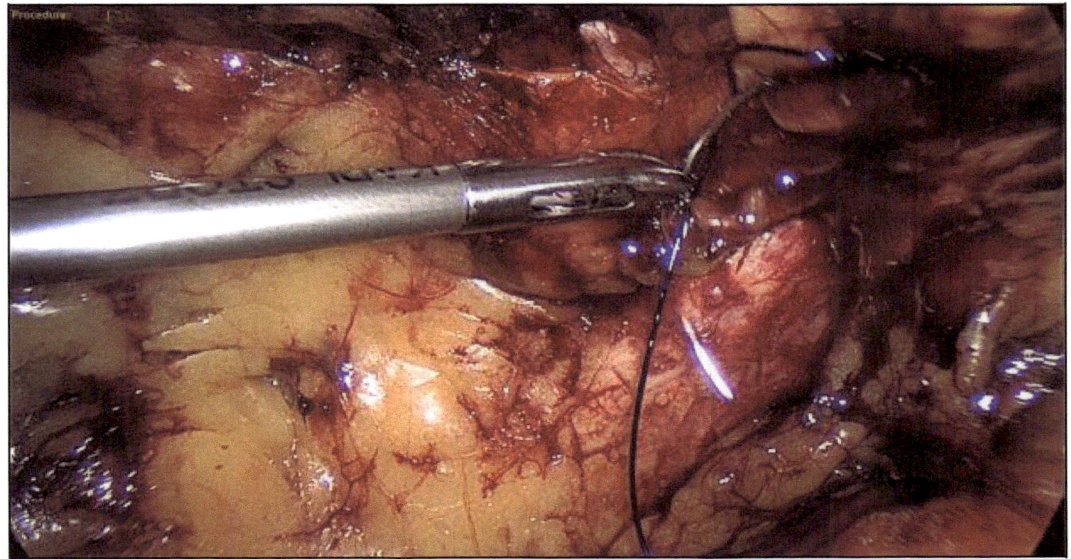
Fig. 7.179. Passing the sutures at the level of Cooper ligament on the left side

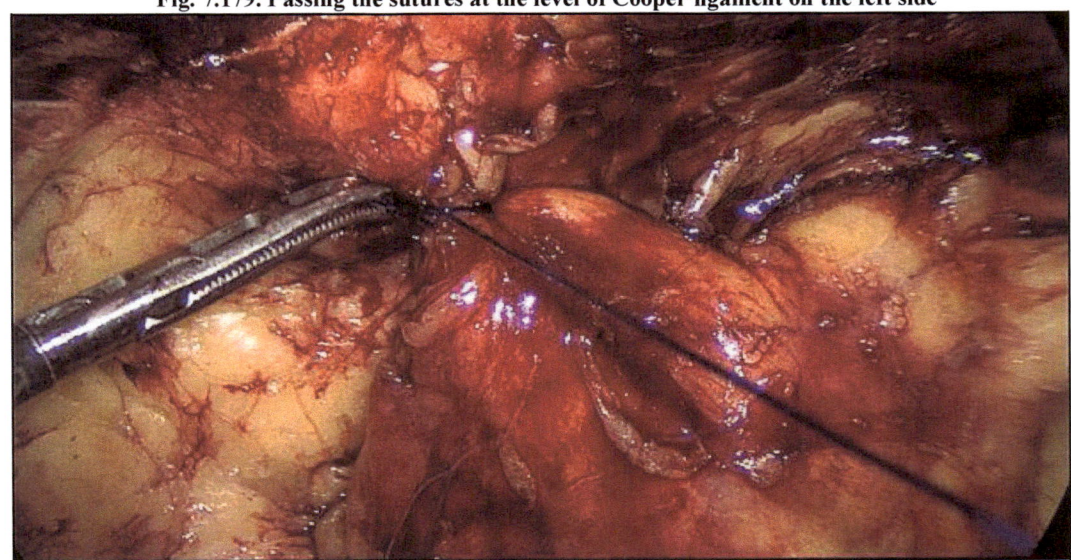
Fig. 7.180. Fixation of the left vaginal fornix at the level of Cooper ligament on the left side

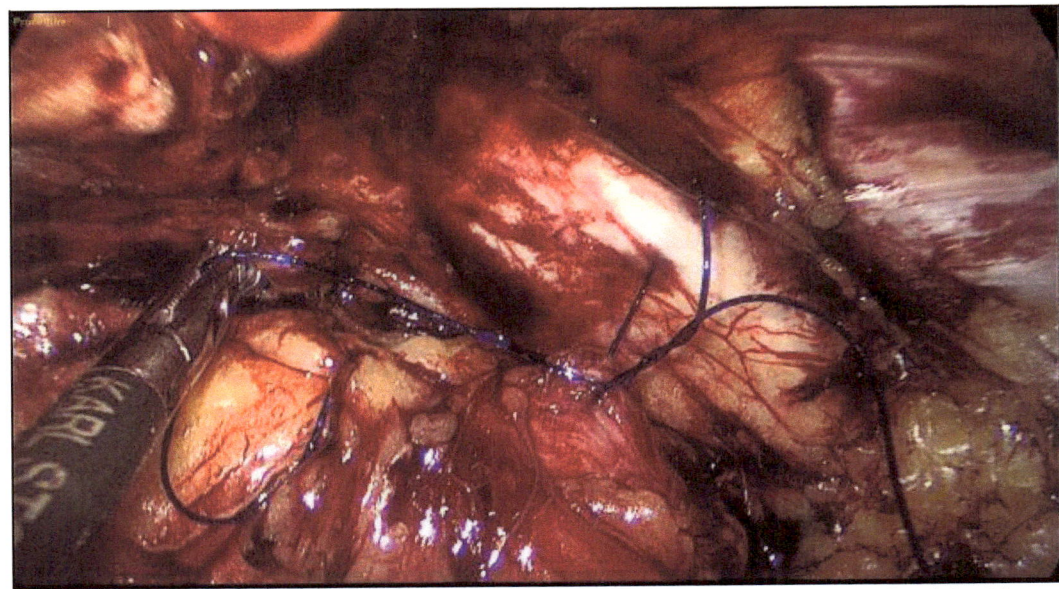
Fig. 7.181. Fixation of the right vaginal fornix at the level of Cooper ligament on the right side

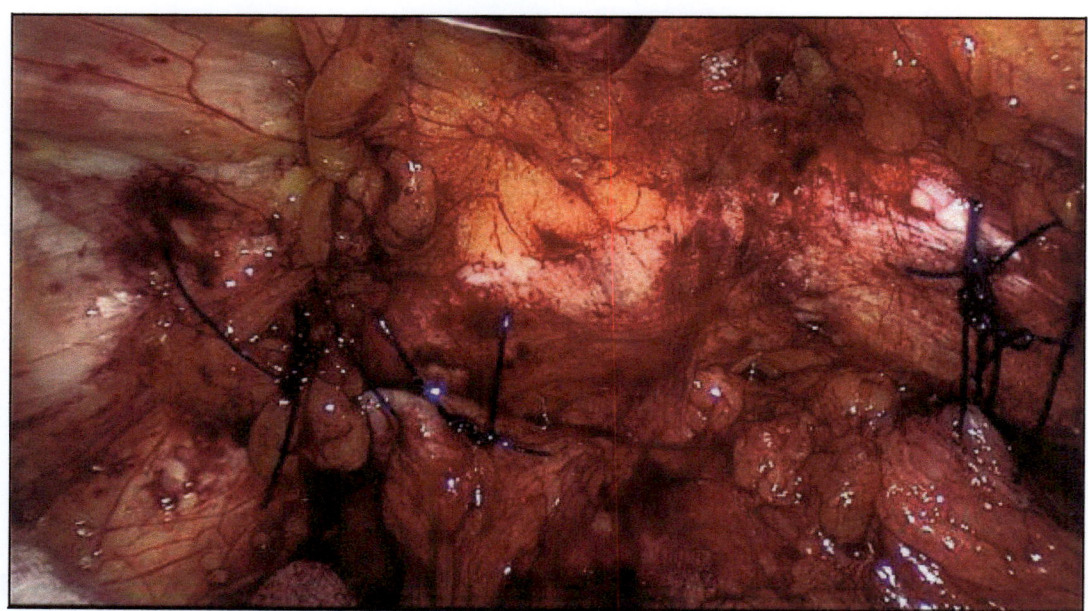
Fig. 7.182. Final aspect after the fixation of the vaginal fornixbilateral to Cooper ligaments

8. Postoperatory complications

It is widely accepted that no surgical technique lacks complications and therefore the same can be affirmed about the pelvic floor disorders surgical corrections. We can distinguish two major categories of complications, regardless of the approach: *complications related to synthetic materials used and complications regarding the surgical technique used* (**Caquant F.,** *et al.,* **2008**). There are many complications whose aetiology is unclear and which are presented in the form of symptoms difficult to classify. A last distinct category, called *syndrome of tethered vagina*, will be treated separately, having a specific etiology and pathophysiology.

8.1. Complications regarding the synthetic materials used

The use of new techniques, using synthetic grafts has opened a new chapter of specific complications. These are due to both new techniques, which often use atypical instruments that go through difficult to explore anatomical spaces and synthetic materials that sometimes cause unexpected reactions. There is also a third category of complications characterized by the appearance of "*de novo*" symptoms without a clear reason.

8.1.1. Erosions

It is the most common complication that occurs because of pelvic reconstruction techniques and they open a completely new chapter in perineal pathology. Their incidence is between 0 - 33% (**Abed H.,** *et al.,* **2011**), although in 2010 Petros did not indicate a rate above 1 - 2%. Probably the very wide range of variation is influenced by the surgeon's experience as well as the technique used.

Recently (**Haylen B.T.,** *et al.* **2011**), IUGA (International Urogynecological Association) and ICS (International Continence Society) published a systematization of the terminology used in this context:

- exposure – the situation in which the alloplastic material is exposed or becomes accessible to exploration, for example through the vaginal mucosa that becomes discontinuous on a given surface, Fig. 8.1.;
- expulsion – the foreign body reaction by excluding a fragment of synthetic material that can be found in the vagina;

- perforation – abnormal passage of a piece of mesh fragment into a cavity organ;

The risk factors that can cause this type of complication may be related to the patient's status and poor response to the synthetic material used: extreme age and local estrogen deficiency, severe vaginal atrophy, scar vaginal mucosa after prior interventions, diabetes, corticosteroid therapy, smoking (**Abed H.,** *et al.,* **2011**). There are authors who have reported an increased incidence of active sexual life (**Kaufman Y.,** *et al.,* **2011**).

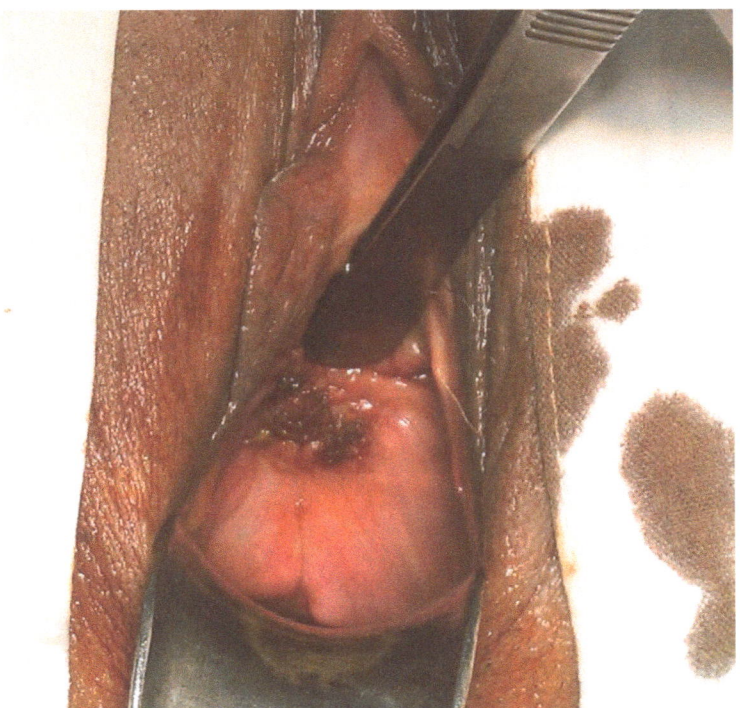

Fig. 8.1. Vaginal erosion with exposure of the mesh fragment
(from the archive of **Enache T.**)

The structure of the materials used may induce erosions, the papers published so far demonstrating that all types used in surgical practice can cause this type of complication (**Zyczynski H.M.,** *et al.,* **2010**), Fig. 8.2. Incriminated mechanisms are the intensity of inflammatory response, an increased aggregation of macrophages perifilamentar associating with the increased incidence of erosions, but an important role of bacterial colonization can also be suspected.

An important risk factor is related to the technique used and surgical experience. The size of incisions and their closing without tension is the most important factor for the reduction of the risk of erosion (**Ganj F.A.,** *et al.,* **2009**). Another factor that can reduce the risk of exposure is the correct anchoring, which prevents plication and agglutination in a certain area. Also, placing the synthetic materials in a too close to the surface of the mucosa area or too deep in the proximity of neighboring organs can lead to exposure or perforation.

Clinical aspect

It varies according to the eroded organ. Vaginal exposure usually occurs with vaginal bleeding, leukorrhea, dyspareunia, or vaginal pain. To the extent that perforation occurs in the urethra or bladder, there are: painful micturition, pollakiuria, urge micturition, hematuria, persistent urinary infections, bladder lithiasis, or even vesicovaginal fistula, as long as the treatment is delayed.

Treatment

It is not yet standardized, due to the small number of cases described. It has to be personalized according to each case. In case of *exposure to the level of vaginal mucosa*, the first therapeutic option is conservative, by applying local antiseptic and estrogen treatment. It is also recommended to stop sexual activity until the complication is solved.

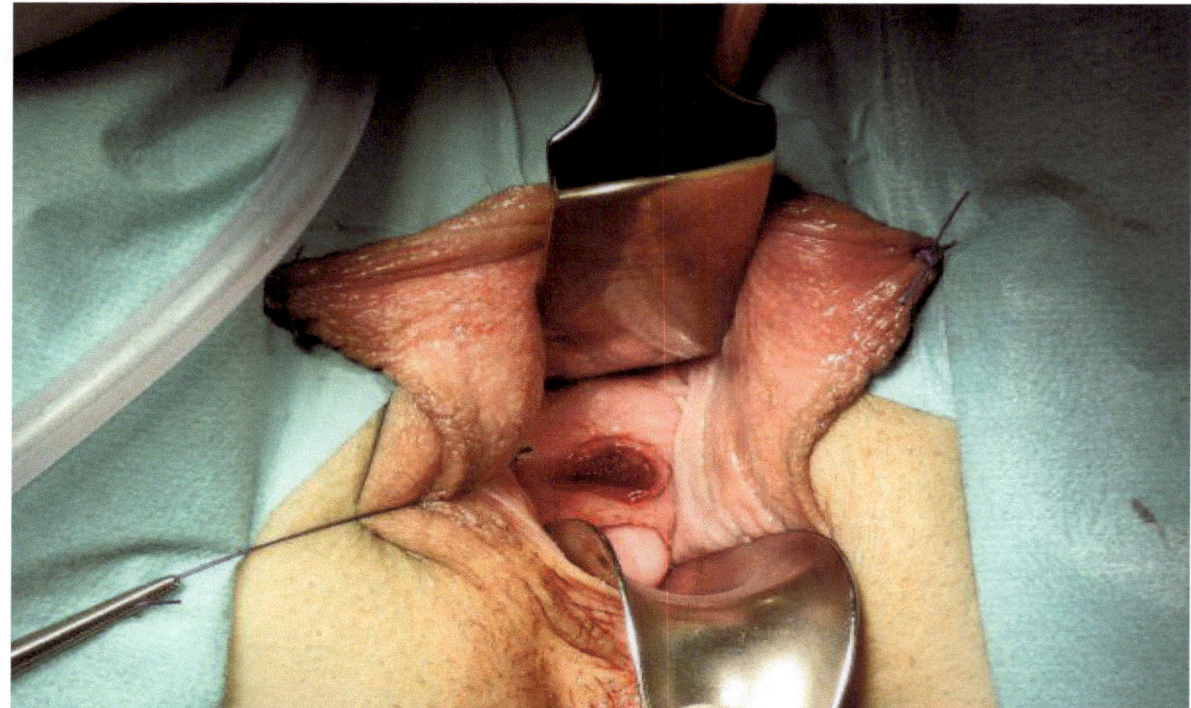

Fig. 8.2. The presence of vaginal erosion after implantation of a preformed mesh
(from the archive of **Mueller-Funogea I.A.**)

A second therapeutic option is the partial or total removal of the alloplastic material fragment, or only the mucosa defect covering. The approach is mainly vaginal, usually under spinal anesthesia or general anesthesia, and most often, the eroded fragment is excised with the closing of mucosa with resorbable sutures that are not tensioned.

The total excision of the mesh is justified only to the extent that the operation is very recent, or is associated with an important septic process; otherwise, the inflammatory reaction process makes the operation virtually impossible.

The laparoscopic approach is reserved for intervention in Retzius space, not being usually used. *Intraurethral and intravesical perforations* should always be surgically treated by extracting mesh fragments. Treatment by open surgery can be done abdominal or vaginal. Bladder lesions are treated by suprapubic or retropubic cystoscopy and the extraction of the eroded fragment. If the lesions of the bladder wall are large, partial cystectomy can be performed.

In the case of urethral lesions by erosion, it is treated by excision of the mesh fragment followed by urethral reconstruction by vaginal approach. In more severe cases, as described by Angulo (**Angulo J.C.,** *et al.,* **2011**), with secondary urethral stenosis, Martius type bladder flap urethroplasty and with graft from *labia majora* was needed. Usually, a multidisciplinary team not lacking an urologist should adopt this treatment.

A very elegant solution is to extract the mesh fragment endoscopically, by ureteroscopy or cystoscopy. Frequently, the eroded fragment is sectioned with the endoscopic scissors and then extracted with the forceps. Some authors proposed the resection with a loop and of a part of bladder muscle, to remove part of the parietal inflammatory process (**Oh T.H.** & **Ryu D.S.,** **2009**). Cases requiring multiple procedures to completely remove the mesh fragment have been described, after each stage, a new portion enveloping the bladder (**Foley C.,** *et al.,* **2010**).

Perforations by erosion of intestinal loops or rectum

Although only few cases have been cited (**Nicolson A. & Adeyemo D., 2008**), so the incidence is extremely low, however, it should be reminded. The most frequent cases quoted were secondary to laparoscopic sacrocolpopexy and the mechanism is uncertain, a possible bacterial contamination, and an intraoperative lesion cannot be totally excluded. In the techniques described, rectal erosions remain only a theoretical possibility; the main clinical manifestation is macroscopic or occult rectalgia, accompanied by diffuse pain and rectal tenesmus.

Their natural evolution is enterovaginal and rectovaginal fistula. Surgical resolution is complex and involves the surgeon's collaboration.

8.1.2. Mesh infections

Present in 0-8% of the cases (**Shah H.N. & Badlani G.H., 2012**), these may or may not associate with the mesh exposure. Colonization is done with both Gram-positive and Gram-negative germs. The important decrease in the rate of colonization is the result of the enforcement of the monofilament polypropylene materials. An important role in the infectious process associated with the synthetic implant is the one of age and associated comorbidities of the patient.

Clinical examination may objectify the erosion of the mesh, but may also indicate the vaginal scar or the granulation tissue. The patient usually presents with leukorrhea or bleeding, dyspareunia, possibly even urinary incontinence or fecal incontinence. Exceptionally, pelvic, urogenital or fistula abscesses may occur. Papers on abscesses that have fused at the level of Scarpa's triangle or even at the level of Hunter's canal to the knee, have been published (**Mueller-Funogea I.A., et al., 2012**).

Treatment is always surgical and involves the extraction of the mesh. Moreover, the drainage of an abscess for several days, depending on the local situation, can be chosen. Intravenous or oral antibiotherapy, possibly guided by the antibiogram obtained from the microbial cultures in the mesh fragments, is mandatory. The local antiseptic cleaning should also be made until the healing of the postoperatory injuries.

8.1.3. Mesh retraction

The incidence of this complication is variable, from 0 - 20% according to some authors (**Lo T.S., 2010**). However, the most important factor in the appearance of mesh retractions is the use of excess synthetic material, which leads to plication, scarring with excessive fibrosis, stiffening of the adjacent vaginal walls and retraction. The main symptoms experienced by the patients include pelvic pain and dyspareunia, associated with urinary disorders and defecation disorders. Over time, prolapse relapse may occur or a degree of urinary incontinence. The clinical examination may reveal a localized thickening of the vaginal walls, with their stiffening, and sometimes a shortening of the length of the vagina, can be observed. Palpation of the scar area can cause pain.

Initially, the treatment is symptomatic, with analgesics and local trophic treatment. The persistence of symptomatology may require surgical intervention with the excision of the scar area and the contracted mesh fragment and the restoration of vaginal elasticity as much as possible (**Feiner B. & Maher C., 2010**).

8.2. Complications regarding the technique used
8.2.1. Hemorrhage and hematoma

Hemorrhage and hematoma are common to all surgical interventions and have a variable impact according to the approach. Vaginal surgery complicates rarely with important intraoperative hemorrhages while the laparoscopic approach involves a higher risk due to the dissection in highly vascularized areas: presacral area, perirectal faucets, etc. As far as it appears, the vascular source should be controlled. Unlike laparoscopic interventions, where the source is accessible, in case of surgeries with perineal approach the access to the vascular source can be difficult or even impossible.

Although rare, the most important vascular complication is the damage to the internal pudendal artery, most commonly in the case of posterior sling or even the patch with sacrospinous fixation. In these cases, the ligation of the source is virtually impossible due to its deep position and the narrow anatomical spaces, often because of digital decollations. Compressible conservative treatment may be tried, possibly with a mesh covered in a diluted dose of adrenalin -1 vial 1 to 1000 diluted in 200 ml serum – and its maintenance for at least 5 minutes. Alternative solutions may be embolization of the artery or ligature of the hypogastric artery laparoscopically, to the extent that there is a significant hemodynamic resonance (**Ko J.K. & Ku C.H., 2014**). The small number of cases described in literature did not imply a standard behavior.

Perineal hematomas are generally self-limiting and are treated conservatively. Even the extensive ones that have fused pararectal and paravesical, symptomatic, can be treated once the hemorrhage is under control. Sometimes, at 2 – 3 days postoperatory, labial, perineal or buttock bruises may occur even spread, but which have a favorable evolution and do not require a special treatment.

A special case is the one in which an extensive hematoma, that generally involves the rectovaginal septum, forms fistulas into the vagina. In this case, after the evacuation, an adequate cleaning of the vaginal incision follows and a *"per secundam"* healing may be attempted. The postoperatory outcome may be partially or totally compromised and may cause relapse.

Strict non-compliance with the anatomical features may theoretically lead to important lesions such as artery or femoral artery lesions, of corona mortis, or of obturator vessel-nerve bundle. The immediate consequences are the formation of extensive hematomas that can even put the patient's life at risk. In the case of femoral vessels, the presence of a vascular surgeon is required, and, in the other two cases, classical or laparoscopic surgical abdominal exploration is required.

8.2.2. Pelvic suppurations

Pelvic suppurations are very rare and may theoretically complicate a fistulized hematoma or may occur in the case of intraoperative contamination. Ischioanal fossa phlegmon may have a very severe evolution, possibly associated with techniques using the intravaginal posterior sling. Their appearance in another context is virtually excluded.

8.2.3. Injuries of adjacent organs

This type of complication is practically synonymous with accidental perforations of the bladder, urethra, rectum, or intestine. The most important aspect is early recognition of the event followed by appropriate treatment. Perforations occur primarily at vaginal insertion of instruments and puncture of various organs. Thus, the removal of the instrument is often sufficient, and the suture of the defect is not necessary. What should be taken into account is that lesions often occur in the subperitoneal space and are very difficult to address. Perforations occurring during laparoscopic interventions can be recognized and repaired during interventions.

Bladder perforations can be treated conservatively if the lesion is punctiform and no trans-bladder alloplastic material remains. In these cases, the instrument is extracted and a new passage is attempted laterally, avoiding as much as possible a new perforation.

Subsequently, a Foley catheter is mounted for 7 days with satisfactory results. If synthetic material remains trans-bladder and cannot be extracted during the intervention, it is possible to choose the cystoscopic approach through which the mesh fragment is sectioned and extracted. The open surgery approach remains just a backup solution.

Bladder perforation can have serious consequences – urethral stricture, urethrovaginal fistula. The first step is to identify the lesion and the therapeutical approach should be decided with the urologist.

Rectum perforations pose particular problems due to septic content and pararectal space rich in adipose tissue susceptible to infection. Most likely, it is damaged during the insertion of posterior sling with the *"tunneller"*. In 2010, Petros was advocating conservative treatment that simply implied the retraction of the instrument, but following different studies that have been made in recent years, the recommendation was to consult a proctologist or a surgeon to establish the optimal approach.

Small intestine perforations are more likely during laparoscopic surgeries, but they are not excluded in vaginal approach either. Thus, they must be taken into consideration in any accidental opening of peritoneal cavity.

The evolution of all perforations undiagnosed in time and untreated is the formation of fistulas: urethrovaginal, cystovaginal, rectovaginal, and enterovaginal.

The indirect damage of the ureters should also be mentioned in this context – *their plication*. Although more frequent during laparoscopic interventions it is also possible after vaginal approach interventions (**Unger C.A.,** *et al.,* **2015**). The consequence is ureterohydronephrosis and the approach is not standardized, with few cases described so far. Urethral catheterization with Cook catheter can be chosen at first, and then, in case of failure, sutures opening or extraction of mesh fragment that compresses the uterus is advisable.

Damage of certain nerve fibers with important consequences is considered lesion of vicinity organs. During laparoscopic interventions, inferior hypogastric plexus may be affected, resulting in bladder, rectal and sexual dysfunctions. However, the risk is minimal if the surgical time and peritoneum dissection is made as superficial as possible. Inferior hypogastric plexus can also be injured during sacrospinous anchoring. The most frequent consequence is sacral, coccydynia pain, sometimes very intense. Pain can be exacerbated by orthostatism. Evolution is usually slow with the disappearance of symptoms up to 6 months. In exceptional cases, the sectioning of sacrospinous sutures is needed for pain remission.

An important risk concerns pudendal nerve lesions in the vaginal approach, especially during the insertion of posterior vaginal sling. Interception of nerve fibers occurs most frequently anterior to the ischial spine, at the entrance of the nerve in the Alcock's canal. Recent studies (**Furtmüller G.J.,** *et al.,* **2014**) have demonstrated the existence of 2 trunks instead of one, and the consequences are not very severe, especially if the lesion is unilateral. Clinical manifestations may manifest as discrete pelvic pain and sexual dysfunction. Treatment is possibly conservative with nonsteroidal analgesics. If the symptoms are intense and persistent, the sectioning of the sling may be done by vaginal approach.

8.3. Other postoperative complications
8.3.1. Dyspareunia

The incidence of this complication results from a meta-analysis in 2011, which was 9.1% (**Murray S.,** *et al.,* **2011**). Generally, dyspareunia occurs as a consequence of erosions, infection or vicious scars. Sometimes, the movement of a sling may induce the appearance of dyspareunia. In these cases, solving the main complication, the excision of eroded fragment, the retraction area, the moved sling, can lead to remission of symptoms.

However, a careful analysis reveals the appearance of dyspareunia also in the absence of clear lesions. The explanation can be the altering of vagina biomechanics by the chance of the vaginal axis. In these cases, it is difficult to initiate a treatment in accordance with the pathogenic visa.

8.3.2. Chronic pelvic pains

Chronic pelvic pains occur in 1.9 - 24.4% of the patients treated for pelvic floor disorder (**Chen X.**, *et al.*, **2011**). Pain can be located in the hypogastrium, in the pelvic area, or may predominate in one or both iliac fossae. During the last years, many references have been made to the surgical technique used and the surgical experience of the surgeon. Because surgical techniques are in a process of development and a standard technique does not exist yet, especially for interventions in case of prolapse, no common element has been found between symptomatology and a specific cause. Keeping the elasticity of vaginal walls intact seems to be a key element.

Treatment is symptomatic, especially with non-steroidal analgesics, but in situations in which it does not work, it is recommended that the alloplastic material is extracted.

8.3.3. Urinary retention

Urinary retention may be acute after the removal of Foley catheter, as a bladder globe, or may occur as post-void residual urine. Most frequently, urinary retention occurs after procedures for stress urinary incontinence treatment. Incidence is considered to be less than 10% of the cases (**Patel B.N.**, *et al.*, **2012**). The bladder globe is treated by bladder catheterization for up to 7 days, and the pathophysiological mechanism is probably a periurethral hematoma with the mechanical blockage of the flow, or perinervous with the obstruction of the reflex arc responsible for micturition. The evolution is favorable and usually without long-term consequences.

Post-void residual urine is defined as the bladder catheterization dependence for at least 28 days, which occurred immediately or shortly after surgery. Transient retention can be treated by intermittent bladder check until the symptoms disappear. For those patients with persistent retention, the surgical means include loosening of the sling as much as possible, meaning before fixation of the sling by fibrosis, sectioning of the sling, extraction of the sling or even complex procedures with labia majora graft.

8.3.4. Other urinary symptoms

After perineal reconstruction surgery, a series of "*de novo*" symptoms can arise: pollakiuria, nocturia, urge incontinence. These may occur because of vicious scars or objectively anatomical complications. However, what should be taken into account is that they may be the consequence of a new vector imbalance resulting from the surgical technique used. Remission of symptoms is related to the ability to establish this diagnosis and the degree of reversibility of the technique used. Some cases may, however, receive medical treatment with anticholinergic drugs such as solifenacin or trospium chloride, over a variable period.

8.3.5. Urinary infection

Urinary infection is often present postoperatory, some studies describing it in 34.69% of the cases (**Mueller-Funogea I.A., 2014**). Antibiotic treatment according to the antibiogram leads to healing in all patients who do not associate other complications: urinary stasis, perforation by erosion, etc.

8.3.6. Relapse of pelvic floor disorders or of stress urinary incontinence

Some authors consider the relapse a late complication that greatly hinders a future reconstruction.

8.3.7. Pelvic deep vein thrombosis

It is common to all interventions in the pelvic area, may also occur in perineal reconstructive surgery, but the incidence is difficult to determine (**Cundiff G.W.,** *et al.,* **2008**; **Kobayashi Y.,** *et al.,* **2014**). The treatment is drug-specific.

General severe, bronchopulmonary, and cardiovascular complications are virtually excluded.

8.4. *"Syndrome of tethered vagina"*

"Syndrome of tethered vagina" (STV) is a clinical entity of iatrogenic origin, not yet fully recognized. It is caused by scar-induced stiffening in the medium third of anterior vaginal wall, Fig. 8.3 a and b. This syndrome has a special place in the concept of Integral Theory. While most of the bladder symptoms are mainly determined by lax connective tissue, the major functional problem in STV is the stiffening of the connective structures.

STV was described by Petros and Ulmsten in 1990 and again in 1993 (**Petros P.E., & Ulmsten U., 1990**; **Petros P.E., 2006**; **Petros P.E., 2010**). It is not yet a distinct notion recognized by the International Continence Society (**Abrams P.,** *et al.,* **2002**).

This problem is somewhat similar to *"motor detrusor instability"* and may occur in patients with multiple surgeries at the vagina level that corresponds to the area of bladder neck. Unlike the classic STV symptomatology, characterized by involuntary loss of urine when the patient walks, symptoms often start with urine loss at the change of position from clinostatic to orthostatic position in the morning, when getting up from the bed. The patient does not have urine loss during sleep. Symptoms are caused by loss of elasticity in the area of the bladder neck: the "critical elasticity area" (CEA), Fig. 8.4.

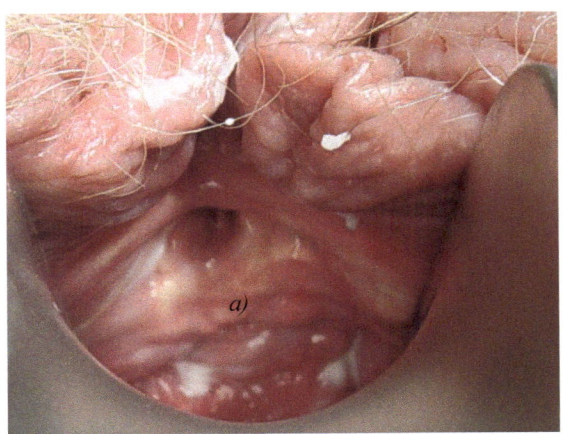 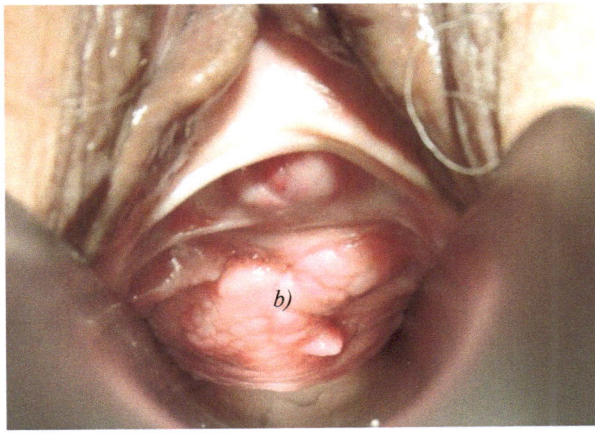

Fig. 8.3. Coarse scar tissue in the vaginal area corresponding to the bladder neck, typical for "syndrome of tethered vagina" (from the archive of **Goeschen, K.**)

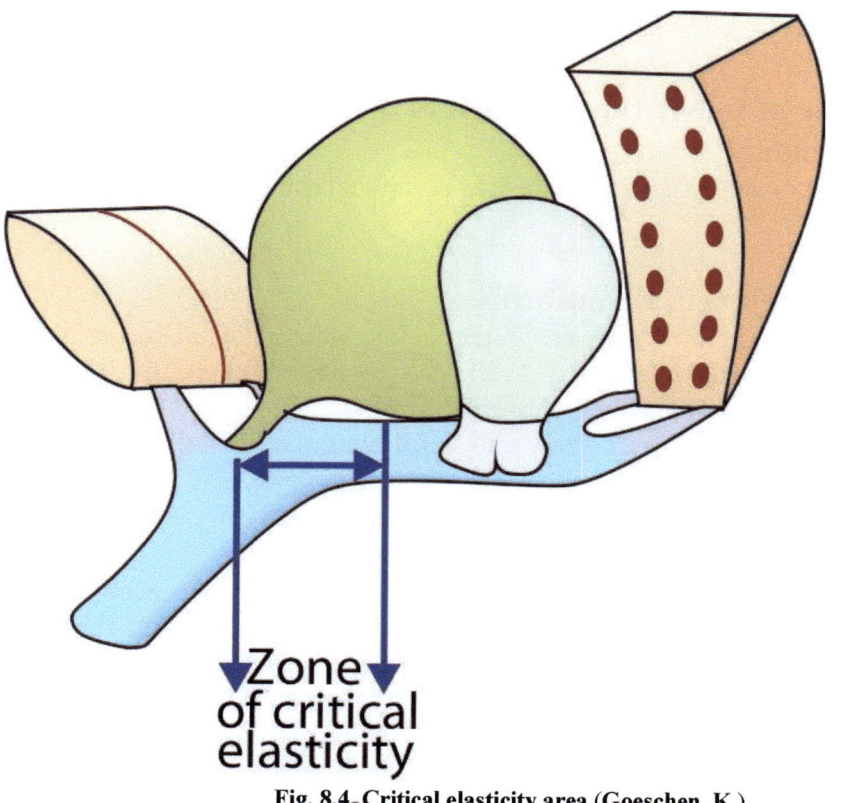

Fig. 8.4. Critical elasticity area (Goeschen, K.)

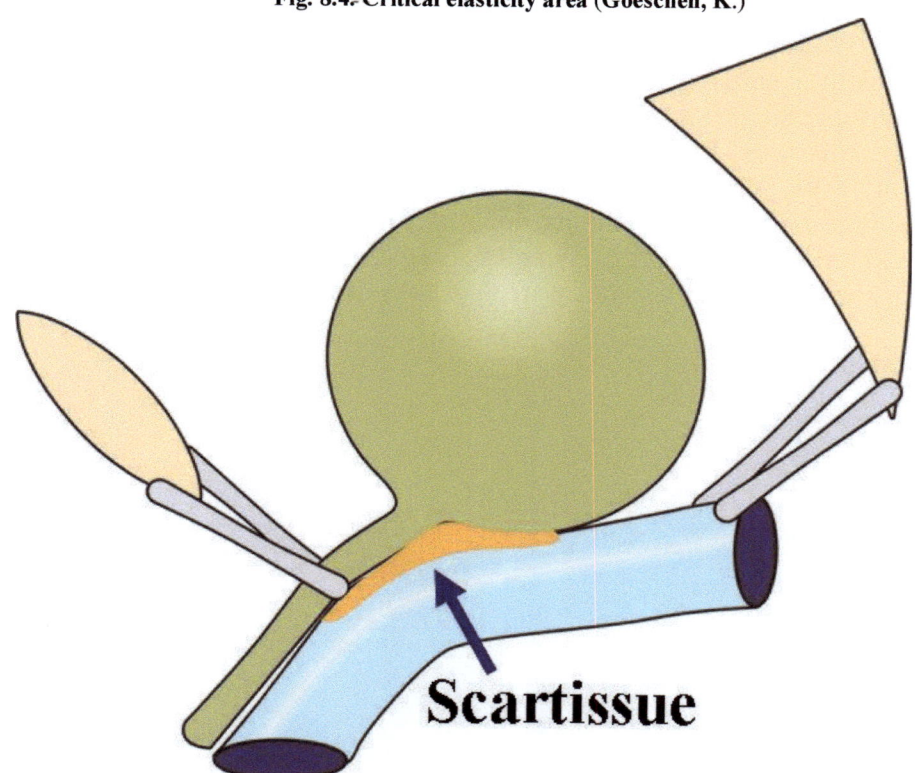

Fig. 8.5. Scar tissue blocks the physiological closing and opening machanism (Goeschen, K.)

Scar tissue in this area, Fig. 8.5., blocks the physiological closing and opening mechanism, because this mechanism is primarily controlled by the pubourethral ligaments (PUL), the green arrow in Fig. 8.6.*a* and not by a so-called sphincter in the area of the bladder neck, the black arrow in Fig. 8.6.*a*. Surgeries at the level of the bladder neck lead to pathological modifications with impact on bladder function, Fig. 8.6.*b* și *c*.

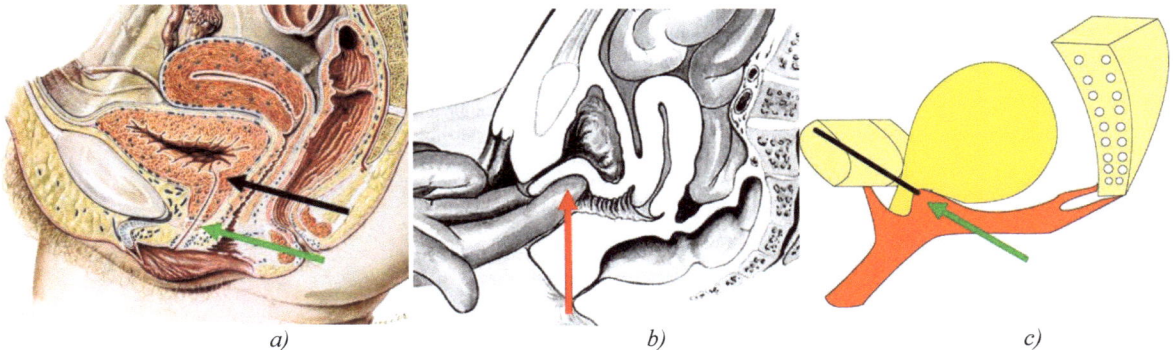

Fig. 8.6. The opening and closing mechanism is mainly located at the level of pubourethral ligaments (PUL) (green arrow) **and not at the level of sphincter area** (black arrow) (**Goeschen, K.**)

Symptomatology

Since scar tissue contracts in time, STV may appear many years after vaginal correction or after bladder neck anchoring. Patients with STV exclusively do not lose urine during sleep. Moreover, they often do not present effort urinary incontinence, or they present a very low degree of incontinence. The reason is that coughing induces short-term rapid contractions, and if CEA maintains minimal elasticity, it prevents urine loss in effort. However, if the vaginal area located immediately behind the scar is gently spotted with a Chaput forceps, the residual elasticity is canceled and the patient will lose urine in coughing effort.

The STV symptomatology is rarely isolated. In most cases, the anterior stiff vaginal wall induces vector redistribution to the posterior compartment, the result being a rectocele/enterocele. This happened in 96% of our cases. Temporary stiffening in CEA occurs sometimes after the insertion of a suburethral sling, resulting in "de novo" appearance of involuntary losses of urine when changing the position from clinostatic to orthostatic. In most cases, elasticity is regained slowly over the next few weeks or months, as tissue tension in the scar tissue decreases. This improves symptomatology without any treatment.

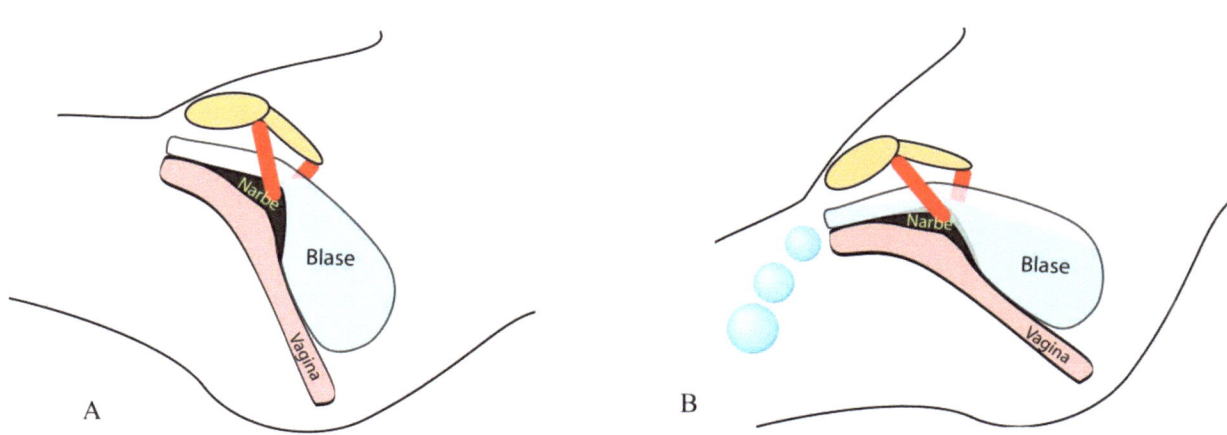

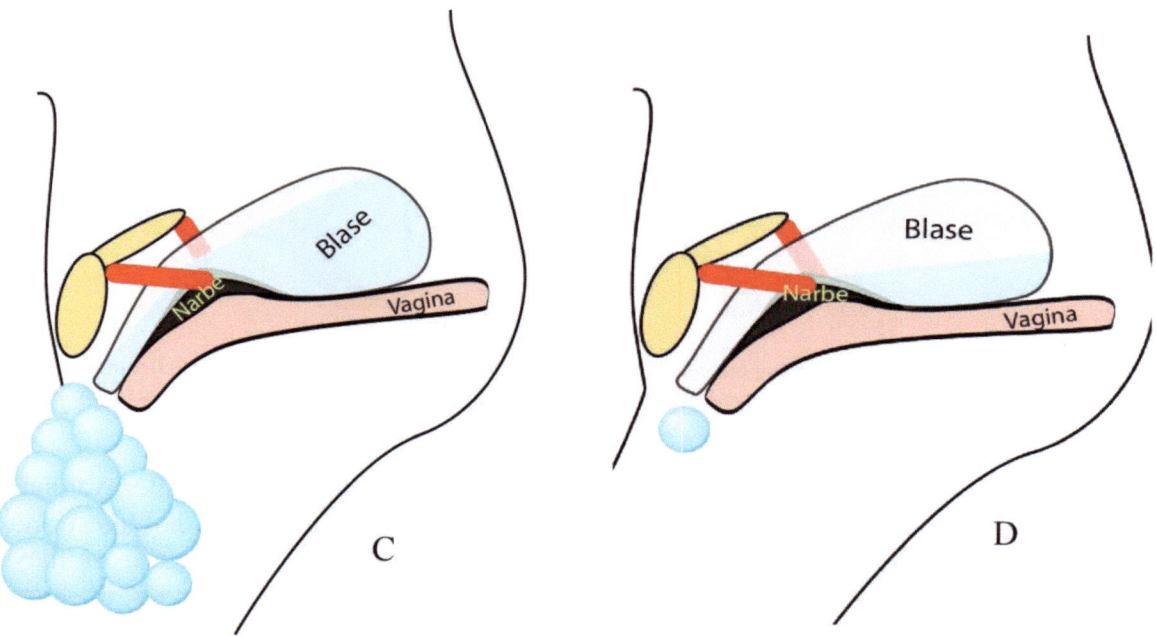

Fig. 8.7. Urine status in the bladder (from the archive of **Goeschen, K.**)
a) The bladder fills into decubitus position. *b)* When rising, the scar prevents the urethral closure.
c) Foot on the floor, massive urine loss. *d)* The patient gets to the toilet, the bladder is almost empty

The explanation of urine loss due to scar tissue at the CEA level is the following: getting out of the bed tensions CEA more than during coughing, because the pelvic muscles need to contract much more to support the intraabdominal organs. Thus, the voiding tract is suddenly opened, resulting in a massive loss of urine as the patient steps on the floor. In the case of scar tissue at CEA level, the bladder neck is like porcelain and behaves like a sprinkler.

In dorsal decubitus position, the bladder fills up, Fig. 8.7.*a*. If the patient rises in sitting position, the levator plate contracts. Scar tissue blocks the effect of contraction of the pubococcygeus muscle and hence an opening of the evacuation tract as it happens during micturition, Fig. 8.7.*b*. Loss of urine occurs while changing from sitting position to orthostatic position, while during orthostatism, the loss of urine is massive, Fig. 8.7.*c*. When the patient reaches the bathroom, the bladder is almost empty, Fig. 8.7.*d*.

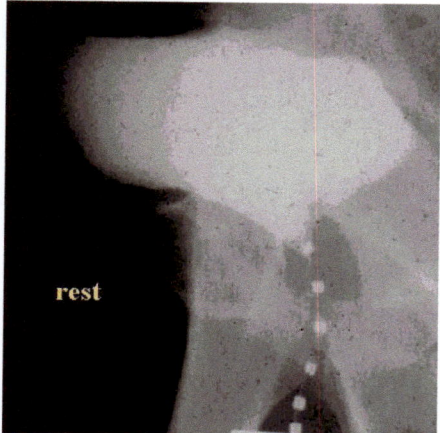

Fig. 8.8. Coarse scar tissue at the level of urethra and in the bladder neck (from the archive of **Goeschen, K.**)

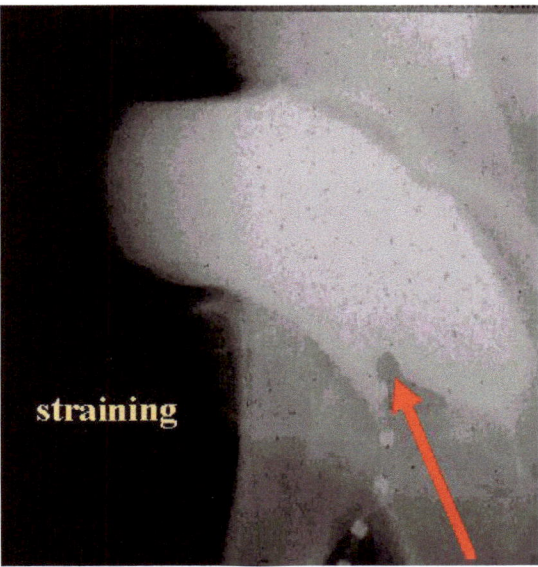

Fig. 8.9. Excessive bladder neck lifting after 8 surgeries in this area (from the archive of **Goeschen, K.**)

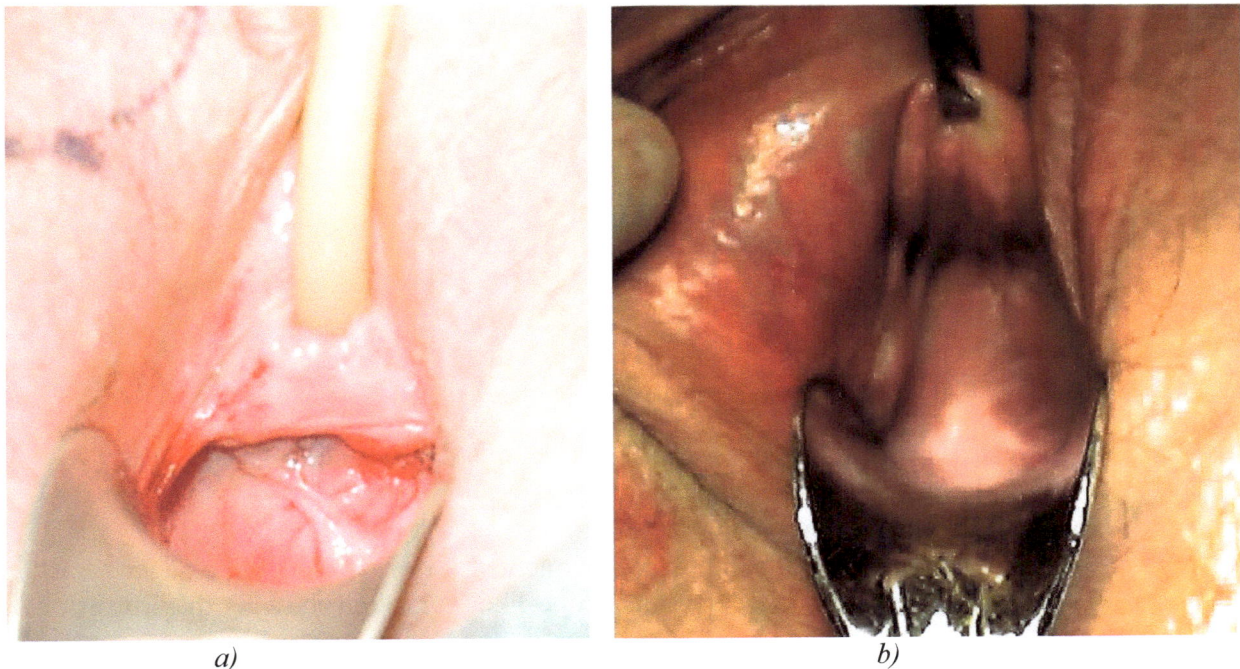

a)   *b)*

Fig. 8.10. Lateral cystogram after Burch colposuspension (from the archive of **Goeschen, K.**)
a) At ease. *b)* During Valsalva manouver when the bladder neck is lifted non-physiologically (red arrow).

Clinical vaginal examination

Usually it is not difficult to observe and feel the scared bladder neck by valves and vaginal tract. It is, however, very important to establish therapy if the scar is responsible for incontinence or not. Effort urinary incontinence and urge incontinence require a completely different approach than the one for stiff vagina.

As mentioned above, coughing and Valsalva maneuver do not cause urine loss in patients with a typical syndrome of tethered vagina. However, if the vagina near the scar is gently tilted posteriorly with a Museux forceps, the residual elasticity disappears from the CEA level and urine is lost during coughing effort.

There are two types of STV patients.

1. Patients after traditional surgery for incontinence surgery, such as:

a) anterior colporrhaphy;

b) Marshall-Marchetti-Kranz urethropexy;

c) Burch colposuspension – can induce a non-physiological lifting of the bladder neck, Fig. 8.8., Fig. 8.9 and Fig. 8.10. *a* and *b*.

d) teflon injection surgeries or periurethral "*macroplastique*", etc.

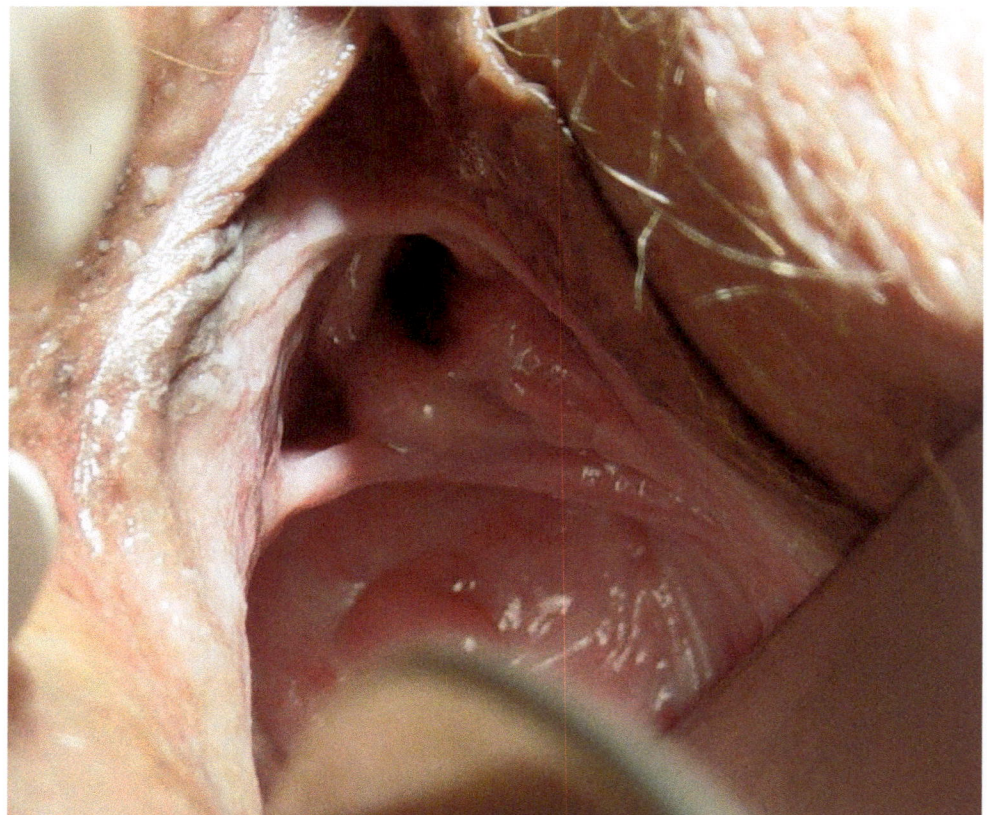

Fig. 8.11. Prominent scar in shape of a rope (from the archive of **Goeschen, K.**)

2. Patients who after the surgeries use autologous or artificial material slings:

a) Narik-Palmrich inguinal-vaginal autologous sling surgery;

b) STRATASIS™ urethral sling;

c) autologous or artificial sling placed erroneously at the level of the bladder neck;

These types of patients present a linear rope-like scar, often showing the protrusion of the mesh fragment, Fig. 8.11.

Diagnosis

Ultrasound

Typical elements of the ultrasound examination are limited movement, funneling or even opening of the bladder neck to straining effort or Valsalva maneuver, Fig. 8.12., Fig. 8.13.*a)* and *b*.

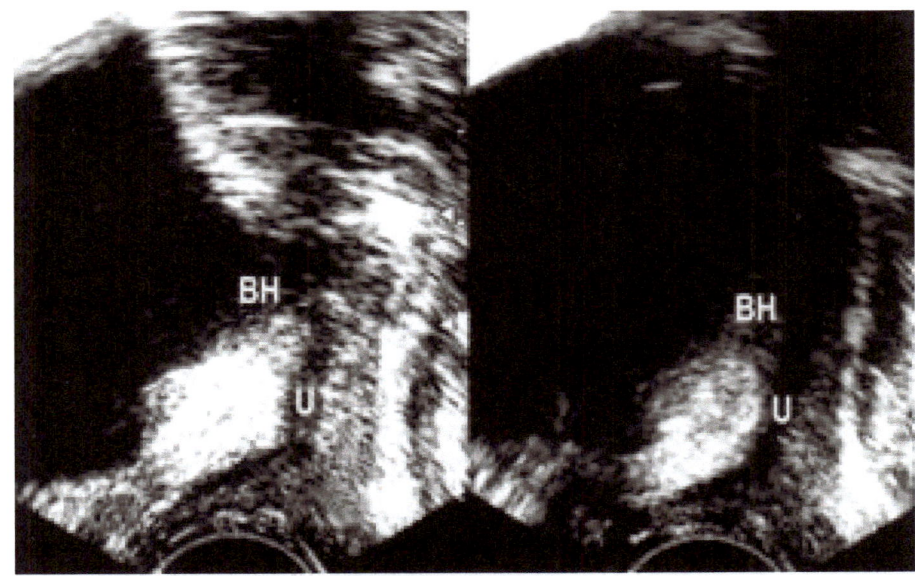

Fig. 8.12. Patient with 8 bladder neck surgeries in her medical history. Bladder neck (BN) at ease (left) is pulled cranial and posterior, while the posterior bladder wall slipped caudally. U = urethra. During strain effort (right), bladder neck keeps its position, while the posterior wall of bladder remains in normal position (from the archive of **Goeschen, K.**)

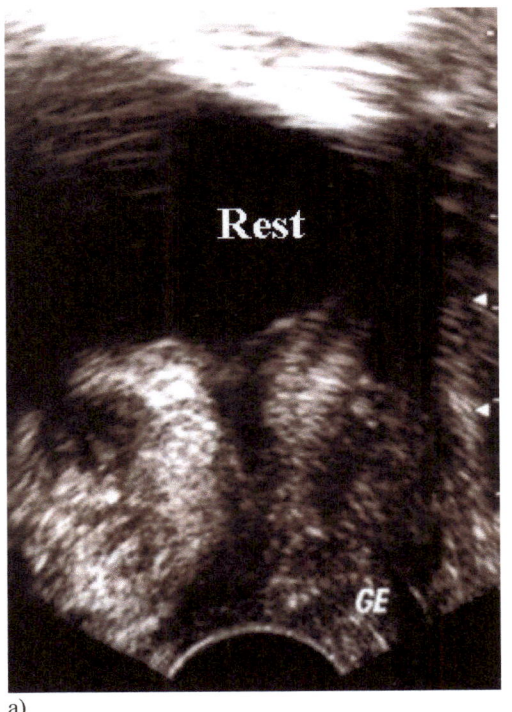
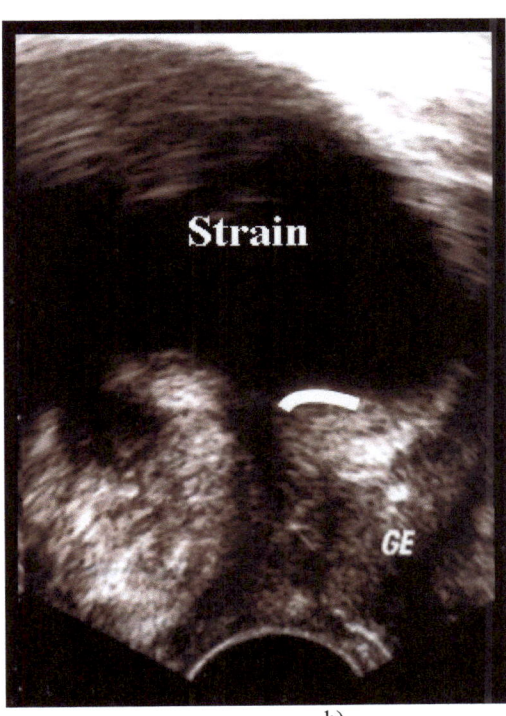

a) b)

Fig. 8.13. Patient with 3 surgeries of the bladder neck in her medical history. (from the archive of **Goeschen, K.**)

Fig. 8.11. No movement of the bladder neck is observed a) during coughing and b) during straining effort

Urodynamics

Urodynamics usually does not reveal a particular pattern when bladder fluid passes through the stiff urethra as passing through a "*sprinkler*". A specific urodynamic aspect may be a low-pressure urethral profile due to stiff tissue, Fig. 8.14.

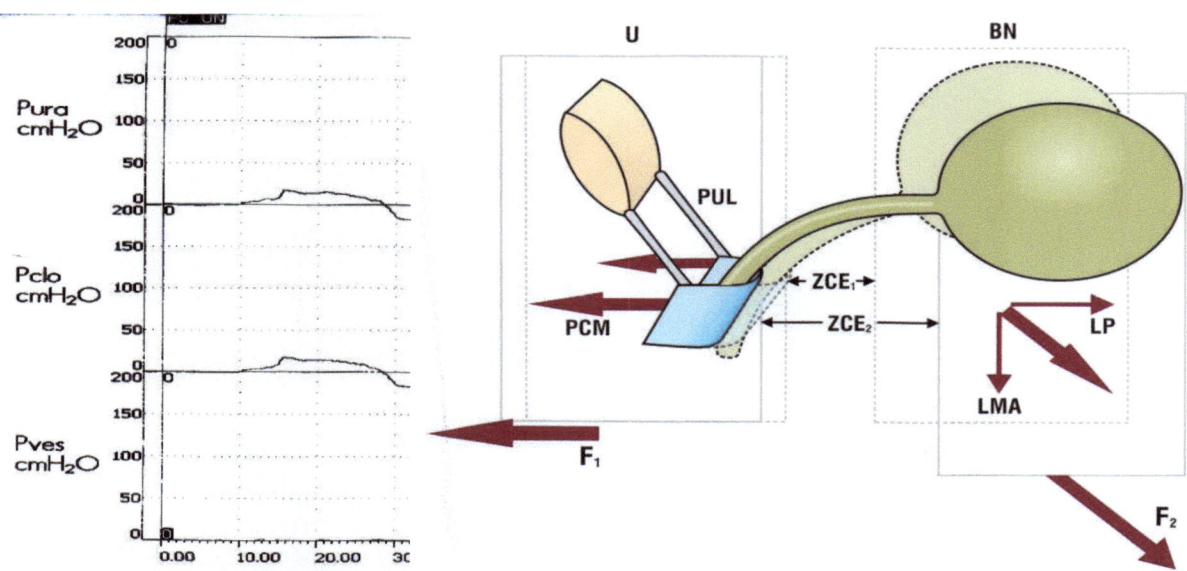

Fig. 8.14. Pressure urethral profile of a patient with STV
Low pressure in the urethra due to stiffness induced by scar

Fig. 8.15. Critical elasticity area: CEA1=CEA at rest; CEA2=CEA during micturition effort
PCM = pubococcygeus muscle; LP = levator plate,
LAM = longitudinal anal muscle.
F1 represents the anterior vector component
F2 represents the resultant of vectors forces represented by LP/ LAM action

Treatment

The periurethral application of microbaloons does not seem to make sense because the bladder neck area is already stiff. This procedure will make the situation worse.

Implanting the artificial sphincter is a very expensive and extremely invasive procedure with countless side effects.

Our strategy consists of two stages.

The first stage is to remove all scar tissue and artificial materials.

The second stage is to restore elasticity in the bladder neck, the *"critical elasticity area"* (CEA), so that *"F1"* and *"F2"* can act independently one from the other Fig. 8.15. An appropriate elasticity of CEA allows the functioning of the closing mechanisms by the antagonistic action of the urethra and bladder neck. *F1* is the anterior vector that tensions the vagina anteriorly from the suburethral area to close the distal urethra, *"urethral closure mechanism"*.

F2 tensions the proximal urethra posteriorly in posterior and lower direction around PUL, to close the *"bladder neck closing mechanism"*. A CEA scar *"stiffens"* the muscle vectors that act antagonistically, so that when applying a prolonged force, as it happens when getting out of bed in the morning, *F2* predominates over *F1* and so the posterior wall of the urethra is pulled behind, exactly in the same way micturition occurs.

Removing all scar tissue and artificial materials

The anatomical basis of our surgeries is the Integral Theory (**Goeschen K., 2006; Goeschen K., et al., 2010**), which attests that an adequate elasticity of the vagina is necessary in the area of the bladder neck so as to allow the muscular forces with different directions to act independently, Fig. 8.15. No matter the surgical technique used to restore elasticity, dissection of vagina at the level of bladder neck and urethra is essential to release all the scar tissue of the urethra, bladder neck, *"urethrovesicolysis"* and of the pubis, Fig. 8.16.*a* and *b*, Fig. 8.17.*a* and *b*, Fig. 8.18.*a* and *b*, Fig. 8.19.*a* and *b*.

Restoration of elasticity in the bladder neck area, CEA

A simple suture of the incision after dissection of the scar will create a new scar tissue with the recurrence of incontinence. To prevent the formation of new scars, healthy tissue must be brought to CEA. Since 1999, we have tested the validity of three different surgeries (**Goeschen K., 2006**; **Goeschen K.,** *et al.,* **2010**), each of which attempting to restore the vaginal elasticity around the bladder neck.

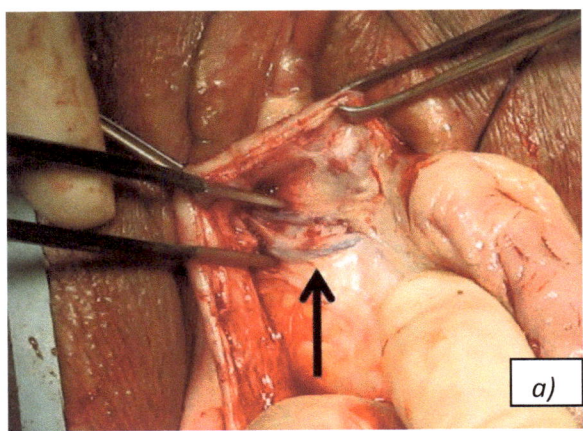

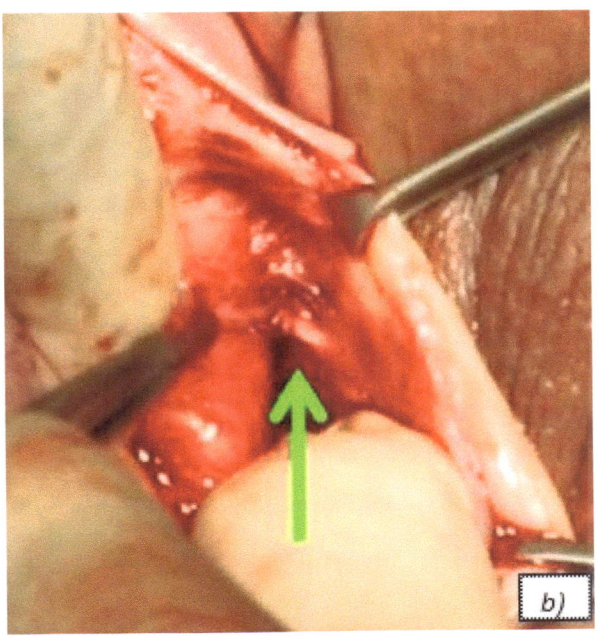

Fig. 8.16. Syndrome of tethered vagina
a) STV secondary to Burch colposuspension
b) STV secondary to Stamey-Pereyra ureterovesical suspension. Vagina is dissected from the bladder and the proximal urethra. Burch sutures (black arrow figure a) and Stamey-Pereyra sutures (green arrow figure b) are still visible "in situ" (from the archive of **Goeschen, K.**)

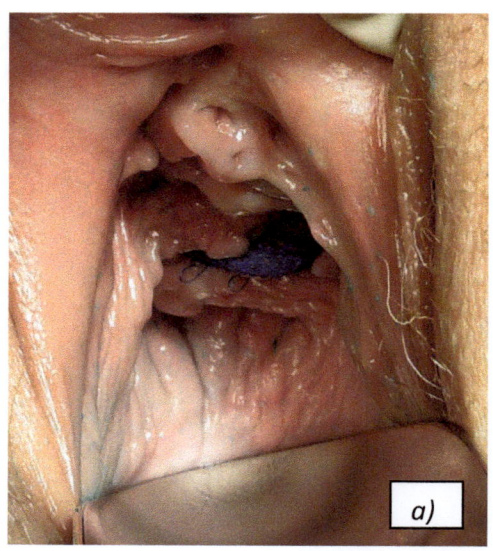 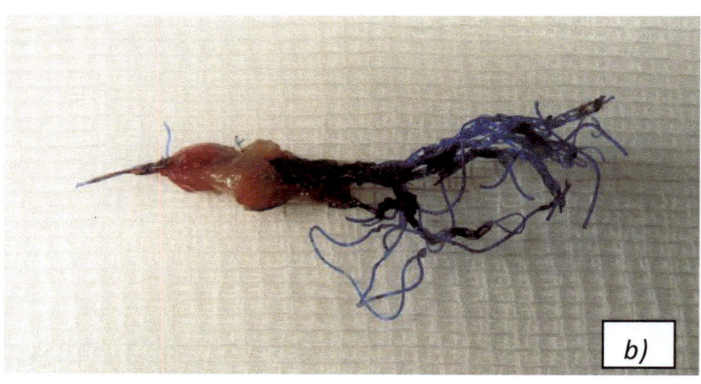

Fig. 8.17. Patient with STV. Vaginal erosion may induce scar stiffness (from the archive of **Goeschen, K.**)
a) "*in situ*" erosion;
b) fragment of eroded mesh after extraction

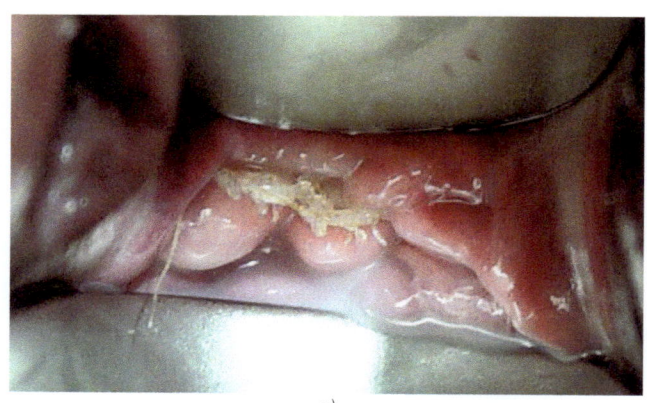 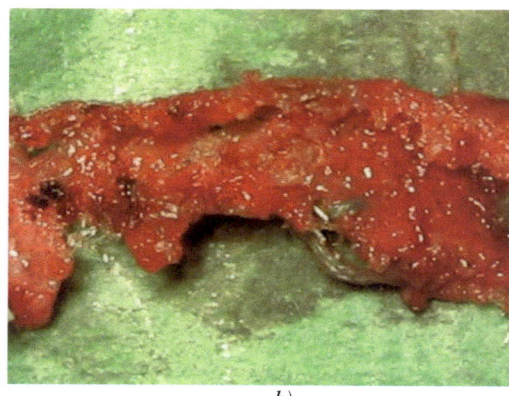

Fig. 8.18. Patient with vaginal erosion (*a*) **and STV** (*b*) (from the archive of **Goeschen, K.**)

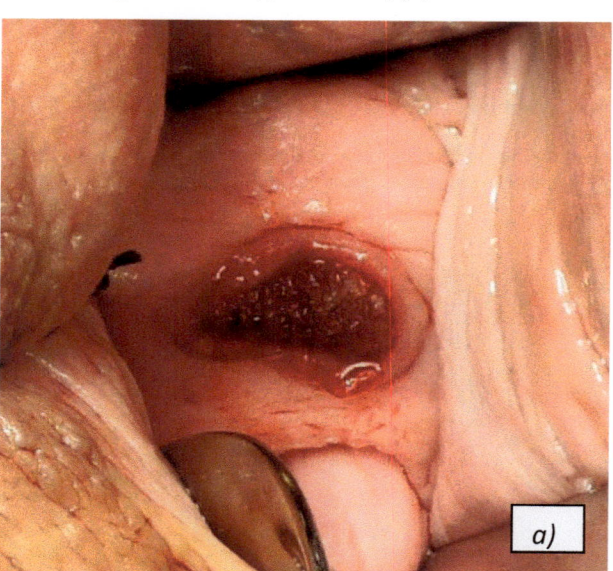

282

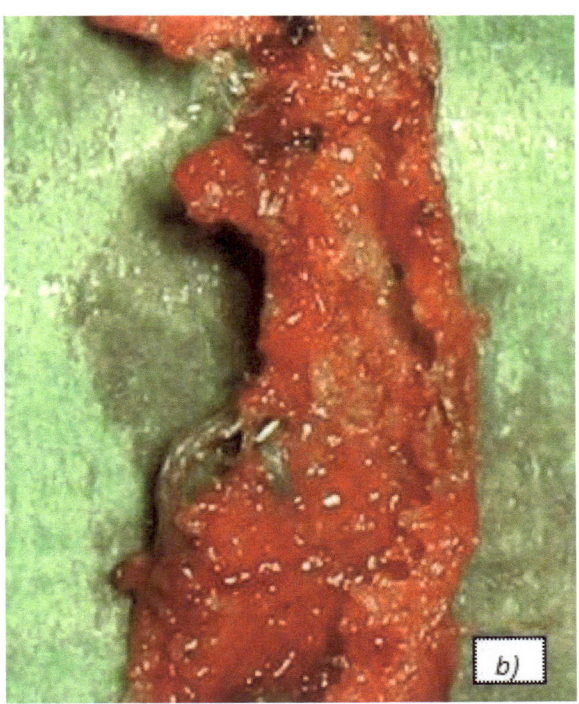

Fig. 8.19. STV due to erosion after mesh insertion (from the archive of **Goeschen, K.**)
 a) *The mesh stretches from the urethra to the cervix*
 b) *Mesh fragment after excision*

"I" shaped plastic surgery

It is shown in Fig. 8.20. It was performed in 13 patients with coexisting cystocele. "I" shaped plastic surgery attempts to increase the tissue volume from the vaginal wall adjacent to the bladder neck, and thus to restore elasticity. In order to achieve this goal, a longitudinal incision is performed, that covers the whole thickness of the vaginal wall, starting from the middle urethra to at least 3-4 cm beyond the bladder neck. The vaginal tissue was dissected from the scar and was extensively mobilized, as far lateral as possible to the edges of urethrovaginal fascia, and posteriorly as far as possible, even to the level of the cervix or the post-hysterectomy scar. The released tissue was brought to CEA and sutured crosswise with separate sutures, thus introducing fresh tissue at the level of the area of interest.

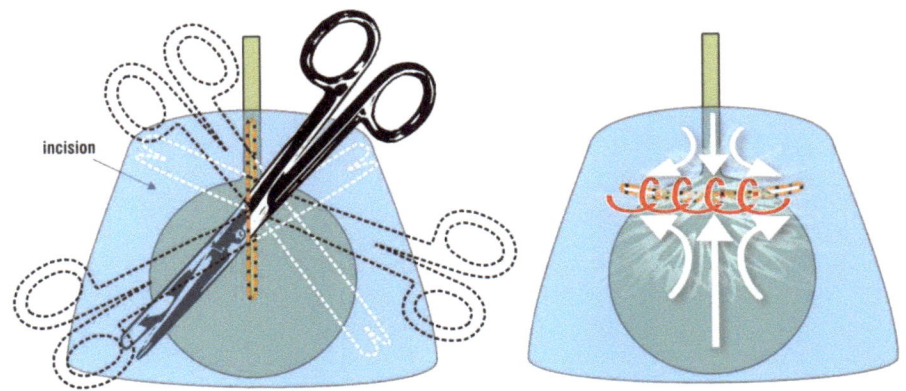

Fig. 8.20. "I" shaped plastic surgery (from the archive of **Goeschen, K.**)

Surgery with skin graft

It is shown in Fig. 8.21. It was performed on 21 patients. After a transversal incision across the whole thickness of the vaginal wall in the area of the bladder neck, the urethra and the bladder neck were released from the scar tissue. The result was a lack of large size vaginal tissue. Rigorous hemostasis was practiced. A 6x4 cm skin graft was sampled from the lower abdominal wall and after removal of the remaining adipose tissue; it was applied at the level of the bladder neck and fixed with "*matelasse stitches*". The graft was then adapted to the size of the gap and then sutured to the adjacent vaginal mucosa with separate Vicryl oo sutures.

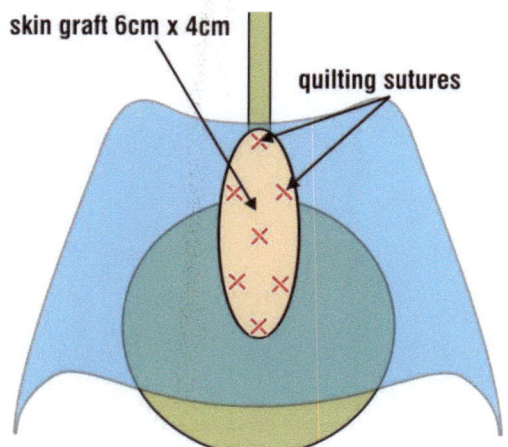

Fig. 8.21. **Skin graft at the level of vagina adjacent to bladder neck, fixed with matelasse stitches** (from the archive of Goeschen, K.)

Bulbocavernosus flap of skin and fat with vascular pedicle

Bulbocavernosus flap of skin and fat with vascular pedicle, Fig. 8.22.*a – f*, was practiced by Goeschen in 105 patients with a lack of vaginal tissue after the dissection of scar.

An ellipsoid incision of 5x3 cm was made at the level of the vulva, from the labia majora, thus achieving a flap, which was transferred with the adjacent adipose and muscular tissue through a tunnel at the level of the dissected area. The tunnel should be wide enough to avoid constriction of the vascular pedicle. The flap was sutured to the remaining vaginal mucosa.

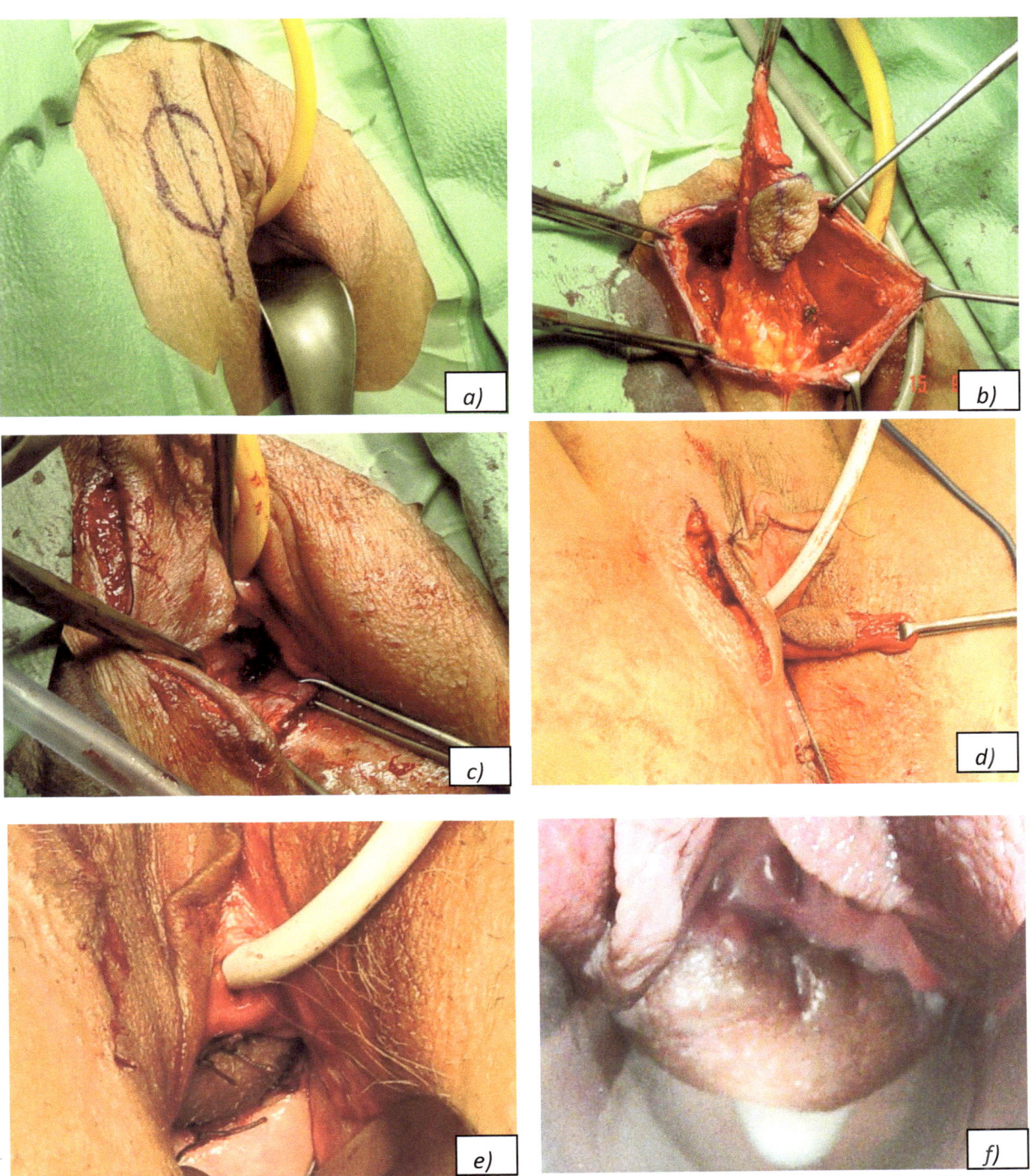

Fig. 8.22. Bulbocavernosus flap of skin and fat with vascular pedicle (from the archive of **Goeschen, K.**)
a) An ellipse of 5x3 cm is delimited with the marker at the level of labia majora. *b)* Preparation of a bulbocavernosus skin-fat-muscle flap with vascular pedicle. *c)* Transversal incision at the level of urethra and bladder neck. The vagina, urethra and bladder neck are mobilized by the scar tissue. *d)* The graft is brought through a tunnel made under the lateral vaginal canal at the level of the dissected area.
e) The graft is sutured at the remaining vaginal mucosa edges. *f)* The graft after 3 months postoperatory

Results

Healing rates, urine losses < 10ml/24 hours, were 3/13 (23%) for "Γ" shaped plastic surgery, 11/21 (52%) for skin graft and 84/105 (80%) for the bulbocavernosus flap.

The average duration of surgery was 62 minutes, ranging from 41 to 98 minutes.

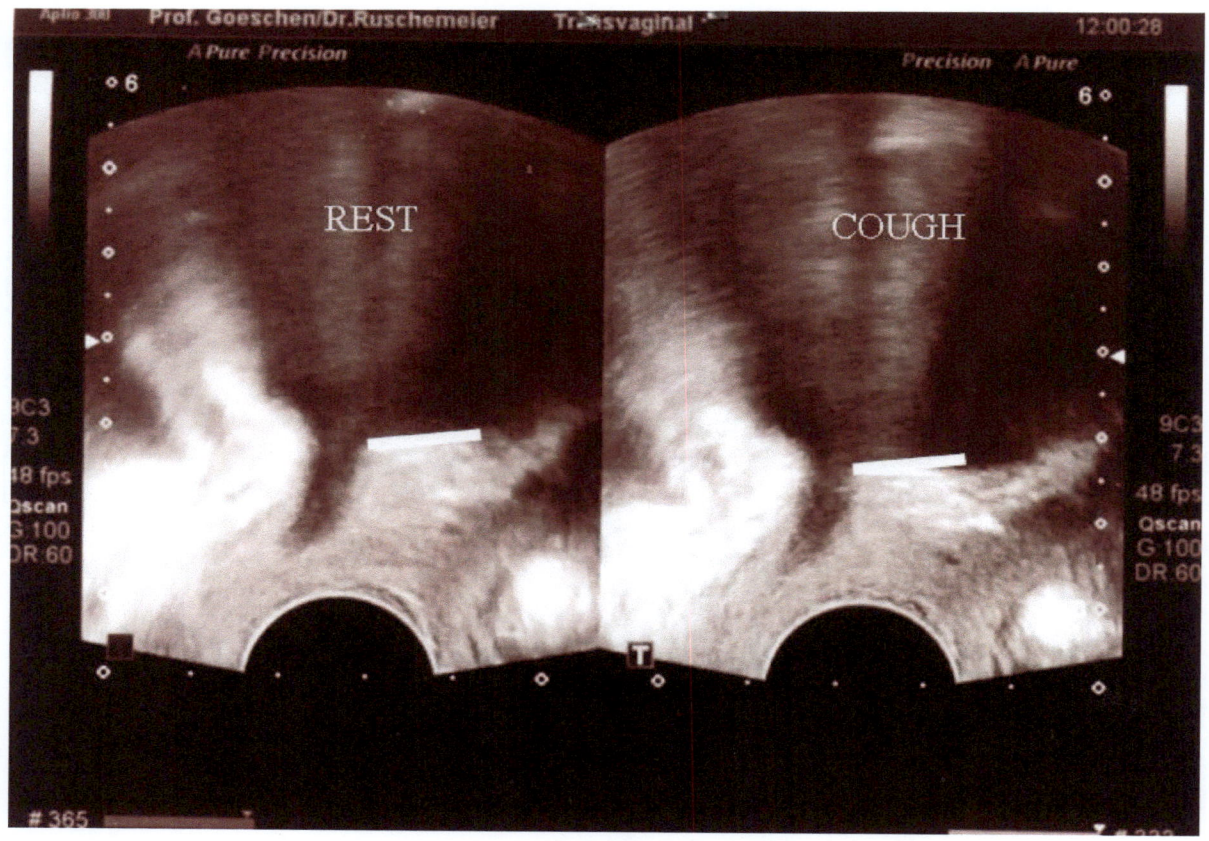

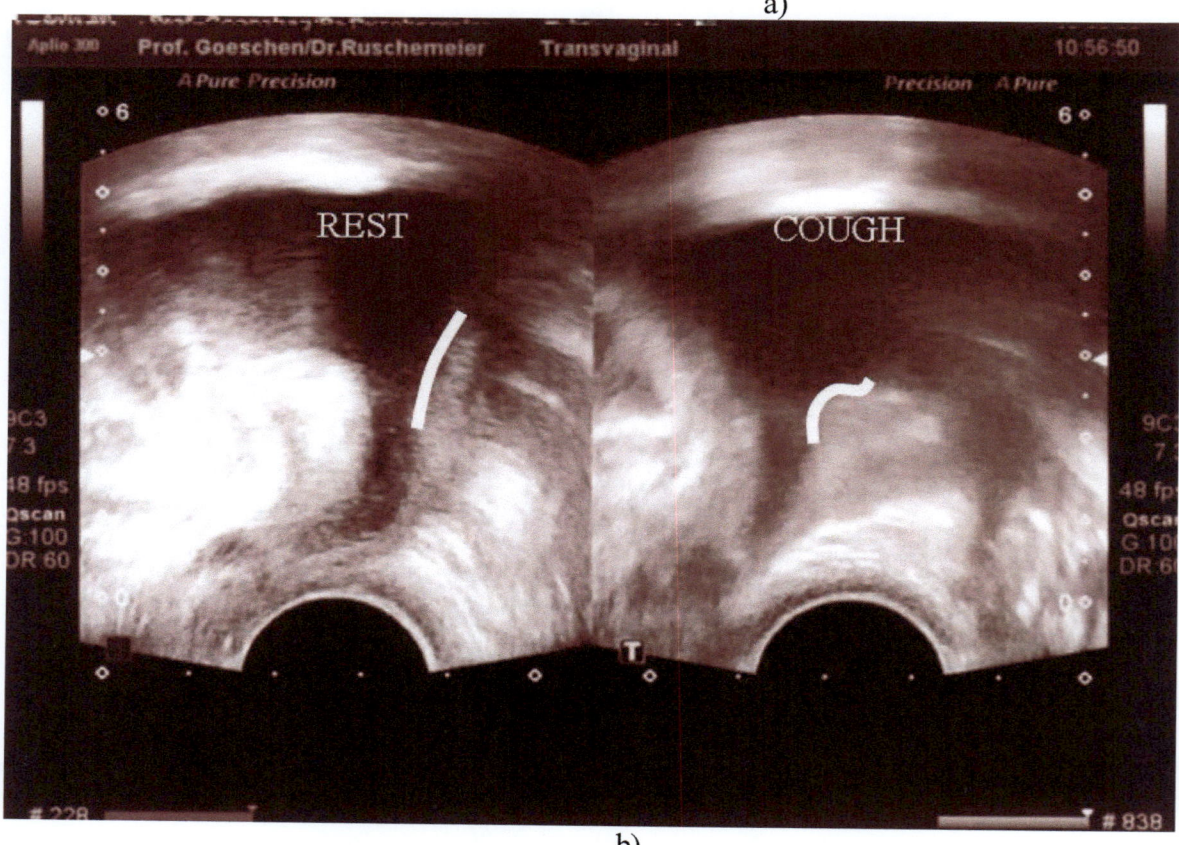

Fig. 8.23. Ultrasound after bulbocavernosus flap (from the archive of **Goeschen, K.**)
a) Before surgery. There is no noticeable mobilization of the bladder neck during coughing or during Valsalva maneuver.
b) After surgery. Normal mobilization of the area of the bladder neck

STV surgery was performed exclusively in 5 patients, 134 of them needed a concomitant treatment of posterior compartment. There was no significant bleeding in any case. The average hospitalization period was 5 days, ranging from 2 to 9 days. All the patients were able to move at least 4 hours postoperatory. Three patients were unable to urinate spontaneously after the removal of Foley catheter at one-day postoperatory and urethral catheterization was necessary for another 24 hours.

Ultrasound after bulbocavernosus flap in patients who were successfully operated, demonstrated a normal movement of the bladder neck and CEA, Fig. 8.23.*a* and *b*.

Thus, with regard to STV treatment, the aim should be the restoration of vagina elasticity around the bladder neck, CEA, so that "*F1*" and "*F2*" can act independently, Fig. 8.15. As a first step, it is essential to dissect the vagina from the urethra and bladder neck and to excise the whole scar tissue, "*urethrovesicolysis*". There must be no residual scar tissue to anchor the bladder neck to the pelvic lateral wall. The second step is to bring healthy tissue at the level of vaginal mucosa around the bladder neck to restore elasticity and to be able to prevent the formation of a new scar at this level.

The "*I*" shaped plastic surgery heals less than a quarter of the patients. That is why we decided not to continue with this method in case in which there is an obvious tissue deficiency. It is still the simplest surgical technique, but keeps its indication only in cases in which there is no major tissue defect. "*I*" shaped plastic surgery works very well in patients whose symptoms cause is the excessive lifting of bladder neck, as for example after Burch colposuspension that coexists with a cystocele. However, if there is a significant lack of vaginal mucosa, it should be covered with a skin graft or a flap.

The results of the technique with a free skin graft are superior to "I" plastic surgery, but a healing rate of about 50% is not convincing. The free skin graft is problematic because there is no blood intake, so in almost one third of the patients, the graft does not take up the vascularization from the adjacent tissues, or it can contract excessively.

Bulbocavernosus flap surgery is more challenging from the technical point of view, but with the advantage of bringing its own source of vascularization. This is, in our opinion, the explanation for the high rate of healing. It is essential to this technique not to compromise the vascular source of the flap. Thus, the pedicle must be sufficiently thick to prevent compression of the vessels in the pedicle, and the space created at the level of the lateral vaginal wall for the flap passage must be adequate.

The explanation for STV healing is to restore the elasticity of this area and refers to a previously described hypothesis (**Petros P.E. & Ulmsten U., 1990**; **Petros P.E. & Ulmsten U., 1993**), Fig. 8.5. There are separate closing mechanisms for the urethra and the bladder neck. For the first one, the anterior vectors tension the vagina adjacent to each side to close the urethra from the posterior side. In the case of the latter, the inferior/ posterior vectors stretch the vagina proximal and the bladder neck posterior and inferior to close the bladder neck.

An appropriate elasticity is required for these separate movements. If fibrosis occurs at this critical point then the possibility of independent movement disappears and the more powerful posterior force prevails over the anterior one. As a result, the urethra is forced to open.

9. 21st century perspectives

The direction in which perineal surgery will develop is hard to predict. In the last ten years, the surgery of uterine prolapse and stress urinary incontinence has seen an important boost.

Abdominal surgical techniques, which are currently more and more replaced by the laparoscopic ones, use polypropylene materials that are placed retroperitoneally and do not have special complications. For this reason, these techniques are internationally accepted and are further developed by finding new fixation points that represent the best anatomical solution. Moreover, there is a special interest also for the robotic technique, which, unfortunately, is still very complex and expensive and cannot become a routine one in the near future.

The issue of the abdominal surgical approach is that it can only coherently solve the problem of prolapse at de Lancey I level and not levels II, cystocele/ rectocele and III, suburethral/ perineal.

These levels remain approachable both on vaginal and classical approach and by using alloplastic materials. The problem of this surgical approach is that it requires a special experience in tactile identifiable topographic anatomy through the so-called *"landmarks"*. Learning this anatomy and implicitly these techniques is hard, these surgeries being performed in virtual spaces that have to be created by the surgeon.

Moreover, the inexperienced use of these techniques with alloplastic materials on vaginal approach by inexperienced surgeons has led to a high rate of complications, noted in 2008 by FDA (Food and Drug Association). This has led to a certain international uncertainty and unfortunately has hindered the evolution of these techniques.

Logically, an urogynecology surgeon should master abdominal/ laparoscopic and vaginal approach techniques. Unfortunately, many surgical specialties do not practice vaginal approach and do not know urology, general surgery, and, the new generations of gynecologists are limited to laparoscopic techniques, which, being handy techniques, are much easier to learn and practice, including the 3D and robotics.

A new impact of perineal surgical treatment is Petros' Integral Theory. It correlates perineal anatomic defects, often discrete, with major functional, urological, and proctologic disorder. From the point of view of this theory, the intention is to repair the anatomical defect and thus to solve the pathophysiological phenomena involved. Therefore, it is a functional surgery with a much more complex concept than the traditional uterovaginal prolapse surgery.

This fascinating multifactorial theory forces the closeness of many specialties that are implicitly bound to think and work together: gynecology, surgery, urology, neurology, and others.

It is quite predictable that in the next decades this new method of diagnosis and therapy, governed by Integral Theory, will unite more medical specialties, which is now happening in the so-called *"pelvic floor units"*, and will place perineal surgery, encompassing the current field of prolapse, which is a simple mechanical disorder. To this end, special education of both physicians and patients is required.

References

Abed H., Rahn D.D., Lowenstein L., Balk E.M., Clemons J.L., Rogers R.G., Systematic Review Group of the Society of Gynecologic Surgeons Int Urogynecol J. **2011** Jul, 22 (7): 789-98.

Abendstein B., Brugger B.A., Furtschegger A., Rieger M., Petros P.E. Role of the uterosacral ligaments in the causation of rectal intussusception, abnormal bowel emptying and fecal incontinence-a prospective study. Pelviperineology, **2008***a*, 27: 118–121.

Abendstein B., Petros P.E.P., Richardson P.A., Goeschen K., Dodero D. The surgical anatomy of rectocele and anterior rectal wall intussusception. Int Urogynecol. J. **2008***b*.

Abrams P. Assessment and treatment of urinary incontinence. Lancet, **2000**, 355: 2153-2158.

Abrams P. Urodynamics. Springer, **2006**.

Abrams P., Cardozo L., Fall M., Griffiths D., Rosier P., Ulmsten U., Van Kerrebroeck Ph., Victor A., Wein A. The standardization of terminology of lower urinary tract function. Neurourol Urodynam **2002**, 21: 167-178.

Abrams P., Cardozo L., Fall M., Griffiths D., Rosier R., Ulmsten U., van Kerrebroeck P., Victor A., Wein A. The Standardisation of Terminology of Lower Urinary Tract Function: ReportfromtheStandardisationSub-committee of the International Continence Society. Neurourology and Urodynamics, **2002**, 21: 167-178.

Abrams P.K., Andersson E., Birder L., Brubaker L., Cardozo L., Chapple C., Cottenden A., Davila W., de Ridder D., Dmochowski R., Drake M., DuBeau C., Fry, C., Hanno P., Hay Smith J., Herschorn S., Hosker G., Kelleher C., Koelbl H., Khoury S., Madoff R,. Milsom I., Moore K., Newman D., Nitti V., Norton C., Nygaard I., Payne C., Smith A., Staskin D., Tekgul S., Thuroff J., Tubaro A., Vodusek D.B., Wein A., Wyndaele JJ., the Members of the Committees, 4th International Consultation on Incontinence Recommendations of the International Scientific Committee: Evaluation and Treatment of Urinary Incontinence, Pelvic Organ Prolapse and Faecal Incontinence. **2009**.

Adekanmi O.A., Freeman R.M., Jackson S., Puckett M., Papapanos P. Prevalence of pubococcygeus muscle detachment from the pubic bone in women with symptomatic anterior vaginal compartment prolapse. J Pelvic Med Surg. **2003**, 9(4): 173–177.

Agarwala N., Hasiak N., Shade M. Laparoscopic sacral colpopexy with Gynemesh as graft material-experience and results. Journal of Minimally Invasive Gynecology, **2007**, Vol. 14, No. 5: 577-583.

Aldridge A.H. Transplantation of fascia for relief of urinary stress incontinence. Am J Obstet Gynecol 44: 398, **1942**.

Amid P.K. Classification of biomaterials and their related complications in abdominal wall hernia surgery, Hernia, May **1997**, Volume 1, Issue 1: 15-21.

Amrute K.V., Eisenberg E.R., Rastinehad A.R., Kushner L., Badlani G.H. Analysis of outcomes of single polypropylene mesh in total pelvic floor reconstruction. Neurourol Urodyn. **2007**, 26 (1): 53-8.

Angulo J.C., Mateo E., Lista F., Andrés G. Reconstructive treatment of female urethral estenosis secondary to erosion by suburethral tape. Actas Urol Esp. **2011** Apr, 35 (4): 240-5.

Araki I., Haneda Y., Mikami T., Takeda M. Incontinence and detrusor dysfunction associated with pelvic organ prolapse: clinical value of preoperative urodynamic evaluation. Int Urogynecol J. **2009**, 20: 1301–1306.

Arthure G.E., Savage D. Uterine prolapse and prolapse of the vaginal vault treated by sacral hysteropexy. The Journalof Obstetrics and Gynaecology of the British Empire, vol. 64, no.3: 355–360, **1957**.

Aukee P., Usenius J.P., Kirkinen P. An evaluation of pelvic floor anatomy and function by MRI. Eur J Obstet Gynecol Reprod Biol, **2004**, 112(1):84–8.

Aungst M.J., Friedman E.B., von Pechmann W.S., Horbach N.S., Welgoss J.A. De novo stress incontinence and pelvic muscle symptoms after transvaginal mesh repair. Am J Obstet Gynecol **2009**, 201: 73.e1–73.e7.

Auwad W., Freeman R.M., Swift S. Is the pelvic organ prolapse quantification system (POPQ) being used? A survey of members of the International Continence Society (ICS) and the American Urogynecologic Society (AUGS). International Urogynecology Journal and Pelvic Floor Dysfunction, **2004** Sep-Oct,15 (5): 324-7.

Baden W.F., Walker T.A. Surgical Repair of Vaginal Defects. Philadelphia: Lippincott, **1992**: 161–174.

Baer J.L., Reis R.A. Laemle R.M. Prolapse of the uterus shifting trends in treatment, American Journal of Obstetrics and Gynecology, **1937**, vol. 34, no. 5: 827–839.

Baessler K., Schuessler B. Abdominal sacropexy and anatomy and function of the posterior compartment. Obstetrics and Gynecology, **2001**, Vol. 97: 678-684.

Baldy J.M. A new operation for retrodisplacement. Am J Obstet, **1902,** 45: 650.

Barrett G, Pendry E, Peacock J, et al (2000) Women's sexual health after childbirth. BJOG 107:186-95.

Bartolo D.C.C., Macdonald A.D.H. Fecal continence and defecation. In: The Pelvic Floor, its functions and disorders. Eds Pemberton J, Swash M, and Henry MM, WB Saunders, London, **2002**: 77-83.

Berek and Novak's Gynecology 15th Edition Lippincott Williams and Wilkins, Hardcover, Rs, **2012**: 1560.

Berghmans L.C.M., Frederiks C.M.A., De Bie R.A., Weil E.H.J., Smeets L.W.H., Van Waalwijk van Doorn E.S.C. Janknegt R.A. Efficacy of biofeedback, when included with pelvic floor muscle exercise treatment, for genuine stress incontinence. Neurourol and Urodyn, **1996**, 15: 37-52.

Berghmans L.C.M., Hendriks H.J.M., Bø K., Hay-Smith De Bie R.A., Van Waalwijk van Doorn E.S.C. Conservative treatment of stress urinary incontinence in women: a systematic review of randomized clinical trials. Br J Urol, **1998**, 82: 181-191.

Berghmans L.C.M., Hendriks H.J.M., De Bie R.A., Van Waalwijk van Doorn E.S.C., Bø K., Van Kerrebroeck Ph.E.V. Conservative treatment of urge urinary incontinence in woman, a systematic review of randomized clinical trials. BJU International, **2000**, 85: 254-263.

Berman I.R. Sutureless laparoscopic rectopexy for procidentia. Technique and implications. Dis Colon Rectum, **1992**, 35: 689-693.

Bissell D. Total hysterectomy, per vaginam, lapping of the anterior vaginal wall fascia and the approximation of the cardinal ligaments, for the cure of extreme procidentia uteri of long standing, The American Journal of Obstetrics and Diseases of Women and Children, vol. 77, **1918**.

Blaisdell F.E. The Anatomy of the Sacrouterine Ligaments. Anat Rec, **1917**, 12: 1-42.

Blaivas J., Marks B., Weiss J. Differential Diagnosis of Overactive Bladder in Men. J Urol. December **2009**, Vol. 182: 2814-2818.

Bø K., Hage R.H., Kvarstein B., Jorgensen J., Larsen S. Plevic floor muscle exercise for the treatment of female stress urinary incontinence. III Effects of two different degrees of pelvic floor muscle exercises. Neurourol Urodyn, **1990**, 9: 489-502.

Bojahr B., Tchartchian G., Waldschmidt M., Ohlinger R., De Wilde R.L. Laparoscopic Sacropexy: A Retrospective Analysis of the Subjective Outcome in 310 Cases. Obstetrics and Gynecology International, **2012**, Article ID 538426, 6: 2012.

Bonney V. The principles that should underlie all operations for prolapse. The Journal of Obstetrics and Gynecology of the British Empire, **1934**, vol. 41, no. 5: 669–683.

Bradley C.S., Nygaard I.E. Vaginal wall descensus and pelvic floor symptoms in older women. Obstet Gynecol **2005**, 106: 759–66.

Breivik H, Collett B., Ventafridda V., Cohen R., Gallacher D. Survey of chronic pain in Europe: prevalence, impact on daily life, and treatment. Eur J Pain. **2006** May, 10(4): 287-333.

Brown J.S., Waetjen L.E., Subak L.L., Thom D.H., Van den E.S., Vittinghoff E. Pelvic organ prolapse surgery in the United States, 1997. Am J Obstet Gynecol, **2002**, 186: 712-716.

Brubaker L., Glazener C., Jacquentin B., Maher C, Melgrem A., Norton P. Surgery for pelvic organ prolapse. In: 4th International Consultation on Incontinence. Recommendations of the International Scientific Committee: evaluation and treatment of urinary incontinence,
pelvic organ prolapse and faecal incontinence. **2008** Jul 5–9, Paris, France: 1273–320.

Bruch H.P., Herold A., Schiedeck T., Schwandner O: Laparoscopic surgery for rectal prolapse and outlet obstruction. Dis Colon Rectum, **1999**, 42: 1189-1194.

Bulent T.M., Sendag F., Dilek U., Guner H: Laparoscopic burch colposuspension: comparison of effectiveness of extraperitoneal and transperitoneal techniques. Eur J Obstet Gynecol Reprod Biol, **2004**, 116: 79-84.

Bump R.C., Mattiasson A., Bo K. The standardization of terminology of female pelvic organ prolapse and pelvic floor dysfunction. American Journal of Obstetrics and Gynecology, **1996,** vol. 175, no. 1: 10-17.

Burch J.C. Urethrovaginal fixation to Cooper's ligament for correction of stress incontinence, cystocele and prolapse. Am J Obstet Gynecol, **1961**, 81: 281-290.

Burrows L.J., Meyn L.A., Walters M.D., Weber A.M. Pelvic symp- toms in women with pelvic organ prolapse. Obstetrics and Gynecology, **2004**, Vol. 104, No. 5 I: 982-988.

Butrick C.W., Sanford D., Hou Q., Mahnken J.D. Chronic pelvic pain syndromes: clinical, urodynamic, and urothelial observations. Int Urogynecol J Pelvic Floor Dysfunct. **2009**, 20: 1047-53.

Caliskan A., Goeschen K., Zumrutbas A.E. Long term results of modified posterior intravaginal slingplasty (P-IVS) in patients with pelvic organ prolapse. Pelviperineology, **2015**, 34: 94-100.

Calomfirescu N., Ambert V., Manu-Marin A.V. Incontinența urinară. Ghid de terapie și tratament. Editura Medicală, **2010**.

Calomfirescu N., Manu-Marin A.V. Urodinamica și Neuro Urologie. Fundamente, tehnici, aplicații. Editura Academiei Române, **2004**.

Campbell R.M. The Anatomy and Histology of the Sacrouterine Ligaments. Am J Obstet Gynecol **1950**, 59: 1-12.

Caruso D., Gomez Ch., Gousse A. Medical management of stress
urinary incontinence:Is there a future? Current Urology Report **2009**, 10 (5): 401-407.

Castaing T., Abello D.E. Prospective study on 185 females with urinary incontinence treated by an outside-in transobturator suburethral sling. Pelviperineology, 1 March **2012**, Issue: Vol. 31 - N.

Chen X., Tong X., Jiang M., Li H., Qiu J., Shao L., Yang X. A modified inexpensive transobturator vaginal tape inside-out procedure versus tension-free vaginal tape for the treatment of SUI: a prospective comparative study. Arch Gynecol Obstet. **2011** Dec, 284 (6): 1461-6.

Choppin S. Removal of the uterus and its appendages in a case of procidentia uteri, by means of the Ecraseur, Southern Journal of the Medical Sciences, **1866**: 841.

CNGOF (2009) Mises à jour en Gynéco Obstétrique, Tome XXXIII, Paris.

Cunningham F., Leveno K., Bloom S., Hauth J., Rouse D., Spong C., Williams Obstetrics. 23rd Edition, **2010**.

Daniels J., Gray R., Hills R.K., Latthe P., Buckley L., Gupta J., Selman T., Adey E., Xiong T., Champaneria R., Lilford R., Khan K.S. On behalf of the LUNA Trial Collaboration. Laparoscopic Uterosacral Nerve Ablation for Alleviating Chronic Pelvic Pain. JAMA, **2009**, 302: 955-961.

Davis K., Kumar D. Posterior pelvic floor compartment disorders. Best Pract Res Clin Obstet Gynaecol. **2005** Dec, 19(6): 941-58.

De Lancey J.O.L. Anatomic aspects of vaginal eversion after hysterectomy. Amer.J.Obstet.Gynecol. **1992**, 166: 1717-1728.

De Lancey JO. (**1994**) Structural support of the urethra as it relates to stress urinary incontinence: the hammock hypothesis. Am J Obstet Gynecol 170:1713-20; discussion 20-3.

De Lancey J.O., Morgan D.M., Fenner D.E.. Comparison of levator ani defects and function in women with and without pelvic organ prolapse. Obstet Gynecol. **2007**, 109: 295-302.

De Lancey J.O. Anatomic aspects of vaginal eversion after hysterectomy, American Journal of Obstetrics and Gynecology, **1992,** vol. 66, no. 6, part 1: 1717–1728.

De Lancey J.O.L. Fascial and muscular abdominalities in women with urethral hypermobility and anterior vaginal wall prolapse; Am J Obstet Gynecol **2002**, 187: 93-8.

De Lancey J.O.L., Hurd W.W. Size of the urogenital hiatus in the levator ani muscles in normal women and women with pelvic organ prolapse. Obstet Gynecol, **1998**, 91: 364–8.

Debodinance P., Delporte P. Miniarc: prospective study and follow up at one year about 72 patients. J Gynecol Obstet Biol Reprod (Paris), **2010**, 39: 25.

Delmas V. La bandelette transobturatrice Uratape dans le traitement de l'incontinence urinaire d'effort de la femme: mécanisme d'action. AFU; **2002**.

Delmas V. The transobturator tape (TOT®): anatomical dangers. EAU, **2003**.

Delorme E. La bandelette trans-obturatrice : un procédé mini-invasif pour traiter l'incontinence urinaire d'effort de la femme., Urologie, Châlon sur Saône, France, Progrès en Urologie, **2001**, 11: 1306-1313.

Delorme E. OPUR treatment of anterior prolapse and mid-segment prolapse of genito-urinary tract through vaginal route [DVD]. Saint Etienne: Abiss Company; **2011**.

Dietz H.P., Franco A.V., Shek K.L., Kirby A. Avulsion injury and levator hiatal ballooning: two independent risk factors for prolapse? An observational study. Acta Obstet Gynecol Scand. **2012** Feb, 91(2): 211-4.

Dietz H.P., Steensma A.B. Posterior compartment prolapse on two-dimensional and three dimensional pelvic floor ultrasound: the distinction between true rectocele, perineal hypermobility and enterocele. Ultrasound Obstet Gynecol, **2005**, 26: 73–7.

Dietz H.P., Steensma A.B., Hastings R. Three-dimensional ultrasound imaging of the pelvic floor: the effect of parturition on paravaginal support structures. Ultrasound Obstet Gynecol, **2003**. 21: 589–95.

Digesu G.A., Hendricken C., Fernando R., Khullar V. Do Women With Pure Stress Urinary Incontinence Need Urodynamics? Urology, **2009**, 74: 278–282.

Douglas J.A. Description of the Peritoneum and of that Part of the Membrana Cellularis Which Lies on its Outside. London: J. Roberts. **1730**.

Downing K.T. Division of Female Pelvic Medicine and Reconstructive Surgery, Department of Obstetrics & Gynecology and Women's Health, Albert Einstein College of Medicine/Montefiore Medical Center, Bronx, NY 10461, USAHindawi Publishing Corporation Obstetrics and Gynecology International Volume, **2012**,

Durnea C.M., Khashan A.S., Kenny L.C., Durnea U.A., Smyth M.M., O'Reilly B.A. Prevalence, etiology and risk factors of pelvic organ prolapse in premenopausal primiparous women. Int Urogynecol J. **2014** Apr 16.

Duthie G.S., Bartolo D.C. Abdominal rectopexy for rectal prolapse: a comparison of techniques. Br J Surg, **1992**, 79: 107-113.

Elterman D., Chughtai B. Long-term Outcomes Following Abdominal Sacrocolpopexy for Pelvic Organ Prolapse. Urology, **2013**, 82(4): 757-8.

Enache T, Enache A., Moisa M. Hypertrophic cervical elongation associated with pelvic organ prolapse – a real concept? ISPP 16th International Pelviperinology Conference. 5-7 september, **2015**, Istanbul, Turcia.

Enache T. Tehnici de reconstrucţie chirurgicală cu material aloplastic a tulburărilor de statică pelviană. Teză de doctorat. Universitatea de medicină şi farmacie *"Carol Davila"* Bucureşti, **2014**.

Enache T., Enache A. Teoria Integrală – O nouă perspectivă asupra problemelor de statică pelviană. Bucureşti, Romania, Analele Medicale Române – Vol I, nr.1, **2011**.

Enache T., Enache A., Moisa M. Hypertrophic cervical elongation associated with pelvic organ prolapse – a real concept? 5-7 september **2015***b*, Istanbul, Turcia.

Enache T., Enache A., Moisa M. Ligament functional reconstruction. 10-12 decembrie, **2015***a*, Ljubljana, Slovenia.

Enache T., Enache A., Moisa M., Ionică M. Pelvic floor disorders – a new perspective. Second MIPS Annual Meeting, November 26-29, **2014**, Nimes, Franţa.

Enache T., Enache A., Moisa M., Ionică M. Surgical management of posterior compartment defect in patients with pelvic floor dysfunction. Italy, Pelviperineology **2016***a*, 35: 37-39.

Enache T., Enache A., Moisa M., Maier T., Iana G., Luchian B., Marinescu B., Neagu C., Albu D. Prolapsul uterin şi simptomatologia urinară – tratament comun. A 10-a Conferinţă Naţională de Obstetrică şi Ginecologie. 25-27 octombrie **2012**, Bucureşti, Romania.

Enache T., Enache A., Mueller-Funogea I.-A., Moisa M., Marinescu B., Puia S., Neagu C., Maier T. Vaginal enterocel repair – a new perspective. Elselvier. International Journal of Gynecology & Obstetrics. 119: S668-S669, october **2012**.

Enache T., Marinescu B., Enache A., Neagu C. Surgical cure of enterocoele and rectocoele – a new perspective (case-report). ObstetricA şi Ginecologia. Cluj Napoca, Romania, Revista Societăţii de Obstetrică şi Ginecologie. Nr. LXI, Nr. 2, Aprilie – Iunie **2013.**

Enache T., Mueller-Funogea I-A., Enache A., Moisa M., Enache T.sr.. Trusă chirurgicală pentru corecţia elitrocelului pe cale vaginală. Brevet de invenţie. OSIM nr.130607/29.11.**2016***b*.

Enache T., Mueller-Funogea, I.A., Enache A., Moisa M., Iana G., Luchian, B. Urgency and nocturia – a posterior compartment defect? The 18th World Congress on Controversies in Obstetrics, Gynecology and Infertility, Viena, Austria, **2013**.

Eriksen B.C. Electrostimulation of the pelvic floor in female urinary incontinence. Thesis University of Trondheim, Norway, **1989**.

Evans S.F.. Editorial. Chronic pelvic pain in Australia and New Zealand Australian and New Zealand Journal of Obstetrics and Gynaecology, **2012**, 52: 499-501.

Falconer C., Ekmanordeberg G., Ulmsten U. Changes in paraurethralconnective tissue at menopause are counteracted by estrogen. Maturitas, **1996**, 24 (3): 197-204.

Fall M., Baranowksi A.P., Fowler C.J. Chronic pelvic pain is non-malignant pain perceived in structures related to the pelvis of either men or women, **2003**.

Fall M., Baranowski A.P., Elneil S., Engeler D., Hughes J., Messelink E.J., Oberpenning F., Williams A.C. EAU Guidelines on Chronic Pelvic Pain, European Urology, **2010**, 57, 3: 5- 48.

Fantl J.A., Newman D.K., Colling J. Urinary incontinence in adults: Acute and chronic management. Rockville Md: US Dept of Health and Human Services, Public Health Service,

Agency for Health Care Policy and Research, March **1996**.

Farnsworth B. Posterior IVS for vault suspension: A re-evaluation, Centre for Pelvic Reconstructive Surgery, Sydney Adventist Hospital, Wahroonga, Australia, **2007**.

Farnsworth B., Goeschen K., Müller-Funogea A. Life-Sugery: Sacrospinous Fixation. Würselen, 28.4.**2008**.

Farnsworth B.N. Posterior intravaginal slingplasty (infracoc- cygeal Sacropexy) for severe posthysterectomy vaginal vault prolapse – a preliminary report on efficacy and safety. Int J Urogynecol, **2001**, 12: 304-308.

Feiner B., Jelovsek J.E., Maher C. Efficacy and safety of transvaginal mesh kits in the treatment of prolapse of the vaginal apex: a systematic review. BJOG **2009**,116: 15–24.

Feiner B., Maher C. Vaginal mesh contraction: definition, clinical presentation, and management. Obstet Gynecol. **2010** Feb, 115 (2 Pt 1): 325-30.

Foley C., Patki P., Boustead G. Unrecognized bladder perforation with mid-urethral slings. BJU Int. **2010** Nov, 106 (10): 1514-8.

Forgács S., Peschka M., Pretterklieber M.L.. Der chronische Beckenschmerz, Wiener Klinisches Magazin 1/2012, Springer Heidelberg-New York, **2012**.

Fothergill W.E. Anterior colporrhaphy and its combination with amputation of the cevixas a single operation. J Obstet Gynaecol Br Emp, **1915,** 27: 146.

Francis W.J., Jeffcoate T.N. Dyspareunia following vaginal operations. J Obstet Gynaecol Br Commonw. **1961** Feb, 68: 1–10.

Frankenhäuser F. Die Nerven der Gebaermutter. Jena, **1867**.

Fritsch H. Beckenhöhle und Beckenboden. In: Drenckhahn D, ed. Benninghoff-Drenckhahn Anatomie. München: Urban & Fischer, **2008**.

Frohme C., Ludt F., Varga Z., Olbert P.J., Hofmann R., Hegele A. TOT approach in stress urinary incontinence (SUI) - outcome in obese female. BMC Urol. **2014**, 14: 20.

Furtmüller G.J., McKenna C.A., Ebmer J., Dellon A.L. Pudendal nerve 3-dimensional illustration gives insight into surgical approaches. Ann Plast Surg, **2014** Dec, 73 (6): 670-8.

Gadonneix P., Ercoli A., Salet-Lizee D., Cotelle O., Bolner B., Van Den A.M., Villet R. Laparoscopic sacrocolpopexy with two separate meshes along the anterior and posterior vaginal walls for multicompartment pelvic organ prolapse. J Am Assoc Gynecol Laparosc, **2004**, 11: 29-35.

Ganatra A.M., Rozet F., Sanchez-Salas R., Barret E., Galiano M., Cathelineau X, Vallancien G. The current status of laparoscopic sacrocolpopexy: a review. Eur Urol. **2009** May, 55(5): 1089-1103.

Ganesh A., Upponi S., Hon L.Q. Chronic pelvic pain due to pelvic congestion syndrome: the orle of diagnostic and interventional radiology. Cardiovasc Intervent Radiol. **2007**, 30: 1105-11.

Ganj F.A., Ibeanu O.A., Bedestani A., Nolan T.E., Chesson R.R. Complications of transvaginal monofilament polypropylene mesh in pelvic organ prolapse repair. Int Urogynecol J Pelvic Floor Dysfunct. **2009** Aug, 20 (8): 919-25.

Goeschen K. Can motor urge incontinence be surgically cured? Pelviperineology, **2007**, 26: 41-42.

Goeschen K. Posterior Fornix Syndrome: Comparison of original (2004) and modified (2015) post-PIVS anatomic and symptomatic results: a personal journey. Pelviperineology, **2015**, 34: 85-91.

Goeschen K. Tethered Vagina. In: PE Papa Petros (ed) The female pelvic floor. Springer, Berlin, Heidelberg, New York, Tokio **2006**.

Goeschen K., Gent H-J. Das posteriore Fornixsyndrom. Frauenarzt, **2004**, 45: 104–112

Goeschen K., Mueller-Funogea A, Petros P. Tethered vagina syndrome: cure of severe involuntary urinaryloss by skin graft to the bladder neck area of vagina Pelviperineology

2010, 29: 100-102.

Goeschen K., Petros P. Der weibliche Beckenboden. Springer, Heidelberg-New York, **2008**.

Gold D.M., Goeschen K. Application of the Pescatori Iceberg to 198 patients presenting with chronic pelvic pain before and after posterior sling surgery. Pelviperineology, **2016**, in press.

Gombrich E.H. A little History of the World, Yale University Press, New Haven, Conn, USA, **2005**.

Guyomard A, Delorme E. Transvaginal treatment of anterior or central urogenital prolapse using six tension-free straps and light mesh. Int J Gynecol Obstet **2016**;133:365–9.

Halban J. Anatomie und Aitologie der Genitalprolapse beim Weibe, Wilhelm Braumuller, Leipzig, Germany, **1907**.

Hannah S.L., Chin A. Laparoscopic retropubic urethropexy. J Am Assoc Gynecol Laparosc, **1996**, 4: 47-52.

Haylen B.T., Freeman R.M., Swift S.E., Cosson M., Davila G.W., Deprest J., Dwyer P.L., Fatton B., Kocjancic E., Lee J., Maher C., Petri E., Rizk D.E., Sand P.K., Schaer G.N, Webb R. An International Urogynecological Association (IUGA)/International Continence Society (ICS) joint terminology and classification of the complications related directly to the insertion of prostheses (meshes, implants, tapes) and grafts in female pelvic floor surgery. International Urogynecological Association, International Continence Society, Joint IUGA/ICS Working Group on Complications Terminology Neurourol Urodyn. **2011** Jan, 30 (1): 2-12.

Hendrix S.L., Clark A., Nygaard I., Aragaki A., Barnabei V., McTiernan A. Pelvic organ prolapse in the Women's Health Initiative: gravity and gravidity. Am J Obstet Gynecol, **2002**, 186: 1160-1166.

Higgs P.J., Chua H.L., Smith A.R.B. Long term review of laparoscopic sacrocolpopexy, BJOG, **2005**, Vol. 112, No. 8: 1134-1138.

Hiroshi Y., Evans F.G. Strength of biological materials, Huntington, New York: Robert E. Krieger Pub. Co, **1973**.

Hoshino K., Yoshimura K., Hachisuga T. How to reduce the operative time of laparoscopic sacrocolpopexy?, Gynecology and Minimally Invasive Therapy, **2016**.

Hsu Y., Lewicky-Gaupp C., DeLancey J.O.L. Posterior compartment anatomy as seen in MRI and 3D reconstruction from asymptomatic nulliparas. Am J Obstet Gynecol, **2008**, 198: 651–7.

Hsu Y., Summers A., Hussain H.K., Guire K.E., DeLancey J.O.L. Levator plate angle in women with pelvic organ prolapse compared to women with normal support using dynamic MR imaging. Am J Obstet Gynecol, **2006**, 194: 1427–33.

Huang W.C., Yang S.H., Yang J.M. Three-dimensional transperineal sonographic characteristics of the anal sphincter complex in nulliparous women. Ultrasound Obstet Gynecol, **2007**, 30: 210–20.

Hyrtl J. Handbuch der topographischen Anatomie. Viena, **1853**.

Ignacio E.A., Dua R., Sarin S. Pelvic congestion syndrome: diagnosis and treatment.
Semin Intervent Radiol. **2008**, 25: 361-8.

Irvin W., Hullfish K. Abdominal techniques for surgical management of vaginal vault prolapse. Operative Gynecology Ninth Edition OBG Manag. **2005** December, 17(12): 19-23.

Judd J.P., Siddiqui N.Y., Barnett J.C., Visco A.G., Havrilesky L.J., Wu J.M. Cost-minimization analysis of robotic-assisted, laparoscopic, and abdominal sacro-colpopexy, Journal of Minimally Invasive Gynecology, **2010**, vol. 17, no. 4: 493–499.

Kaiwa Y., Kurokawa Y., Namiki K., Myojin T., Ansai M., Satomi S: Outcome of laparoscopic rectopexy for complete rectal prolapse in patients older than 70 years versus younger patients. Surg Today, **2004**, 34: 742-746.

Kamina P. Anatomie Operatoire, Gynecologie et Obstetrique, Maloine, Paris, **2000**.

Karam J.A., Vazquez D.V., Lin V.K., Zimmern P.E. BJU Elastin expression and elastic fibre width in the anterior vaginal wall of postmenopausal women with and without prolapse. Int. **2007** Aug, 100(2): 346-50.

Kato T., Murakami G., Yabuki Y Does the cardinal ligament of the uterus contain a nerve that should be preserved in radical hysterectomy. Anat Sci Int, **2002**, 77: 161-8.

Kaufman Y., Singh S.S., Alturki H., Lam A. Age and sexual activity are risk factors for mesh exposure following transvaginal mesh repair. Int Urogynecol J. **2011** Mar, 22 (3): 307-13.

Kellokumpu I.H., Vironen J., Scheinin T. Laparoscopic repair of rectal prolapse: a prospective study evaluating surgical outcome and changes in symptoms and bowel function. Surg Endosc, **2000**, 14: 634-640.

Kelly C.E., Evaluation of Voiding Dysfunction and Measurement of Bladder Volume, Rev Urol. **2004**, 6(Suppl 1): S32–S37.

Kelly H.A. Incontinence of urine in women. Urologic and Cutaneous Review, **1913**, 17: 291-329.

Kennelly M.J., Moore R., Nguyen J.N. Prospective evaluation of a single incision sling for stress urinary incontinence. Int Urogynecol J, **2010**. 184: 604.

Kerkhof M.H., Ruiz-Zapata A.M., Bril H., Bleeker M.C., Belien J.A., Stoop R., Helder M.N. Changes in tissue composition of the vaginal wall of premenopausal women with prolapse. Am J Obstet Gynecol. **2014** Feb, 210(2): 168. e1-9.

Kiilholma P., Haarala M., Polvi H., Makinen J., Chancellor M.B. Sutureless endoscopic colposuspension with fibrin sealant. Tech Urol, **1995**, 1: 81-83.

Ko J.K., Ku C.H. Embolization for pelvic arterial bleeding following a transobturator tape procedure. J Obstet Gynaecol Res. **2014** Mar, 40 (3): 865-8.

Kobayashi Y., Kuroda K., Shibuya H., Nishigaya Y., Momomura M., Matsumoto H., Iwashita M. Preoperative evaluation of deep venous thrombosis in patients with pelvic organ prolapse. J Obstet Gynaecol Res. **2014** Jun, 40 (6): 1754-8.

Krause H.G., Goh J.T., Sloane K., Higgs P., Carey M.P: Laparoscopic sacral suture hysteropexy for uterine prolapse. Int Urogynecol J Pelvic Floor Dysfunct, **2006**, 17: 378-381.

Kwok S.P., Carey D.P., Lau W.Y., Li A.K. Laparoscopic rectopexy. Dis Colon Rectum, **1994**, 37: 947-948.

Langenbeck C.J.M. Geschichte einer von mir glucklich verichteten extirpation der ganger gebarmutter. Biblioth Chir Ophth Hanover, **1817**, 1: 557.

Latthe Pm. Review of transobturator and retropubic tape procedures for stress urinary incontinence. Curr Opin Obstet Gynecol, **2008**, 20 (4): 31-6.

Lazarou G. Uterine prolapse. http://emedicine.medscape.com/article/264231-overview#a0199 – dec. **2013**.

Lazarou G., Grigorescu B.A., Olson T.R.. Int Urogynecol J Pelvic Floor Dysfunct. **2007** Nov 24.

Lee K.S., Lee Y.S., Seo J.T. A prospective multicenter randomized comparative studybetween the U- and H-type methods of TVT SECUR procedure for the treatment of female stress urinary incontinence: 1-year follow-up. Eur Urol, **2010**, 57: 973.

Lee Y.-S., Han D.H., Lee J.Y., Kim J.C., Choo M.-S., Lee K.-S. Anatomical and Functional Outcomes of Posterior Intravaginal Slingplasty for the Treatment of Vaginal Vault or Uterine Prolapse: A Prospective, Multicenter Study Korean J Urol. **2010** Mar,

51(3): 187-192.

Liu C.Y., Paek W. Laparoscopic retropubic colposuspension (Burch procedure). J Am Assoc Gynecol Laparosc, **1993**, 1: 31-35.

Lo T.S. One-year outcome of concurrent anterior and posterior transvaginal mesh surgery for treatment of advanced urogenital prolapse: case series. J Minim Invasive Gynecol. **2010** Jul-Aug, 17 (4): 473-9.

Luijendijk R.W. Acomparison of suture repair with mesh repair for incisional hernia, New England Journal of Medicine, **2000**, vol. 343, no. 6: 392–398.

Lupu G. Anatomia omului. Aparatul genital. Ed. Universitară „*Carol Davila*", București **2005.**

Lyons T.L. Minimally invasive retropubic urethropexy: the NolanLyons modification to the Burch procedure. Gynecol Endosc, **1994**, 3: 40–52.

Mackenrodt A. Uber dieUrsachen der normalen und pathologischen Lagen des Uterus. Arch Gynak, **1895**, 48: 394-421.

Maher C.F., Feiner B., Baessler K., Schmid C. Surgical management of pelvic organ prolapse in women. Cochrane Database Syst Rev. **2010**, (4): CD004014.

Maher C.F., Qatawneh A.M., Dwyer P.L., Carey M.P., Cornish A., Schluter P.J. Abdominal sacral colpopexy or vaginal sacrospinous colpopexy for vaginal vault prolapse: a prospective randomized study, The American Journal of Obstetrics & Gynecology, **2004**, Vol. 190, No. 1: 20-26.

Maher C.M., Feiner B., Baessler K., Glazener C.M. Surgical management of pelvic organ prolapse in women. Cochrane Database of Systematic Reviews **2010**, Issue 4.

Maher C.M., Feiner B., Bassler K., Glazener C.M. Surgical management of pelvic organ prolapse in women: the updated summary version Cochrane review Int Urogynecol J, **2012**, 22: 1445-1457.

Markovsky O. Pelvic pain caused by apical prolapse: cure by Elevate anterior/apical and Elevate posterior/apical. International Society for Pelviperineology, Munich, Germany 12th- 15th Sept. **2014.**

Marshall V.F., Marchetti A.A., Krantz K.E. The correction of stress incontinence by simple vesicourethral suspension. Surg Gynecol Obstet, **1949,** 88: 509.

Martius H. Die Gynäkologischen Operationen. Thieme Stuttgart.

1936. Martius H. Lehrbuch der Gynäkologie. Thieme, Stuttgart **1946.**

Martius H. U"ber einen häufigen gynäkologischen Symptomkomplex. Archives of Gynecology and Obstetrics, **1938**, 166: 332-335.

Mathias S.D., Kuppermann M., Liberman R.F., Lipschutz R.C., Steege J.F. Chronic pelvic pain: prevalence, health-related quality of life, and economic correlates. Obstetrics and Gynecology, **1996**, 87: 321-7.

Maurer M. 3D Finite Element Pelvic Floor Modeling, The Institute of Mechanical Systems. Conference paper. Conference: 11th World Congress on Computational Mechanics (WCCM XI), 5th European Conference on Computational Mechanics (ECCM V), 6th European Conference on Computational Fluid Dynamics (ECFD VI), July 20-25 **2014**, Barcelona, Spain.

Mayer E.A., Naliboff B.D., Craig A.D. Neuroimaging of the brain–gut axis: from basic understanding to treatment of functional GI disorders. Gastroenterology, **2006**, 131: 1925–1942.

Mayo C.H. Uterine prolapse associated with pelvic relaxation, Journal of Surgery, Gynecology and Obstetrics, **1915,** vol. 20: 257.

McCall M.L. Posterior culdeplasty: surgical correction of enterocele during vaginal hysterectomy; a preliminary report. Obstet Gynecol, **1957**, 10: 595.

Mengert W.F. Mechanics of uterine support and position. I. Factors influencing uterine support (an experimental study), American Journal of Obstetrics and Gynecology, **1936,** vol. 31, no. 5: 775–782.

Messelink B. The standardization of terminology of pelvic floor muscle function and dysfunction. Report from the pelvic floor clinical assessment group of the International Continence Pelvic Care Centre Prinsengracht, Neurourol Urodyn. **2005.** 24(4): 374-80.

Messner-Pellenc L., Moron C. A Mechanical Model For the Opening of the FemaleUrethr, The University of Western Australia School of Mechanical Engineering, **2004. Miller D.,** Lucente V., Babin E., Beach P., Jones P., Robinson D. Prospective clinical assessment of the transvaginal mesh technique for treatment of pelvic organ prolapse-5-year
results. Female Pelvic Med Reconstr Surg **2011,** 17: 139–43.

Miller N.F. A new method of correcting complete inversion of the vagina, Journal of Gynecology and Obstetrics, vol. 44: 550–554.

Moore R.D., Mitchell G.K., Miklos J.R. Single-center retrospective study of the technique, safety and 12-month efficacy of the MiniarcTM single-incision sling: a new minimally invasive procedure for treatment of female SUI. Surg Technol Int, **2009,** 18: 175.

Morgan D.M, DeLancey JO, Guire KE, Fenner DE. Symptoms of anal incontinence and difficult defecation among women with prolapse and a matched control cohort. Am J Obstet Gynecol. **2007,**197(5): 509.e1–509.e6.

Morren G.L., Beets-Tan R.G.H., van Engelshoven J.M.A. Anatomy of the anal canal and perianal structures as defined by phased-array magnetic resonance imaging. Br J Surg, **2001,** 88: 1506–12.

Moschcowitz A.V. The pathogenesis, anatomy and cure of prolapse of the rectum. Surg Gynecol Obstet, **1927,** 15: 7.

Mouritsen L., Larsen J.P. Symptoms, bother and POPQ in women referred with pelvic organ prolapse. International Urogynecology Journal and Pelvic Floor Dysfunction, **2003.,** Vol. 14, No. 2: 122-127.

Mueller-Funogea I.A. Sindromul de fornix posterior, o nouă entitate uroginecologică. Mecanism etiopatogenic și propunere de terapie chirurgicală. Teză de doctorat. UMF „*Carol Davila*", București, **2014.**

Mueller-Funogea I.A., Goeschen K., Linn C., Meid P. Managing an incidental abscess after secondary insertion of transobturator tape, Pelviperineology, June **2012,** Vol. 31 - N.

Muir T.W., Stepp K.J. Adoption of the pelvic organ prolapse quantification system in peer-reviewed literature .Am J Obstet Gynecol. **2003,**189: 1632–1635.

Müller-Funogea A. Posterior fornix syndrome: a new urogynecologic entity. Ethiopathogenesis and proposal for surgical therapy. Thesis, Medical University of Bucharest, Romania, **2014.**

Murphy M. Clinical practice guidelines on vaginal graft use from the society of gynecologic surgeons. Society of Gynecologic Surgeons Systematic Review Group. Obstet Gynecol **2008,** 112: 1123–30.

Murray S., Haverkorn R.M., Lotan Y., Lemack G.E. Int Urogynecol J. Mesh kits for anterior vaginal prolapse are not cost effective. **2011** Apr; 22 (4): 447-52.

Musset R. (1997) Vaginal aplasia with a functional uterus; surgical results and comments. Apropos of 10 case reports. J Gynecol Obstet Biol Reprod 7:316-33.

Myung-Jae J., Hyun-Joo J., Sue-Min C., Sei-Kwang K., Sang-Wook B. Comparison of the treatment outcome of pubovaginal sling, tension-free vaginal tape, and transobturator tape for stress urinary incontinence with intrinsic sphincter deficiency American Journal of Obstetrics & Gynecology, July **2008,** Vol. 199, Issue 1, Pages 76.e1-76.e4.

Narducci F., Occelli B., Hautefeuille J., Cosson M., Francke J.-P., Querleu D., Crepin G. L'arc tendineux du fascia pelvien: etude anatomique; J Gynecol Obstet Biol, **2000,** 29:

644- 649.

Nicolson A., Adeyemo D. Colovaginal fistula: a rare long-term complication of polypropylene mesh sacrocolpopexy. J Obstet Gynaecol. **2009** Jul, 29 (5): 444-5.

Normand L. LE, de Nantes Chu, Cosson Nantes M., de Lille Chu, Cour Lille F., Hôpital Foch, Suresnes … Recommandations pour la pratique clinique Synthèse des recommandations pour le traitement chirurgical du prolapsus génital non récidivé de la femme par l'AFU, le CNGOF, la SIFUD-PP, la SNFCP, et la SCGP.

Nunoo-Mensah J.W., Efron J.E., Young-Fadok T.M. Laparoscopic rectopexy. Surg Endosc, **2007**. 21: 325-326.

Nygaard I.E., McCreery R., Brubaker L., Connolly A., Cundiff G., Weber A.M., Zyczynski H. Abdominal sacropexy: a comprehensive review. Obstetrics and Gynecology, **2004**, Vol. 104, 805-823.

O Sullivan O.O., Reilly B. Difficult sacrocolpopexy, Gynecologic and Obstetric Surgery – challenges and management options – Ed Wiley Blackwell, **2016**.

Oh T.H., Ryu D.S. Transurethral resection of intravesical mesh after midurethral sling procedures. J Endourol. **2009** Aug, 23 (8): 1333-7.

Olsen A.L., Smith VJ., Bergstrom J.O.., Colling J.C., Clark A.L. Epidemiology of surgically managed pelvic organ prolapse and urinary incontinence. Obstet Gynecol, **1997**. 89: 501-506.

Ou C.S., Rowbotham R. Five-year follow-up of laparoscopic bladder neck suspension using synthetic mesh and surgical staples. J Laparoendosc Adv Surg Tech A, **1999**, 9: 249-252.

Panzer J. A mechanical model of the female urethra, Diploma Thesis, University of Western Australia, **2003**.

Pardo JS, Sola VD, Ricci PA, et al (2006) Colpoperineoplasty in women with a sensation of a wide vagina. Acta Obstet Gynecol Scand 85:1125-7.

Papilian V. Anatomia omului. Vol. II, Splanhnologia, ed. VII-a, revizuită şi adăugită de Prof. Dr. Ion Albu, Ed. All, **1993**: 285-208; 337-350.

Par´e A. The Workes of That Famous Chirurgion Ambrose Par´e, Richard Cotes andWilli Du-Gard, London, UK, **1649**.

Paradisi G., Petros P.E.P. Cure of haemorrhoids following a TFS posterior sling and TFS perineal body repair - a case report. Pelviperineology, **2010**, 29: 62-63.

Park G.S., Miller E.J. Jr. Surgical treatment of stress urinary incontinence: a comparison of the Kelly plication, Marshall-Marchetti-Krantz and Pereyra procedures. Obstet Gynecol, **1988**, 71: 575-579.

Patel B.N., Kobashi K.C., Staskin D. Iatrogenic obstruction after sling surgery. Nat Rev Urol. **2012** Aug, 9 (8): 429-34.

Pereyra A.J. A simplified surgical procedure for the correction of stress incontinence in *women*. West J Surg, **1959**, 67: 223–226.

Persu C., Chapple C.R., Cauni V., Gutue S.,. Geavlete P. Pelvic Organ Prolapse Quantification System (POP–Q) – a new era in pelvic prolapse staging Journal of Medicine and Life January, **2011**.

Perumal S., Antipova O., Orgel J.P. Collagen fibril architecture, domain organization, and triple-helical conformation govern its proteolysis. PNAS, **2008**, 105 (8): 2824–2829.

Petros P., Inoue H. Transvaginal perineal body repair for low rectocele. Tech Coloproctol. **2013** Aug, 17 (4): 449-54.

Petros P. Pelvic pain caused by apical prolapse: cure by TFS surgery. International Society for Pelviperineology, Munich, Germany 12th-15th Sept. **2014**.

Petros P. Severe Chronic Pelvic Pain in Women May Be Caused By Ligamentous Laxity in the Posterior Fornix of the Vagina Aitsr. NZ J 0hsrt.r Gyoecol, **1996**, 36, 3: 35.

Petros P. The Female Pelvic Floor – Function and Dysfunction According to the Integral Theory, Second Edition. Springer Medizin Verlag Heidelberg, **2011**a.

Petros P. The Female Pelvic Floor Function, Dysfunction and management According to the Integral theory. Second Edition, Springer Medizin Verlag Heidelberg, **2007**.

Petros P. The Female Pelvic Floor, Function, Dysfunction and Management according to the Integral Theory. Springer, Heidelberg, 3rd Ed. **2010**: 1-330.

Petros P. The Female Pelvic Floor. Function and Dysfunction According to the Integral Theory, Second Edition. Springer Medizin Verlag Heidelberg, **2011**b.

Petros P. The Integral System. Cent European J Urol. **2011**a, 64(3): 110-9.

Petros P. The Integral System. Central European Journal of Urology. **2011**c, 64: 3.

Petros P. Vault prolapse I: Dynamic supports of the vagina, Int J Urogynecol, **2001**a, 12: 292-295.

Petros P. Vault prolapse II: Restoration of dynamic vaginal supports by infracoccygeal sacropexy, an axial daycase vaginal procedure. Int J Urogynecol, **2001**b, 12: 296-303.

Petros P., Richardson P.A. TFS posterior sling improves overactive bladder, pelvic pain and abnormal emptying, even with minor prolapse. A prospective urodynamic study Pelviperineology, **2010**, 29: 52-55.

Petros P., Swash M. A Musculo-Elastic Theory of anorectal function and dysfunction in the female. Pelviperineology, **2008**, 27: 86-87.

Petros P., Swash M. Experimental Study No. 1: Directional muscle forces activate anorectal continence and defecation in the female Pelviperineology, **2008**, 27: 94-97.

Petros P. Influence of hysterectomy on pelvic floor dysfunction. Lancet, **2000**, 356: 1275.

Petros P. New ambulatory surgical methods using an anatomical classification of urinary dysfunction improve stress, urge, and abnormal emptying. Int J Urogynecol, **1997**, 8: 270-278.

Petros P. Reconstructive Pelvic Floor Surgery According to the Integral Theory. In: Petros PE, The Female Pelvic Floor. Springer Heidelberg **2006**, 135-141.

Petros P. Severe chronic pelvic pain in women may be caused by ligamentous laxity in the posterior fornix of the vagina, Aust NZ J Obstet Gynaecol. **1996**, 36:3: 351-354.

Petros P. The female pelvic floor – function, dysfunction and management according to the Integral Theory – third edition – Springer Verlag, **2010**.

Petros P. The integral theory system: A simplified clinical approach with illustrative case histories. Pelviperineology, **2010**, 29: 37-51.

Petros P. Vault prolapse I: dynamic supports of the vagina. Int Urogynecol J Pelvic Floor Dysfunct **2001**, 12: 292–5.

Petros P. The anatomy and dynamics of pelvic floor function and dysfunction In: The female pelvic floor [Internet]. Springer, Berlin, Heidelberg; **2004** [cited 2018 Feb 9]. p. 14–47. Available from https://link.springer.com/chapter/10.1007/978-3-662-05445-1_2.

Petros P., Ulmsten U. An Integral Theory and its Method for the Diagnosis and Management of Female Urinary Incontinence. Scand J Urol Nephrol, **1993**, Suppl 153: 1-93.

Petros P., Ulmsten U. An Integral Theory and its Method, for the Diagnosis and Management of female urinary incontinence. Scandinavian Journal of Urology and Nephrology, **1993**. Vol 27, Suppl. No 153: 1-93.

Petros P., Ulmsten U. An Integral Theory of Female Urinary Incontinence, Acta Obst Gynecol Scand, **1990**, Suppl 153: 1-79.

Petros P., Ulmsten U. Role of the pelvic floor in bladder neck opening and closure: I muscle forces, II vagina. Int. J Urogynecol Pelvic Floor **1997**, 8: 69-80.

Petros P., Ulmsten U. The posterior fornix syndrome: a multiple symptom complex of pelvic pain and abnormal urinary symptoms deriving from laxity in the posterior fornix. Scandinavian Journal of Urology and Nephrology, **1993**, Vol 27 Supplement No 153, PART IV: 89-93.

Petros P., Ulmsten U. The tethered vagina syndrome, post surgical incontinence and I-plasty operation for cure. Act Obstet Gynecol Scand, **1990**, Suppl 153, 69: 63-67.

Petros P., Ulmsten U., Papadimitriou J. The Autogenic Neoligament procedure: A technique for planned formation of an artificial neo-ligament. Acta Obstetricia et Gynecologica Scandinavica, **1990**, Supplement 153, Vol 69: 43-51.

Petros P., Ulmsten U.I. An integral theory of female urinary incontinence. Experimental and clinical considerations. Acta Obstet Gynecol Scand Suppl. **1990**, 153: 7-31.

Petros P. The female pelvic floor – function, dysfunction and management according to the Integral Theory –, third edition – Springer Verlag, **2010**.

Petros P., Richardson P.A. TFS posterior sling improves overactive bladder, pelvic pain and abnormal emptying, even with minor prolapse - a prospective urodynamic study. Pelviperineology, **2010**, 29: 52-55.

Petros P. Vault prolapse II: restoration of dynamic vaginal supports by infracoccygeal sacropexy, an axial day-case vaginal procedure, International Urogynecology Journal andPelvic Floor Dysfunction, **2001**, vol. 12, no. 5: 296–303.

Petros P., von **Konsky B.R.** Anchoring the Midurethra Restores Bladder-Neck Anatomy and Continence, The Lancet, Volume 354, Number 9183, 18 September, **1999**: 997-998.

Petros P., Ulmsten U. Natural volume handwashing urethrocystometry: a physiological technique for the objective diagnosis of the unstable detrusor. Gynecol Obstet Invest, **1993**, 36: 42–46.

Pickens R.B., Klein F.A., Mobley J.D. 3rd, White W.M. Single incision mid-urethral sling for treatment of female stress urinary incontinence. Urology, **2011**, 77: 321.

Price N., Jackson S. Uterine suspension procedures: laparoscopic hysteropexy. Gynecologic and Obstetric Surgery – challenges and management options – Ed Wiley Blackwell, **2016**.

Rahmanou P., Price N., Jackson S. Laparoscopic hysteropexy: a novel technique for uterine preservation surgery. Int Urogynecol J, **2014**, 25: 139-140.

Rardin C.R., Washington B.B. New considerations in the use of vaginal mesh for prolapse repair. J Minim Invasive Gynecol, **2009**, 16: 360–4.

Rechberger T., Futyma K., Jankiewicz K., Adamiak A., Skorupski P. The Clinical Effectiveness of Retropubic (IVS-02) and Transobturator (IVS-04) Midurethral Slings: Randomized Trial. Eur Urol, **2009**.

Rechberger T., Uldbjerg N., Oxlund H, Connective tissue changes in the cervix during normal pregnancy and pregnancy complicated by a cervical incompetenceObstets & Gynecol., **1988**, 71: 563-567.

Retzius A.A. Uber das ligamentum Pelvoprostaticum oder den apparat, durch welchen die Harnblasee, die Prostata und die Harnrohre an den untern Beckenoffnung befestigt sind. Muller's Arch Anat Physiol Wiss Med, **1849**, 11: 182.

Ricci J.V. The Genealogy of Gynaecology: History of the Development of Gynaecology Throughout the Ages, 2000 B.C. - 1800 A.D., **1950**.

Richter K. The surgical anatomy of the vaginaefixatio sacrospinalis vaginalis. A contribution to the surgical treatment of vaginal blind pouch prolapse, Geburtshilfe und Frauenheilkunde, **1968**, vol. 28, no. 4: 321–327.

Robinson B. The abdominal and pelvic brain. In: David Mcmillin. Lifeline Press, **1997**.

Rock J., Howard W.J-III. Te Linde's Operative Gynecology, 9th edition, **2003**.

Roemer H. Methoden der Geburtserleichterung. In: Gynäkologie und Geburtshilfe.

Hrsg.
O. Käser et al. Thieme, Stuttgart, **1967**, Bd.II, 672.

Rosenman A.E. Pelvic organ prolpase. Healthy women. **2017**.

Roshanravan S.M., Wieslander C.K., Schaffer J.I., Corton M.M. Neurovascular anatomy of the sacrospinous ligament region in female cadavers: Implications in sacrospinous ligament fixation. Am J Obstet Gynecol. 2007, Dec **1976**: 660.

Rosier P.F., Bosch J.R. A prospective study to find evidence for the ICS definition of urgency, ICS, **2002.**

Ross J.W. Laparoscopic Burch Repair Compared to Laparotomy Burch for Cure of Urinary Stress Incontinence. Int Urogynecol J, **1995**, 6:323-328.

Ross J.W., Preston M. Laparoscopic sacrocolpopexy for se- vere vaginal vault prolapse: five-year outcome. Journal of Minimally Invasive Gynecology. **2005,** Vol. 12, No. 3: 221-226.

Saidi M.H., Sadler R.K., Saidi J.A. Extraperitoneal laparoscopic colposuspension for genuine urinary stress incontinence. J Am Assoc Gynecol Laparosc, **1998**, 5: 247-252.

Schafer W., Abrams P., Liao L., Mattiasson A., Pesce F., Spangberg A.,. Sterling A.M., Zinner N.R., van Kerrebroeck P. Good Urodynamic Practices: Uroflowmetry, Filling Cystometry, and Pressure-Flow Studies. Neurourology and Urodynamics, **2002**, 21: 261-274. **Schellart R.P.,** Oude Rengerink K., Van der Aa F.. A randomized comparison of a single- incision midurethral sling and a transobturator midurethral sling in women with stress urinary
incontinence: results of 12-mo follow-up. Eur Urol, **2014**, 66: 1179.

Schimpf M.O., Rahn D.D., Wheeler T.L. Sling surgery for stress urinary incontinence in women: a systematic review and metaanalysis. Am J Obstet Gynecol, **2014**, 211: 71: e1.

Sederl J. Surgery in prolapse of a blind-end vagina, Geburtshilfe Frauenheilkd, **1958**, vol. 18, no. 6: 824–828.

Sekiguchi Y., Kinjyo M., Inoue H. Outpatient mid urethral tissue fixation system sling for urodynamic stress urinary incontinence: 1-year results. J Urol, **2009**, 182: 2810.

Sellheim H. Schwebende Pein, ein typisches gynäkologisches Krankheitsbild. Vortrag auf der 88. Versammlung der Gesellschaft deutscher Naturforscher und Ärzte in Düsseldorf vom
19. bis 26. September, **1926**.

Serati M., Topazio L., Bogani G., Costantini E., Pietropaolo A., Palleschi G., Carbone A., Soligo M., Del Popolo G., Li Marzi V., Salvatore S., Finazzi A. Urodynamics Useless Before Surgery For Female Stress Urinary Incontinence: Are You Sure? Neurourology and Urodynamics, **2015**.

Serati M., Topazio L., Bogani G., Costantini E., Pietropaolo A., Palleschi G., Carbone A., Soligo M., Del Popolo G., Li Marzi V., Salvatore S., Finazzi A. Urodynamics Useless Before Surgery For Female Stress Urinary Incontinence: Are You Sure? Neurourology and Urodynamics, **2015**.

Serels S., Douso M., Short G. Preliminary findings with the Solyx single-incision sling system in female stress urinary incontinence. Int Urogynecol J, **2010**, 21: 557.

Serrand M, Lefebvre A, Delorme E. Bilateral plication of the puborectal muscles: A new surgical concept for treating vulvar widening J Gynecol Obstet Hum Reprod. **2017** Sep;46(7):545-550. doi: 10.1016/j.jogoh.2017.06.008. Epub 2017 Jul 8.

Shafik A, Sibai OE, Shafik AA, Shafik IA (2007) A novel concept for the surgical anatomy of the perineal body. Dis Colon Rectum 50:2120-5.

Shah H.N., Badlani G.H. Mesh complications in female pelvic floor reconstructive surgery and their management: A systematic review. Indian J Urol. **2012** Apr-Jun, 28 (2): 129–153.

Sinelnikov R.D. Atlas of Human Anatomy, vol. II, MIR Publisher, Moscow, **1981**.

Sivaslioglu A.A., Unlubilgin E., Aydogmus S., Keskin L., Dolen I. A Prospective Randomized Controlled Trial of the Transobturator Tape and Tissue Fixation Mini-Sling in Patients with Stress Urinary Incontinence: 5-Year Results, J Urol, July **2012**, Vol. 188: 194-199.

Sîrbu P., Chiricuță I., Pandele A., Seatlacec D. Chirurgia Ginecologică. Vol. 1. Ed. Medicală București, **1981**.

Sîrbu P. Chirurgia ginecologică, vol. I, **1981**, București

Speert H. Iconographia Gyniatrica. A pictorial History of Gynecology and Obstetrics, F.A. Davis, Philadelphia, Pa, USA, **1973**.

Spinosa J.P., Dubuis P.Y., Riederer B. Transobturator surgery for female urinary continence: from outside to inside or from inside to outside: a comparative anatomic study]. Prog Urol, **2005**, 15: 700.

Stoeckel W. The use of the pyramidal muscle in the surgical treatment of urinary incontinence. Zbl Gynack 41: 11, **1917**.

Stoica R.A., Enache T. Acomparative study between laparoscopic sacrocolpopexy and transvaginal approach for genital prolapse. 20th International EAES Congress, Brussels, Belgium, 20-23 June **2012**.

Stones W., Cheong Y.C., Howard F.M. Interventions for treating chronic pelvic pain in women, Cochrane review **2007**.

Strohbehn K., DeLancey J.O.L. The anatomy of stress incontinence. Oper Tech Gynecol Surg, **1997**.

Strohbehn K., Ellis J.H., Strohbehn J.A., DeLancey J.O.L. Magnetic resonance imaging of levator aniwith anatomic correlation. Obstet Gynecol, **1996**, 87(2): 277–85.

Sundaram C.P., Venkatesh R., Landman J., Klutke C.G. Laparoscopic sacrocolpopexy for the correction of vaginal vault prolapse. Journal of Endourology, **2004**, Vol. 18, No. 7: 620-623.

Sung V.W., Rogers R.G., Schaffer J.I., Balk E.M., Uhlig K., Lau J. Graft use in transvaginal pelvic organ prolapse repair: a systematic review. Society of Gynecologic Surgeons Systematic Review Group. Obstet Gynecol **2008**, 112: 1131–42.

Sutton C. Hysterectomy: a historical perspective. Baillieres Clin Obstet Gynaecol, **1997**, 11: 1-22.

Swash M., Henry M.M., Snooks S.J. A unifying concept of pelvic floor disorders and incontinence. J Roy Soc Med, **1985**, 78: 906-912.

Symington J. Splanchnology. In: Schäfer EA, Symington J, Bryce TH, ed. Quain's Elements of Anatomy. London: Longmans, Green & Co., **1914**.

Tanagho E.A. Colpocystourethropexy: the way we do it. JUrol, **1976**, 116: 751-753.

Tan-Kim J.M.M., Shawn A., Luber K.M. Robotic assisted and laparoscopic sacrocolpopexy: comparing operative times, costs and outcomes. Female Pelvic Medicine andReconstructive Surgery, **2011,** vol. 17, no. 1: 44–49.

Tapp A.J.S., Hills B., Cardozo L.D. Randomized study comparing pelvic floor physiotherapy with the Burch colposuspension. Neurourol Urodyn, **1989**, 8: 356-57.

Terminologica Anatomica de Kearney et al 2004.

Thompson J.D. Surgical correction of defects in pelvic support. In: Rock JR, Thompson JD, eds. TeLinde's Operative Gynecology. 8th ed. Philadelphia, Pa: Lippincott-Raven, **1997**.

Thompson J.R., Gibb J.S., Genadry R., Burrows L., Lambrou N., Buller J.L. Anatomy of pelvic arteries adjacent to the sacrospinous ligament: importance of the coccygeal branch of the inferior gluteal artery. Obstet Gynecol, **1999** Dec, 94(6): 973-7.

Thompson P. On the levator ani, or ischio-anal muscle of ungulates, with special reference to its morphology. Journal of Anatomy and Physiology, **1989,** vol. 33, part 3: 423-433.

Tiny A., de Boer, Marijke C.P., Slieker-ten H., Mark E. Vierhout The prevalence and risk factors of overactive bladder symptoms and its relation to pelvic organ prolapse symptoms in a general female population Int Urogynecol J. **2011** May, 22(5): 569–575.

Ulmsten U., Henriksson L., Johnson P., Varhos G. An ambulatory surgical procedure under local anesthesia for treatment of female urinary incontinence. Int Urogynecol J Pelvic Floor Dysfunct. **1996**, 7: 81–5.

Ulmsten U., Petros P. Intravaginal slingplasty (IVS): an ambulatory surgical procedure for treatment of female urinary incontinence. Scand J Urol Nephrol, **1995**, 29: 75-82.

Unger C.A., Walters M.D., Ridgeway B., Jelovsek J.E., Barber M.D., Paraiso M.F. Incidence of adverse events after uterosacral colpopexy for uterovaginal and posthysterectomy vault prolapse. Am J Obstet Gynecol. **2015** May, 212 (5): 603.e1-7.

Velemir L., Amblard J., Fatton B., Savary D., Jacquetin B. Transvaginal mesh repair of anterior and posterior vaginal wall prolapse: a clinical and ultrasonographic study. Ultrasound Obstet Gynecol **2010**, 35: 474–80.

Verheyn P. Anatomie oder Zerlegung des menschlichen Leibes. Leipzig: Th. Fritschen, **1708.**

Von Theobald P., Labbe E. Posterior intravaginal slingplasty: Feasibility and preliminiary results in a prospective obsternational study of 108 cases. Pelviperineology, **2008**, 27: 12-16.

Wagenlehner F. Pelvic pain in men and women: an overview. International Society for Pelviperineology, Munich, Germany 12th-15th Sept. **2014.**

Wagenleuhner F., Petros P., Gunnemann A., Richardson P.A., Sekiguchi Y., Cardinal ligament: a live anatomical study, Pelviperineology, **2013**, 32: 72-76.

Wang A.C., Wang Y.Y., Chen M.C. Single-blind, randomized trial of pelvic floor muscle training, biofeedback-assisted pelvic floor muscle training, and electric stimulation in the management of overactive bladder. Urology, **2004**, 63(1): 61-66.

Watkins T.J. The treatment of cystocele and uterine prolapse after the menopause. Am J Obstet Dis Wom, **1899**, 15: 420.

Wei JT, De Lancey JOL. Functional anatomy of the pelvic floor and lower urinary tract. Clin Obstet Gynecol 2004;47:3–17.

Wells T.J., Brink C.A., Diokno A.C., Wolfe R., Gillis G.L. Pelvic muscle exercise for stress urinary incontinence in elderly women. JAGS, **1991**, 39: 785-91.

Wheeless C.R.Jr., Roenneburg M.L. Abterior Repair and Kelly Plication. Atlas of Pelvic Surgery, **2017.**

Whitehead W.E., Wald A., Diamant N.E., Enck P., Pemberton J.H., Rao S.S. Functional disorders of the anus and rectum. Gut **1999**, 45 (Suppl II): II55-II59.

Wilson P.D., Bø K., Hay-Smith J., Nygaard I., Staskin D., Wyman J. Conservative treatment in women. . In: Abrams P, Cardozo L, Khoury S, Wein A (eds). Incontinence. Plymouth, UK. Health Publication Ltd, **2002**:573-624.

Woodward AP, Matthews CA (2010) Outcomes of revision perineoplasty for persistent postpartum dyspareunia. Female Pelvic Med Reconstr Surg.

Wu J.M., Matthews C.A., Conover M.M., Pate V., Jonsson F.M. Lifetime risk of stress urinary incontinence or pelvic organ prolapse surgery. Obstet Gynecol, **2014**, 123: 1201-1206.

Wu Q., Luo L., Petros P. Case report: Mechanical support of the posterior fornix relieved urgency and suburethral tenderness. Pelviperineology, **2013**, 32: 55-56.

Yamada H. Aging rate for the strength of human organs and tissues. Strength of Biological Materials, Williams & Wilkins Co, Balt. (Ed) Evans FG. **1970**: 272-280.

Yamanishi T., Yasuda K., Sakakibara R., Hattori T., Suda S. Randomized, double blind study of electrical stimulation for urinary incontinence due to detrusor overactivity. Urology, **2000**, 55: 353-357.

Yildiz G., Ceylan Y., Ucer O. Safety and efficacy of single-incision sling for female stress urinary incontinence: 3 years' results. Int Urogynecol J, **2016**, 27: 1667.

Zabihi N., Mourtzinos A., Maher M.G., Raz S., Rodriguez. L.V. Short-term results of bilateral S2–S4 sacral neuromodulation for the treatment of refractory interstitial cystitis, painful bladder syndrome, and chronic pelvic pain, International Urogynecology Journal, April **2008**, Volume 19, Issue 4: 553-557.

Zabihi N., Mourtzinos A., Maher M.G., Raz S., Rodriguez. L.V. Short-term results of bilateral S2–S4 sacral neuromodulation for the treatment of refractory interstitial cystitis, painful bladder syndrome, and chronic pelvic pain, International Urogynecology Journal, April **2008**, Volume 19, Issue 4: 553-557.

Zacharin R.F. The suspensory mechanism of the female urethra. JAnat. **1963**, 97: 423–7.

Zetkin M., Schaldach H. Parametropathia spastica In: Zetkin M, Schaldach H, ed. Lexikon der Medizin. München: Elsevier, **2005**.

Zetkin M., Schaldach H. Parametropathia spastica In: Zetkin M, Schaldach H, ed. Lexikon der Medizin. München, Elsevier, **2005**.

Zweifel P. Vorlesungen ¨uber Klinische Gyn¨akologie. Hirschwald, **1892**.

Zyczynski H.M., Carey M.P., Smith A.R., Gauld J.M., Robinson D., Sikirica V., Reisenauer C., Slack M. Prosima Study Investigators. One-year clinical outcomes after prolapse surgery with nonanchored mesh and vaginal support device. Am J Obstet Gynecol. **2010** Dec, 203 (6): 587.e1-8.

***. **FDA.** US Food and Drug Administration, Public health notification: serious complications associated with transvaginal placement of surgical mesh in repair of pelvic organprolapse and stress urinary incontinence, in US Food and Drug Administration, **2008**.

***. **FDA.** US Food and Drug Administration, Safety Communication: UPDATE on Serious Complications Associated with Transvaginal Placement of Surgical Mesh for Pelvic Organ Prolapse, **2011**.

***. **ICS** Pelvic Floor Clinical Assessment Group. Terminology of pelvic floor function and dysfunction. ICS report **2001**.

***. **ICS**. International Continence Society. Epidemiology of urinary and faecal incontince and pelvic organ prolapse. **2010**.

***. Oxford Gynaecology and Pelvic Floor Centre, **2017**.

***. Transvaginal mesh procedures for pelvic organ prolapse. SOGC Technical Update No. 254. Society of Obstetricians and Gynaecologists of Canada. J Obstet Gynaecol Can, **2011**, 33: 168–74.

Bei Fragen zur Produktsicherheit wenden Sie sich bitte an:
If you have any questions regarding product safety,
please contact:

Walter de Gruyter GmbH
Genthiner Straße 13
10785 Berlin
productsafety@degruyterbrill.com